I0072268

Pharmaceutical Science: Current Research

Pharmaceutical Science: Current Research

Edited by Ralph Hahn

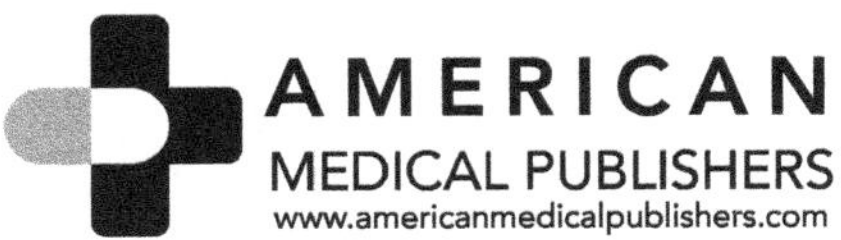

American Medical Publishers,
41 Flatbush Avenue,
1st Floor, New York,
NY 11217, USA

Visit us on the World Wide Web at:
www.americanmedicalpublishers.com

ISBN: 978-1-63927-545-8

Cataloging-in-Publication Data

Pharmaceutical science : current research / edited by Ralph Hahn.
p. cm.
Includes bibliographical references and index.
ISBN 978-1-63927-545-8
1. Pharmacy. 2. Drugs. 3. Pharmacology. 4. Pharmaceutical industry. I. Hahn, Ralph.
RS92 .P43 2022
615.1--dc23

Table of Contents

Preface

Pharmaceutical sciences include the various areas of study that focus on the action, design, delivery and disposition of drugs. It applies knowledge from different biological fields such as anatomy, physiology, biochemistry, cell and molecular biology. It also uses tools from other subjects such as physics, chemistry, mathematics, chemical engineering and epidemiology. There are four main branches of pharmaceutical sciences- pharmacology, pharmaceutical chemistry, pharmaceutics, and pharmacognosy. The biochemical and physiological effects of drugs on humans are studied under pharmacology. Pharmaceutical chemistry studies the drug design to optimize pharmacokinetics and pharmacodynamics and synthesis of new drug molecules. Pharmaceutics focuses on the study and design of drug formulation for the best delivery, pharmacokinetics, stability and patient acceptance. Pharmacognosy is related to the study of medicines derived from natural sources. This book contains some path-breaking studies in the field of pharmaceutical sciences. It presents researches and studies performed by experts across the globe. Researchers and students in this field will be assisted by this book.

This book is a comprehensive compilation of works of different researchers from varied parts of the world. It includes valuable experiences of the researchers with the sole objective of providing the readers (learners) with a proper knowledge of the concerned field. This book will be beneficial in evoking inspiration and enhancing the knowledge of the interested readers.

In the end, I would like to extend my heartiest thanks to the authors who worked with great determination on their chapters. I also appreciate the publisher's support in the course of the book. I would also like to deeply acknowledge my family who stood by me as a source of inspiration during the project.

Editor

Analysis of Piroxicam in Pharmaceutical Formulation and Human Urine by Dispersive Liquid–Liquid Microextraction Combined with Spectrophotometry

Ahad Bavili Tabrizi[1]*, Nakisa Seyyedeh Tutunchi[2]

[1] *Department of Medicinal Chemistry, Faculty of Pharmacy & Biotechnology Research Center, Tabriz University of Medical Sciences, Tabriz, Iran.*

[2] *Students' Research Committee, Tabriz University of Medical Sciences, Tabriz, Iran.*

ARTICLE INFO

Keywords:
Dispersive liquid–liquid-microextraction
Piroxicam
Pharmaceutical preparation
Spectrophotometry
Urine

ABSTRACT

Purpose: Piroxicam, is non–steroidal anti–inflammatory and analgesic agent, which is widely used in the treatment of patients with rheumatologic disorders. A new analytical approach based on the dispersive liquid–liquid microextraction (DLLME) has been developed for the extraction and determination of PX in pharmaceutical preparation and human urine. ***Methods***: From the PX standard solution or solutions prepared from real samples, aliquot volumes were pipetted into centrifuge tubes and mixed with acetate buffer at pH 3.0 and NaCl solution. The contents were subjected to the DLLME, so 700 µL of methanol containing 70 µL of chloroform was injected rapidly into a sample solution. A cloudy solution was rapidly produced and the PX extracted into dispersed fine droplets. The mixture was centrifuged, thus these fine droplets of chloroform were settled. The supernatant aqueous phase was readily decanted, then the remained organic phase was diluted with ethanol and the absorbance measured at 355 ± 3 nm against a reagent blank. ***Results***: The main factors affecting the extraction efficiency such as pH, extraction and disperser solvent types and *etc.* were studied and optimized systematically. Under optimized conditions, the calibration graphs were linear over the range of 0.2 to 4.8 µg/mL. The limit of detection and relative standard deviation were found to be 0.058 µg/mL and 2.83%, respectively. Relative recoveries in the spiked samples ranged from 97 to 110%. ***Conclusion***: Using the developed method PX can be analyzed in pharmaceutical formulation and human urine sample in a simpler, cheaper and more rapid manner.

Introduction

Piroxicam, 4–hydroxy–2–methyl–N–2–pyridinyl–2H–1,2–benzothiazine–3–carboxamide 1,1–dioxide (PX), is non–steroidal anti–inflammatory, and analgesic agent belonging to a new class of compounds called oxicams. It is widely used in the treatment of patients with rheumatologic disorders.[1]

PX is readily absorbed after oral or rectal administration. After a single oral dose of 20 mg of PX, its peak plasma concentration and plasma half–life were 4.5 µg/mL and 35–60 h, respectively. PX is extensively metabolized to 5–hydroxypiroxicam (5–HP) and the hydroxylated metabolite undergoes subsequent glucuronidation. About 2–5% of an oral dose is excreted unchanged in urine, and under steady state conditions, 75% of a dose is excreted as either 5–HP or 5–HP glucuronide in urine and feces.[2]

The employment of several analytical methods such as membrane sensors,[1] potentiometric titration,[3] spectrophotometry,[3–7] spectrofluorimetry,[8–11] luminescence[12] and chromatography[5] has been proposed for the determination of PX in pharmaceutical preparations. On the other hand, different analytical methods such as derivative spectrophotometry,[2] spectrofluorimetry[10,13] and high performance liquid chromatography (HPLC)[14–20] have been reported for the determination of PX in different biological fluids.

In general, HPLC has been the most employed method to measure PX in different biological fluids. Most of these methods require liquid–liquid extraction (LLE) with consecutive evaporation.[15–19] The extraction procedure is prone to complications because it involves several separate steps, which not only make the method tedious and time consuming but also increase the potential of introducing a bias in the results.[20]

Simple, effective and environmentally–friendly extraction procedures are still in demand. Nowadays, a new mode of liquid–phase micro–extraction (LPME) named DLLME as a high–performance, powerful, rapid

***Corresponding author:** Ahad Bavili Tabrizi, Department of Medicinal Chemistry, Faculty of Pharmacy & Biotechnology Research Center, Tabriz University of Medical Sciences, Tabriz, Iran. E–mail: a.bavili@tbzmed.ac.ir

and inexpensive ME method has been proposed.[21] The basic principles of this method is dispersion of extraction solvent (immiscible in water) assisted with disperser solvent (miscible in both water and extraction solvents) within aqueous solution which lead to very high contact area between aqueous phase and extraction solvent.[22] The ease of the operation, speed, lower sample volume, low cost, high recovery and high enhancement factor are some advantages of DLLME.

With the development of DLLME, the principles and the applications of this new technique have been reviewed recently[23,24] and its application extended to separation, pre–concentration and determination of organic[21,25–27] and inorganic[22,28–30] compounds in different samples. However, to the best of our knowledge, this is the first report concerning PX extraction using the DLLME method.

In this work a DLLME methodology has been developed and optimized for the extraction of PX from human urine and pharmaceutical formulation. The extracted PX was analyzed by using spectrophotometry and this method was used due to ease and low cost of operation. Potential parameters affecting the DLLME and analytical performance were studied and optimized systematically. Using the developed method PX can be analyzed in pharmaceutical formulation and human urine sample in a simpler, cheaper and more rapid manner.

Materials and Methods

Apparatus

Spectral measurements were carried out with Shimadzu UV–visible Recording Spectrophotometer (UV–160 model) using 1–cm path length and 1.5 mL quartz cells. A Hettich centrifuge (EBA 20 model/ Andreas Hettich GmbH & Co. KG, Föhrenstr. 12, D–78532 Tuttlingen, Germany) with 15 mL calibrated centrifuge tubes (Hirschmann, EM techcolor, Germany) was used to accelerate the phase separation process. A Corning M120 pH–meter (Halstead, Essex, England CO9 2DX) was used for checking the pH of solutions.

Reagents

All solvents containing chloroform, dichloromethane, carbon tetrachloride, acetone, acetonitrile, ethanol and methanol were obtained from Merck (Darmstadt, Germany). The β–glucuronidase, Type HP–2 from *Helix pomatia* (116,400 units/mL), was from Sigma–Aldrich.

A stock solution of 500 μg/mL of PX was prepared by dissolving appropriate amounts of pure drug (obtained from Zahravi, Tabriz, Iran) in ethanol and was kept away from the light in a refrigerator at approximately 4°C. Working standard solutions were obtained by appropriate dilution of this stock standard solution.

The acetic acid/acetate buffer (1 mol/L, pH 3.0) was prepared from sodium acetate trihydrate (Riedel–De Haën) and acetic acid (Merck). A 20% (w/v) solution of NaCl (Merck) was prepared. All other reagents were of analytical reagent grade or higher. Ultrapure water (Milli–Q Advantage A 10 system, Millipore) was used throughout the work.

Procedure for DLLME

From the PX standard solution (10 μg/mL) aliquot volumes, in the range 0.2–4.8 μg/mL, were pipetted into 15–mL centrifuge tubes and mixed with 0.5 mL of 1.0 mol/L acetate buffer at pH 3.0 and 2.0 mL of 20% NaCl solution. The contents were diluted to 5.0 mL and subjected to the DLLME. Seven hundred microlitres of methanol (as disperser solvent) containing 70 μL of chloroform (as extraction solvent) was injected rapidly into a sample solution using a 2.0–mL syringe. A cloudy solution was rapidly produced, resulting from fine droplets, and the PX was extracted into these fine droplets. The mixture was centrifuged at 3500 rpm for 3 min and the dispersed fine droplets of chloroform were settled. The supernatant aqueous phase was readily decanted with a Pasteur pipette. The remained organic phase was diluted to 700 μL with ethanol–water (1:1 v/v) and the absorbance measured at 355 ± 3 nm against a reagent blank.

Procedure for pharmaceutical preparation

The contents of ten capsules (Pursina Pharm. Co., Tehran, Iran), each containing 10 mg PX, were accurately weighed individually and finely powdered. Powdered sample containing 10 mg PX was weighed and placed into a 15–mL glass tube dissolved in 10–mL methanol and was vigorously shaken on a vortex mixer for 30 sec. The solution was then filtered and transferred into a 50–mL volumetric flask. The residue was washed in enough methanols and the solution was finally made up to the mark with water. Thus, a 200 μg/mL solution of PX was obtained. This solution was diluted quantitatively to yield concentrations in the range of working standard solution and then the PX content was analyzed by the procedure proposed above.

Procedure for urine sample

Urine sample was obtained from healthy male volunteer who took single oral dose of 10 mg PX capsule. After administration, the samples were collected between 0–24 h and frozen at –20 °C until analysis. The frozen urine samples were thawed at room temperature, centrifuged for 15 min at 4000 rpm and then the supernatants were transferred to clean glass tubes. Enzymatic deconjugation was performed according to the literature,[14,16] with some modifications. For this purpose, 2.0 mL of urine sample was transferred into 10–mL centrifuge tube and 300 μL of sodium acetate buffer (1.0 mol/L, pH 5.0) and 200 μL of β–glucuronidase/aryl sulphatase (116400–1015 IU/mL) were added. The tubes were mixed vigorously and incubated at 56°C for 6 h. Then tubes were centrifuged at 3000 rpm for 15 min and 0.5 mL aliquots of the supernatant solutions were subjected to the above mentioned procedure.

Results and Discussion

A literature survey reveals that both spectrophotometric and spectrofluorimetric techniques have been the most employed methods for the determination of PX in pharmaceutical preparations. By taking into account that the extracted PX didn't show any significant and sensitive fluorescence in the studied conditions, spectrophotometric detection was adopted for its monitoring after DLLME.

The spectrophotometric methods used for the determination of PX are generally based on the oxidation of PX with different agents, such as potassium iodate,[3] ferric salts,[6] ceric ammonium sulfate[31] and indirect spectrophotometric determination of the reaction products, solid–phase spectrophotometry[4] and or chelating with ferric ion.[5] In this study, quantitative determination of PX in different real samples was performed by direct spectrophotometry in order to avoid of slow derivatization reactions, specific or toxic agents, large sample volumes and/or excess use of organic solvents. Figure 1 shows the absorption spectrum of the target analyte after DLLME which exhibits an absorption band peaking at 355 ± 3 nm. To obtain higher extraction efficiency, the effect of different factors such as pH, type and volume of dispersive and extraction solvents, salt addition and *etc.* were tested using the one variable at a time method.

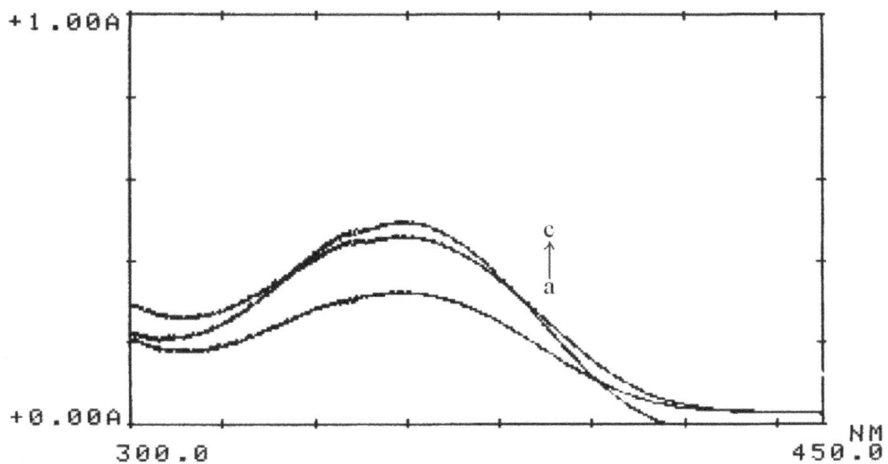

Figure 1. Absorption spectra of PX after DLLME: a) Standard solution of PX (2.0 µg/mL) (b) sample "a" after addition of NaCl (8% w/v), (c) 0.5 mL urine sample spiked with PX (2.0 µg/mL); other conditions: 0.5 mL of 1.0 mol/L acetate buffer at pH 3.0; extraction with 500 of methanol µL containing 50 µL of chloroform.

Effect of pH

It is well known that the pH of the sample solution was one of the important factors affecting the states of analytes (as ions or neutral forms). Figure 2 shows the effect of pH on the absorption signal of the target analyte. As can be seen, the signal intensity of PX improved with the increasing of pH from 3.0 to 3.5, and then decreased in pH 3.5–12.0. This can be explained by the following reasons: Analytes in neutral forms are much easier to be extracted by extraction solvent than those in ion forms due to their strong affinity. According to the literature,[8,32] the pK_a values of PX are 1.81 and 5.12. By considering these values, below pH 1.8 both the pyridyl and enolic groups are mostly prorogated (LH^{2+}, positive global charge) and above pH 5.1 these groups are deprotonated (L^-, negative global charge). In the pH range 1.8–5.1, a tautomeric equilibrium between the neutral molecule (LH^0) and the zwitterions ($LH^{\pm}$) is established.[8] Hence, when the pH of the solution was between 1.8–5.1, the analyte is neutral form in aqueous solution which has a greater tendency to be extracted into the extraction solvent. Accordingly, the pH of samples was controlled at 3.0 by acetate buffer for subsequent study.

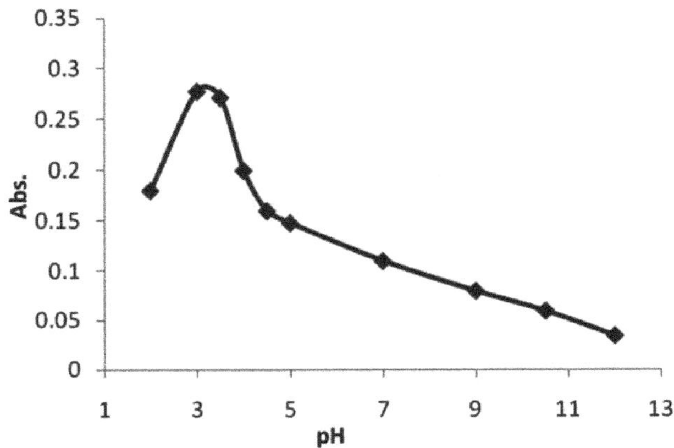

Figure 2. Effect of pH on the analytical responses, PX (1.2 µg/mL); other conditions: 2.0 mL of 20% NaCl; 0.5 mL of 1.0 mol/L acetate buffer at pH 3.0; extraction with 500 of methanol µL containing 50 µL of chloroform.

Effect of the extraction and disperser solvent type

The type of extraction solvent used in DLLME is an important factor for efficient extraction. The solvent should be denser than water. Moreover it should have more capability for the extraction of interested compounds and lower solubility in water. Thus, chloroform, dichloromethane and carbon tetrachloride were studied as extraction solvent. On the other hand, the selection of a dispersive solvent is limited to solvents such as methanol, ethanol, acetonitrile and acetone, that are miscible with both water and extraction solvents.

In this study, all combinations of dichloromethane, chloroform and carbon tetrachloride as extraction solvents (50 μL) and methanol, ethanol, acetonitrile and acetone as dispersive solvents (500 μL) were tested. The results shown in Figure 3 indicated that, when dichloromethane was used as extraction solvent, no cloudy state was observed and also no sediment droplet of extract was found on the bottom of the tube after centrifuging. With carbon tetrachloride and chloroform, a two–phase system was formed with all four dispersive solvents but in the case of carbon tetrachloride low signals was observed, probably due to little extractability of the analyte in this solvent. While in the case of chloroform with methanol more stable two–phase systems and higher signals were observed. Thus chloroform and methanol was selected as extraction and disperser solvents, respectively, in subsequent experiments.

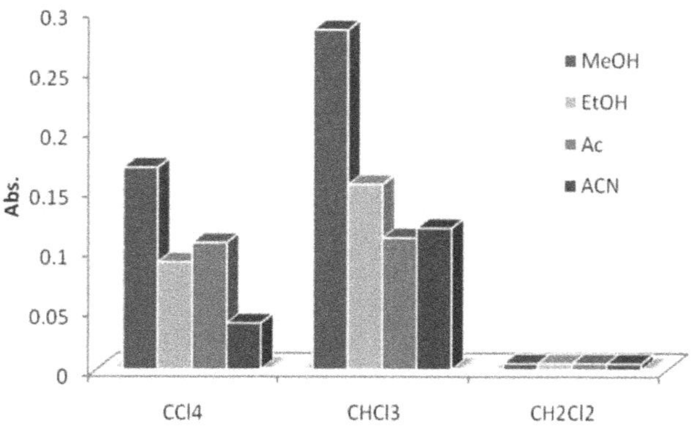

Figure 3. Effect of the type of extraction and dispersant solvents on the analytical responses, EtOH: ethanol, MeOH: methanol, Ac: acetone, ACN: Acetonitrile, PX (1.8 μg/mL); other conditions have been mentioned in Figure 2.

Effect of the extraction and disperser solvent volume

The effect of the volume of the extraction solvent on the analytical signals was investigated. Experiments were performed with different volumes of chloroform (in the range of 30–90 μL) as the extraction solvent by fixing the volume of the methanol at 500 μL. Figure 4 indicates that the absorbance increased by increasing the volume of the chloroform to 70 μL and then remained approximately constant by further increasing of its volume between 70 and 90 μL. Thus 70 μL of chloroform was used in other experiments. In order to examine the effect of the disperser solvent volume, solutions containing different volumes of methanol (in the range of 400–800 μL) containing 70 μL of chloroform were subjected to the same DLLME procedure. As shown in Figure 5, the absorbance reached to its maximum value at 700 μL of the methanol. Thus this volume was used in other experiments.

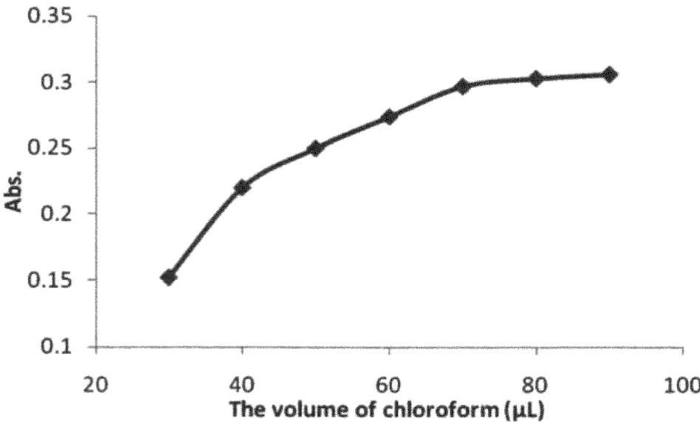

Figure 4. Effect of the extraction solvent ($CHCl_3$) volume on the analytical signals, PX (1.8 μg/mL); other conditions have been mentioned in Figure 2.

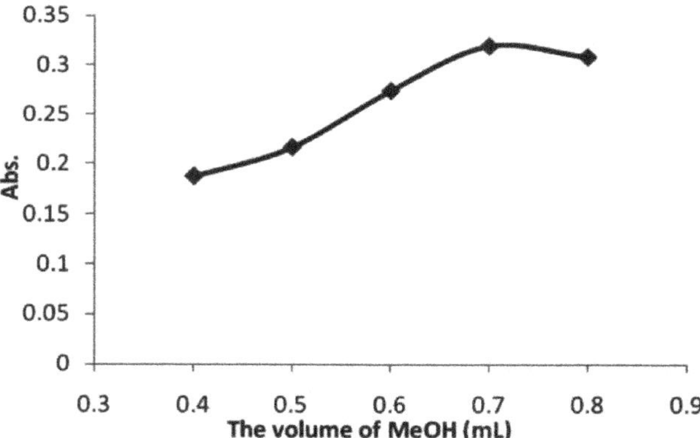

Figure 5. Effect of the dispersant solvent (MeOH) volume on the analytical signals, PX (1.8 μg/mL); other conditions have been mentioned in Figure 2.

Effect of salt addition

For investigating the influence of ionic strength on the extraction efficiency of DLLME, various experiments were performed by adding different amount of NaCl (0–15%, w/v) when other experimental conditions were kept constant. It was found that the absorbance was increased by increasing the amount of NaCl from 0 to 8%, and then decreased gradually by further increase of the salt concentration (see Figure 6). Based on these results, 8% (w/v) NaCl was chosen as the optimal salt concentration in the DLLME procedure.

Method validation

The optimized DLLME–spectrophotometric method was validated according to ICH guidelines.[33]

Calibration graphs were obtained by DLLME of 5 mL of standard solutions containing known amount of the PX and under the experimental conditions specified in the procedure. The remained phase (≈100 μL) was diluted to 0.7 mL with ethanol: water (1:1 v/v) and the absorbance measured. Thus, the theoretical and experimental preconcentration factors of 50 and ≈7 were achieved. The calibration curve for the detection of PX was linear over the concentration range 0.2 to 4.8 μg/mL and the corresponding regression equation was: Abs. = 0.1711C – 0.0154 (r = 0.9965), where Abs. is the absorbance intensity, C is the concentration of PX as μg/mL and r is correlation coefficient.

Table 1 indicates the analytical characteristics of the proposed method. Limit of detection (LOD) was calculated as $3\sigma_s/R$, where σ_s is the standard deviation of the blank and R the slope of the calibration curve, and found to be 0.058 μg/mL. This LOD was sufficiently low to be valuable for the determination of PX in different biological fluids. In addition, obtained linear range, LOD and RSD were comparable with those reported in other extractive methods (see Table 1).

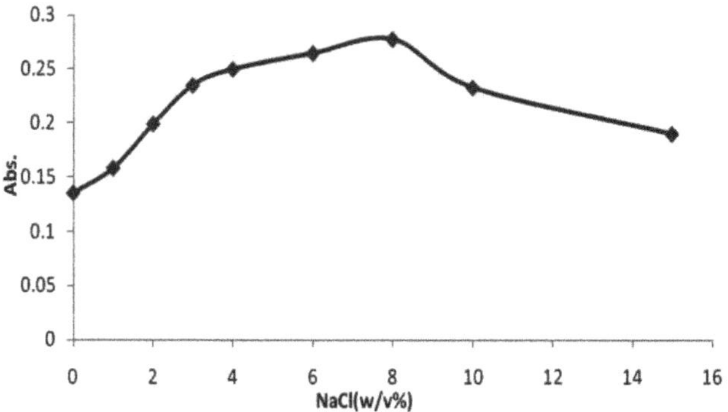

Figure 6. Effect of salt amount on the analytical signals, PX (1.8 μg/mL); other conditions have been mentioned in Figure 2.

Table1. Analytical characteristics of the different extractive methods.

Method	Sample & Ex. method	Concentration range (μg/mL)	Slope	Intercept	r	RSD%	LOD (μg/mL)	Mean recovery (%)	Ref.
E.C sensor	P.P	5.2×10^{-5}-10^{-2}	55.8	22.5	-	0.83-1.4	0.795	98.8-102	1
S	B.S	0.50-12	0.348	-0.014	0.9998	0.13-2.0	0.290[a]	89.4	2
S	P.P	0.05-1.1	1.07	-0.033	-	0.62-2.6	0.012[b]	99.7-100	3
Solid phase S	P.P	0.5-10	5.10×10^{-2}	0.013	0.9950	1.8	0.100	95.7-104	4
Derivative S	P.P	2.4-20	5.20×10^{-3}	-4.04×10^{-4}	0.9986	1.29	-	99.7	5
HPLC	–	5.0-20	1.14×10^{4}	2.72×10^{3}	0.9996	0.82	-	-	-
S	P.P	0.20-6.5	0.112	0.021	0.9993	0.93	8.35-8.75[b]	98.9-99.6	6
		0.05-6.5	0.112	0.032	0.9989	0.88	-	98.9-99.5	-
F	P.P	0.02-1.0	28.6	2.90	0.9990	1.6	0.020	100	8
F	P.P	0.03-0.20	42.3	1.02	0.9930	2.9	0.010	100	9
F	P.P and B.S & LLE	0.05-1.5	18.0	3.29	0.9993	1.3-1.6	0.015	99-104	10
Luminescence	P.P and B.S	0.2-1.0	1.83	-0.024	0.9955	0.5-3.9	0.029	97.5-100.8	12
S	B.S	1.0-10	-	-	0.9777-0.9975	1.0(S.D)	0.030-0.040	99-114	13
HPLC	B.S & LLE	0.05-20	0.463	-4.70×10^{-3}	0.9999	0.6-2.9	0.050	88-99	16
HPLC	B.S & LLE	7.2×10^{-4}-0.6	0.727-1.44	-0.197-0.574	0.9960	3.2	7.20×10^{-4}[a]	57.8-67.8	18
HP–TLC	B.S & LLE	0.1-15	0.689	0.046	0.9970	3.1-4.9	0.050	94.8	19
HPLC	B.S & P.P	0.1-6.0	0.972	0.011	0.9998	4.2-5.4	0.020	100	20
S	-	0.2-4.8	0.171	-0.015	0.9965	2.8	0.058	97-110	This work

E. C=Electrochemical; S.D=standard deviation; S=Spectrophotometry; F=Spectrofluorimetry; Pharmaceutical preparation=P.P; Biological sample=B.S; P.P=protein precipitation; a LOQ has been reported; b sensitivity has been reported.

The interferences

As can be seen from Figure 1, the analytical signals in the presence of urine are higher than that obtained in the absence of it. This can be attributed to the chemical composition of the urine and present salts which can contribute at higher extraction efficiencies of PX, due to salting out effect. It was found that the addition of NaCl to the standard solutions of PX, up to concentrations of 8% (w/v), can increase its extraction efficiency due to salting out effect, therefore remove this interference effect.

The validation and application of the method

Application to the commercial formulation

The proposed method was successfully applied to the analysis of PX in its pharmaceutical dosage form (10 mg per capsule) and the results are shown in Table 2. The data in this table show that the PX content measured by the proposed method was in excellent agreement with those obtained by an independent spectrofluorimetric method.[10] A comparison using t–test at 95% confidence interval demonstrates that there isn't any significant difference among the achieved results using these two methods.[34] The accuracy of the proposed method was further tested by performing recovery experiments on the solutions prepared from PX formulation. The results are summarized in Table 3 and recoveries ranged from 104–110%. These recoveries indicate that no significant matrix effect was observed in the proposed procedure.

Table 2. Results of recoveries of spiked samples.

Sample	PX added (μg/mL)	†PX found (μg/mL)	Recovery (%)
PX solution* (μg/mL)	0.5	0.52 ± 0.015	104
	1.0	1.07 ± 0.031	107
	1.5	1.65 ± 0.048	110
Human urine▾	0.5	0.51 ± 0.015	102
	1.0	0.97 ± 0.029	97
	1.5	1.62 ± 0.048	108

*Prepared from drug formulation.
▾A 0.5 mL portion of urine sample was used for recovery experiments.
†Average of three determinations ± standard deviation.

Table 3. Determination of PX in pharmaceutical preparation.

Method	*PX concentration (μg/mL)	†The tabulated t & F values
Spectrofluorimetry [10]	11.0 ± 0.170	t = 1.78 (2.78)
Spectrophotometry (this work)	10.5 ± 0.350	F = 4.24 (19)

*Average of three determinations ± standard deviation.
†Figures between parenthesis are the tabulated *t* and F values at p = 0.05.[34]

Application to the human urine

Drug–free urine sample obtained from healthy volunteer was used for recovery experiments. Aliquots of 0.5 mL of urine sample was spiked with certain concentrations of PX and subjected to the recovery experiments. The obtained recoveries ranged from 97 to 108%, as shown in Table 2, and seem to be satisfactory. Typical spectra of a standard solution of PX, blank urine and a urine sample taken from a volunteer after β-glucuronidase treatment are illustrated in Figure 7. No additional picks due to interferences were observed at the analytical absorption wavelength. Thus the coincidence of absorption spectra along with reasonable recoveries indicated that no significant matrix effect was encountered in the proposed method.

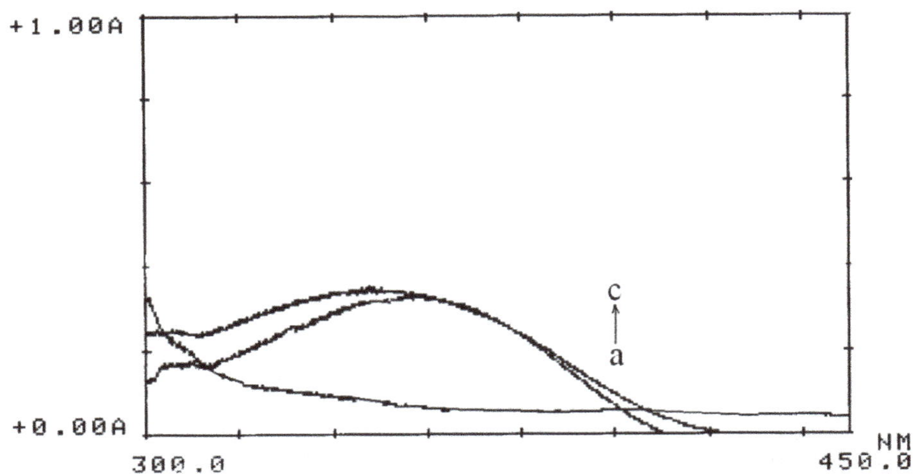

Figure 7. Absorption spectra of (a) urine blank, (b) Standard solution of PX (1.8 μg/mL) (c) collected urine after oral administration of 10 mg of PX and β–glucuronidase treatment; other conditions have been mentioned in Figure 2.

The proposed method was successfully applied to the determination of PX in human urine. For this purpose, urine was collected for 24 h after a single oral dose of 10 mg of PX to one volunteer. It must be mentioned that according to the literature,[2] there is an extensive overlap of the spectral bands of PX and 5–HP. Therefore the total excreted drug, *i.e.* unchanged PX and its metabolites, can be determined as PX after β–glucuronidase treatment and performing the analysis in the analytical absorption wavelength of PX.

The average concentration of PX was found to be 2.99±0.09 μg/mL in a total volume of 0.79 L of urine. In the present study, approximately 23.6% of the PX dose was recovered in urine as the 5'–hydroxy metabolite and its glucuronide conjugate, which was in accordance with values reported in the literature.[35,36] Also, urinary excretion of unchanged PX was negligible and below the detection limit of the assay.

Conclusion

The feasibility of employing DLLME as a simple and effective tool for the extraction of PX from different real samples has been studied. The method was validated using real samples and applied to the determination of PX in human urine. Compared to the HPLC, the proposed method allows carrying out the analysis of PX with low operational costs, simplicity of instrumentation and without further sample clean–up steps. Thus, the time and cost of analysis can be significantly decreased in addition to other well–known advantages of DLLME methodology. The method can be further developed by combining DLLME methodology with the proper HPLC method for the separation and determination of each PX and its metabolites.

Acknowledgments

Authors are grateful to the Research Office of Tabriz University of Medical Sciences for Financial support.

Conflict of interest

There is no conflict of interest in this work.

References

1. Khalil S, Borham N, EL-Ries MA. PX and tenoxicam selective membrane sensors. *Anal Chim Acta* 2000;414:215-9.
2. Klopas A, Panderi I, Parissi–Poulou M. Determination of PX and its major metabolite 5–hydroxyPX in human plasma by zero–crossing first–derivative spectrophotometry. *J Pharm Biomed Anal* 1998;17:515-24.
3. El-Ries MA, Mohamed G, Khalil S, El-Shall M. Spectrophotometric and Potentiometric Determination of PX and Tenoxicam in Pharmaceutical Preparations. *Chem Pharm Bull* 2003;51(1):6-10.
4. Pascual-Reguera MI, Ayora-Canãda MJ, Castro Ruiz MS. Determination of PX by solid–phase spectrophotometry in a continuous flow system. *Eur J Pharm Sci* 2002;15:179-83.
5. Basan H, Göğer NG, Ertas N, Tevfik Orbey M. Quantitative determination of PX in a new formulation (PX–β–cyclodextrin) by derivative UV spectrophotometric method and HPLC. *J Pharm Biomed Anal* 2001;26:171-8.
6. Nagaralli BS, Seetharamappa J, Melwanki MB. Sensitive spectrophotometric methods for the determination of amoxycillin, ciprofloxacin and PX in pure and pharmaceutical formulations. *J Pharm Biomed Anal* 2002;29:859-64.
7. Hejaz Azmi SN, Iqbal B, Mohad Jaboob MA, Said Al Shaharia WA, Rahman N. Spectrophotometric Determination of PX via Chelation with Fe(III) in Commercial Dosage Forms. *J Chin Chem Soc* 2009;56:1083-91.
8. Escandar GM, Bystol AJ, Campiglia AD. Spectrofluorimetric method for the determination of PX and pyridoxine. *Anal Chim Acta* 2002;466:275-83.
9. Escandar GM. Spectrofluorimetric determination of PX in the presence and absence of β-cyclodextrin. *Analyst* 1999;124:587-91.
10. Manzoori JL, Amjadi M. Spectrofluorimetric Determination of PX in Pharmaceutical Preparations and Spiked Human Serum Using Micellar Media. *Microchim Acta* 2003;143:39-44.
11. Tabrizi AB. A Simple Spectrofluorimetric Method for Determination of PX and Propranolol in Pharmaceutical Preparations. *J Food Drug Anal* 2007;15:242-8.
12. Al-Kindy SMZ, Suliman FEO, Al-Wishahi Haidar AA, Al-Lawati AJ, Aoudia M. Determination of PX in pharmaceutical formulations and urine samples using europium-sensitized luminescence. *J Lumin* 2007;127:291-6.
13. Arancibia JA, Escandar GM. Two different strategies for the fluorimetric determination of PX in serum. *Talanta* 2003;60:1113-21.
14. McKinney AR, Suann CJ, Stenhouse AM. The detection of PX, tenoxicam and their metabolites in equine urine by electrospray ionisation ion trap mass spectrometry. *Rapid Commun Mass Sp* 2004;18:2338-42.
15. Ji HY, Lee HW, Kim YH, Jeong DW, Lee HS. Simultaneous determination of piroxicam, meloxicam and tenoxicam in human plasma by liquid chromatography with tandem mass spectrometry. *J Chromatogr B* 2005;826(1-2):214-9.
16. Milligan PA. Determination of PX and its major metabolites in the plasma, urine and bile of humans by high performance liquid chromatography. *J Chromatogr* 1992;516:121-8.
17. Tsai Y-H, Hsu L-R, Naito S-I. Simultaneous determination of PX and its main metabolite in plasma and urine by high–performance liquid chromatography. *Int J Pharm* 1985;24:101-8.
18. De Jager AD, Ellis H, Hundt HK, Swart KJ, Hundt AF. High-performance liquid chromatographic determination with amperometric detection of piroxicam in human plasma and tissues. *J Chromatogr B Biomed Sci Appl* 1999;729(1-2):183-9.
19. Riedel K-D, Laufen H. High-performance thin–layer chromatographic assay for the routine determination of PX in plasma, urine and tissue. *J Chromatogr* 1983;276:243-8.
20. Dadashzadeh S, Vali AM, Rezagholi N. LC determination of PX in human plasma. *J Pharm Biomed Anal* 2002;28:1201-4.

21. Rezaee M, Assadi Y, Milani Hosseini MR, Aghaee E, Ahmadi F, Berijani S. Determination of organic compounds in water using dispersive liquid–liquid microextraction. *J Chromatogr A* 2006;1116:1-9.
22. Pajand Birjandia A, Bidaria A, Rezaeia F, Milani Hosseinia MR, Assadi Y. Speciation of butyl and phenyltin compounds using dispersive liquid–liquid microextraction and gas chromatography-flame photometric detection. *J Chromatogr A* 2008;1193:19-25.
23. Anthemidis AN, Ioannou K-IG. Recent developments in homogeneous and dispersive liquid–liquid extraction for inorganic elements determination. A review. *Talanta* 2009;80(2):413-21.
24. Nuhu AA, Basheer C, Saad B. Liquid-phase and dispersive liquid-liquid microextraction techniques with derivatization: Recent applications in bioanalysis. *J Chromatogr B* 2011;879:1180-8.
25. Zeeb M, Ganjali MR, Norouzi P. Dispersive liquid–liquid microextraction followed by spectrofluorimetry as a simple and accurate technique for determination of thiamine (vitamin B_1). *Microchim Acta* 2010;168:317-24.
26. Zgoła-Grześkowiak A. Application of DLLME to Isolation and Concentration of Non-Steroidal Anti-Inflammatory Drugs in Environmental Water Samples. *Chromatographia* 2010;72:671-8.
27. Tabrizi AB, Rezazadeh A. Development of a dispersive liquid–liquid microextraction technique for the extraction and spectrofluorimetric determination of fluoxetine in pharmaceutical formulations and human urine. *Adv Pharm Bull* 2012;2(2):157-64.
28. Tabrizi AB. Development of a dispersive liquid–liquid microextraction method for iron speciation and determination in different water samples. *J Hazard Mater* 2010;183:688-93.
29. Mashkouri Najafi N, Tavakoli H, Alizadeh R, Seidi S. Speciation and determination of ultra–trace amounts of inorganic tellurium in environmental water samples by dispersive liquid–liquid microextraction and electrothermal atomic absorption spectrometry. *Anal Chim Acta* 2010;670:18-23.
30. Abdolmohammad-Zadeh H, Sadeghi GH. Combination of ionic liquid-based dispersive liquid–liquid micro-extraction with stopped-flow spectrofluorometry for the pre-concentration and determination of aluminum in natural waters, fruit juice and food samples. *Talanta* 2010;81(3):778-85.
31. Godwa BG, Seetharamappa J, Melwanki MB. Indirect spectrophotometric determination of propranolol hydrochloride and PX in pure and pharmaceutical preparations. *Anal Sci* 2002;18:671-4.
32. Takács-Novák K, Tam KY. Multiwavelength spectrophotometric determination of acid dissociation constants: Part V: microconstants and tautomeric ratios of diprotic amphoteric drugs. *J Pharm Biomed Anal* 2000;21:1171-82.
33. Islambulchilar Z, Ghanbarzadeh S, Emami S, Valizadeh H, Zakeri-Milani P. Development and Validation of an HPLC Method for the Analysis of Sirolimus in Drug Products. *Adv Pharm Bull* 2012;2(2):135-9.
34. Miller JC, Miller JN. Statistics for Analytical Chemistry. New York: Wiley; 1984.
35. Verbeeck RK, Richardson CJ, Blocka KLN. Clinical pharmacokinetics of piroxicam. *J Rheumatol* 1986;13:789-96.
36. Richardson CJ, Blocka KLN, Ross SG, Verbeeck RK. Piroxicam and 5'-Hydroxypiroxicam Kinetics Following Multiple Dose Administration of Piroxicam. *Eur J Clin Pharmacol* 1987;32:89-91.

2

Development and Application of an HPLC Method for Erlotinib Protein Binding Studies

Soheila Bolandnazar[1,2], Adeleh Divsalar[1], Hadi Valizadeh[3], Arash Khodaei[4], Parvin Zakeri-Milani[5]*

[1] *Department of Biological Sciences, Kharazmi University, Tehran, Iran.*

[2] *Biotechnology Research Center, Tabriz University of Medical Sciences, Tabriz, Iran.*

[3] *Research Center for Pharmaceutical Nanotechnology and Faculty of Pharmacy, Tabriz University of Medical Sciences, Tabriz, Iran.*

[4] *Department of biological sciences, Institute for Advanced Studies in Basic Sciences, Zanjan, Iran.*

[5] *Drug Applied Research Center and Faculty of Pharmacy, Tabriz University of Medical Sciences, Tabriz, Iran.*

ARTICLEINFO

Keywords:
Erlotinib
HPLC
Protein binding
Ultrafilteration

ABSTRACT

Purpose: The aim of the present study was to develop a simple and rapid reversed-phase high performance liquid chromatographic method with UV detection for erlotinib hydrochloride quantification, which is applicable for protein binding studies. ***Methods:*** Ultrafilteration method was used for protein binding study of erlotinib hydrochloride. For sample analysis a simple and rapid reversed-phase high performance liquid chromatographic method with UV detection at 332 nm was developed. The mobile phase was a mixture of methanol, acetonitril and potassium dihydrogen phosphate buffer (15:45:40 %v/v) set at flow rate of 1.3 ml/min. ***Results:*** The run time for erlotinib hydrochloride was approximately 6 minutes. The calibration curve was linear over the range of 320-20000 ng/ml with acceptable intra- and inter-day precision and accuracy. The intra-day and inter-day precisions were less than 10% and the accuracies of intra and inter-day assays were within the range of 97.20-104.83% and 98.8-102.2% respectively. ***Conclusion***: Based on the obtained results, a simple, accurate and precise reversed-phase isocratic HPLC method with UV detection has been optimized and validated for the determination of erlotinib hydrochloride in biological samples.

Introduction

Lung cancer is the leading cause of cancer mortality in the world.[1-3] The epidermal growth factor receptor (EGFR) is mutated and over expressed in many human cancers, such as head and neck, breast, ovarian and non-small cell lung cancers (NSCLC).[4] Epidermal growth factor receptor-tyrosine kinase inhibitors (EGFR-TKIs) are used as first-line and efficient therapy in the treatment of advanced non-small cell lung cancer patients.[2,5] The family of epidermal growth factor receptor (HER1/EGFR), containing four members, are essential in modulating cell proliferation, cell differentiation, and cell survival in many tissue types.[6] Erlotinib is a quinazolinamine with the chemical name of N-(3- ethynylphenyl)- 6,7- bis(2-methoxyethoxy)- 4- quinazolinamine.[7] The chemical structure of erlotinib is shown in Figure 1.

Plasma protein binding of erlotinib is reported to be approximately 93% and it has an apparent volume of distribution of 232 liters.[3,8,9] It is a white powder, slightly soluble in water, soluble in organic solvents such as ethanol, DMSO, and dimethyl formamide (DMF), which should be purged with an inert gas.[10] Erlotinib is almost a new drug used for the treatment of non-small cell lung cancer after the failure of more than one or two courses of previous chemotherapy. It is an orally available low molecular weight EGFR inhibitor that binds competitively to the ATP binding site at the kinase domain of EGFR and inhibits EGFR tyrosine kinase autophosphorylation by inhibition of the intracellular domain.[3,6] Erlotinib is metabolised by the hepatic cytochromes in humans, primarily CYP3A4/CYP3A5 and to a lesser extent by CYP1A2 and the pulmonary isoform CYP1A1.[11,12] On the other hand, binding of drugs to plasma and tissue proteins significantly affects the pharmacokinetic and pharmacodynamic behaviors of drugs. The pharmacologic effect of a drug in the body is related to the free drug concentration at the target site. Because the bound drug is kept in the blood stream while the unbound components of the drug, may be distributed or metabolized, making them the active part of the drug. Therefore protein binding studies would be of great

***Corresponding author:** Parvin Zakeri-Milani, Department of Pharmaceutics, Faculty of Pharmacy, Tabriz University of Medical Sciences, Tabriz, Iran. 51664. E-mail: pzakeri@tbzmed.ac.ir

importance in clinical and pharmaceutical sciences. For this purpose drug analysis in study samples is the main issue. Although several HPLC techniques have been developed for the assay of erlotinib, like liquid chromatography – tandem mass spectrometry (LC/MS/MS) methods, there is still no simple and rapid HPLC method available for its quantification in clinical and pharmaceutical samples.[13-18] Therefore in the present study a simple, sensitive, rapid and effective HPLC method was developed and validated for quantification of erlotinib hydrochloride with the application to protein binding studies.

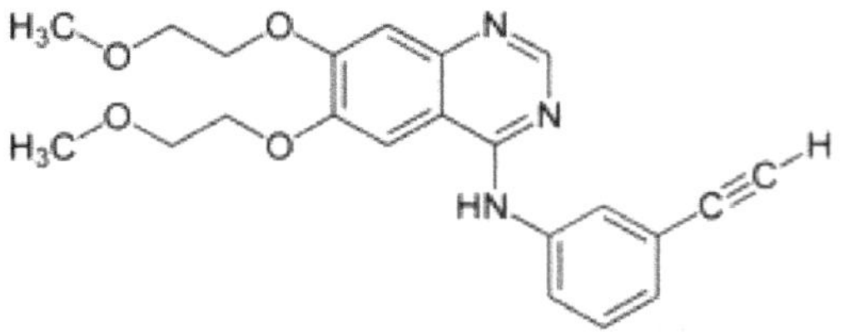

Figure 1. Chemical structure of Erlotinib.

Materials and Methods

Chemicals

Dialysis membranes and dialyzers were obtained from Harvard (Harvard, USA). HPLC grade solvents, such as methanol and acetonitril were purchased from Merck (Darmstadt, Germany). Triethylamine, potassium dihydrogen phosphate, sodium hydroxide, and orthophosphoric acid were also provided from Merck (Darmstadt, Germany). Pharmaceutical-grade human albumin 20% was purchased from CSL Behring GmbH, Germany. Double-distilled water was used during the experiments.

Chromatographic system

Analysis was performed with a knauer high performance liquid chromatography system (Berlin, Germany). Analytical column used for analysis was a reversed-phase Symmetry C18 column shimadzu, Shim-pack VP ODS (250 mm × 4.6 mm, 5 μm) at room temperature. Injection volume was 20μl which was injected into the column using a Hamilton (Bonaduz, Switzerland) injector syringe and the flow rate was set at 1.3 ml/min. Erlotinib hydrochloride was detected by UV absorption at 332 nm. The mobile phase was a mixture of 15% (v/v) methanol, 45% (v/v) acetonitril and 40% (v/v) potassium dihydrogen phosphate buffer with pH adjusted to 4.5 with orthophosphoric acid.

Preparation of stock and standard solutions

The stock solution of erlotinib was prepared by dissolving 10 mg erlotinib hydrochloride in potassium phosphate buffer, adjusted to pH 7.4 with NaOH 0.2 M, in a 50 ml volumetric flask to provide a concentration of 200 μg/ml. Then, working standard solutions were prepared by serial dilution using potassium phosphate buffer (pH 7.4) solution to obtain erlotinib hydrochloride concentrations of 0.3, 0.62, 1.25, 2.5, 5, 10 and 20 μg/ml for demonstration of calibration curve.

Method Validation

Validation of the assay consisting of linearity, lower limit of detection and quantitation (LOD and LOQ), intra-day and inter-day accuracy and precision of the method was performed. To assess linearity, known concentrations of erlotinib hydrochloride in PBS buffer were prepared. The accuracy and precision data were obtained by analyzing four aliquots of samples at different concentrations. Intraday reproducibility was determined using four aliquots of samples and inter-day reproducibility was determined over a 3- day period (n=4). Accuracy was evaluated by calculating the percentage deviation of the calculated concentration and the theoretical concentration while the precision was assessed via calculating the coefficient of variation percentage (CV %) for intra- and inter-day runs. The acceptable value for accuracy is less than ±15% deviation from the nominal values and, CV% ≤ ±15% for precision.[19] There are three different methods for determination of LOD and LOQ as indicated in ICH guidelines. However in this study, to determine the LOD, the signal to noise ratio was used by comparing test results from samples with known concentrations to blank samples. The LOQ is also defined as the lowest concentration that can be quantitate with acceptable precision and accuracy under the stated experimental condition.[20,21]

Stability test

The stability of working standard samples was determined at ambient temperature by analyzing the solutions over a period of 8 hours (considering the approximate time required for preparation of samples and analysis by HPLC method). The aim was to ensure that the preparation of samples and analysis time did not contribute to the degradation of drug to indicate that the samples will remain stable during the course of the analysis.[19,21,22]

Protein binding study

Ultrafiltration (UF) method which is a simple and reliable procedure for measuring the protein unbound fraction of a drug in plasma was used in this investigation. Aqueous solutions containing 2, 4, 6, 8, 10 μg/ml of erlotinib hydrochloride and 0.04 g/ml of human serum albumin were prepared. After a period of 1 hour, to produce ultrafiltrates containing unbound drug, the samples were added in the ultrafiltration system (cellulose acetate membrane with 25KDa molecular weight cut-off). Centrifugations were performed at 37°C, for 10 min at 4000 rpm, resulting in filtrate volumes of 0.3–0.4 mL. The fraction of unbound drug was calculated as the ratio of the ultrafiltrate (free) concentration and the total concentration determined in the HPLC analysis. The drug concentrations were plotted according to

Scatchard where the abscissa represents the binding r (the number of molecules of drug bound per molecule of albumin), and the ordinate r/D_f (D_f is free drug concentration). The data of r and D_f were fitted by linear least squares regression analysis. Then the number of binding sites and association constants were calculated.[23]

Results and Discussion

Linearity

Six standard samples (0.3, 0.6, 1.2, 2.5, 5, 10 and 20 µg/ml) were prepared to generate the calibration curve for linearity of the method. Representative chromatogram of consecutively concentrations of erlotinib hydrochloride is shown in Figure 2. Statistical analysis using least square regression indicated excellent linearity for erlotinib hydrochloride in the mentioned range. A good correlation between erlotinib hydrochloride peak heights and drug concentration was observed with $r^2 \geq 0.99$ for all standard curves (Table 1). Concentration curves for erlotinib hydrochloride had a mean slope, intercept and r^2 of 0.33, -22.8 and 0.996 respectively. The retention time was approximately 6 min.

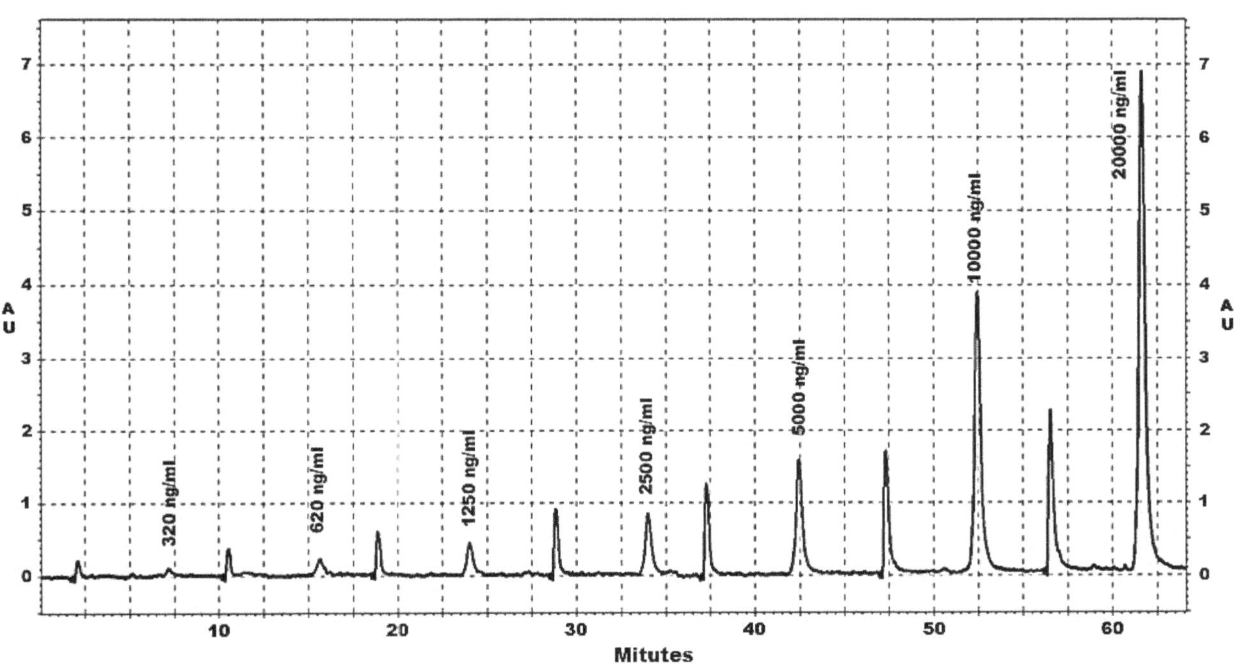

Figure 2. Representative chromatogram of erlotinib hydrochloride standard samples with different concentrations.

Table 1. Analytical parameters of erlotinib hydrochloride calibration curves on three consecutive days.

Standard curve	Slope	Intercept	r^2
Day 1	8861.0	2053.0	0.9979
Day 2	9010.6	1776.1	0.9970
Day 3	9019.2	1343.0	0.9976
Mean	8963.6	1724.0	0.9970
RSD	0.009	0.207	0.0004

LOD and LOQ

The LOD was defined as the analyte concentration that gives a signal equal to $y_b+3.3s_b$, where y_b is the signal of the blank and s_b is its standard deviation. Similarly, the LOQ was defined as y_b+10s_b. In the unweiged least-squares method it is quite suitable in practice to use s_{xy} (Residual standard deviation) instead of s_b and the value of the calculated intercept instead of y_b. Thus LOD = 3.3 s_{xy} / b and LOQ = 10 s_{xy} /b, Where b is the slope of the regression line. Based on the above equations, the calculated LOD and LOQ values for erlotinib hydrochloride were 46 and 150 ng/ ml respectively.

Accuracy and Precision

The intra- and inter-day precision and accuracy was shown as percent of coefficient of variation (CV %) and mean percentage of analyte recovered in the assay, respectively. The Intra-day precision, accuracy and relative errors range were calculated to be 1.91-3.07%, 97.2-104.83% and 0.6- 4.83, respectively. The same parameters for inter-day evaluations were 1.56-9.91%, 98.8-100% and 0-2.2%, respectively. Precision (CV %) and relative error percent acquired at all of concentrations do not exceed ±15% (Table 2) which is required by guidelines.

Table 2. Intra-day and inter-day accuracy and precision obtained from calibration curves with four levels of QC samples.

Added concentration (µg/ml)	Intra-day				Inter-day			
	Measured concentration (mean ± SD, µg /ml)	Precision (CV %)	Accuracy (%)	Relative Error %	Measured concentration (mean ± SD, µg /ml)	Precision (CV %)	Accuracy (%)	Relative Error %
0.62	0.65±0.02	3.07	104.83	4.83	0.62±0.05	8.06	100	0.0
2.5	2.43±0.19	7.81	97.2	2.8	2.47±0.24	9.91	98.8	1.2
10	9.93±0.26	2.61	99.3	0.7	10.22±0.16	1.56	102.2	2.2
20	19.88±0.38	1.91	99.4	0.6	19.92±0.56	2.81	99.6	0.4

Stability

The stability of erlotinib hydrochloride standard samples was tested at room temperature by testing the solutions over a period of 8 hours (Table 3). The purpose of this test was to confirm that erlotinib hydrochloride in both standard and protein binding samples were stable during the course of analysis. The solutions were considered stable if the variability in the assay results was less than 15 % of initial. Results indicated that erlotinib hydrochloride was quite stable during sample preparation and analysis period.

Table 3. Erlotinib Stability during 8h at ambient temperature.

Added concentration (µg/ml)	Measured concentration (mean ± SD, µg /ml)	Standard Deviation (%)
0.62	0.627±0.02	0.04
5	4.99±0.05	0.05
20	19.55±0.12	0.20

Protein binding studies

The free drug concentrations in ultrafiltrates and mean protein binding percentages were in the range of 0.027-0.26 µg/ml and 95.6-98.6% respectively. ν, the number of binding sites and K , the association constant was calculated according to the regression line equation as 0.0328 and 5×106 respectively (Figure 3). Based on the results, the protein binding percentage of erlotinib hydrochloride reduced with increasing the drug concentration. Concentration-dependent protein binding has been observed for many drugs such as some macrolides and beta-lactams. As the concentration of drug increases, binding sites on proteins are increasingly saturated, resulting in higher percentages of unbound drug.[23]

Conclusion

The mentioned method described in this paper has acceptable linearity, accuracy, and precision. Therefore the validated method can be used for routine analysis of erlotinib hydrochloride in samples of different studies like plasma protein binding investigations which are of great importance in clinical and pharmaceutical sciences.

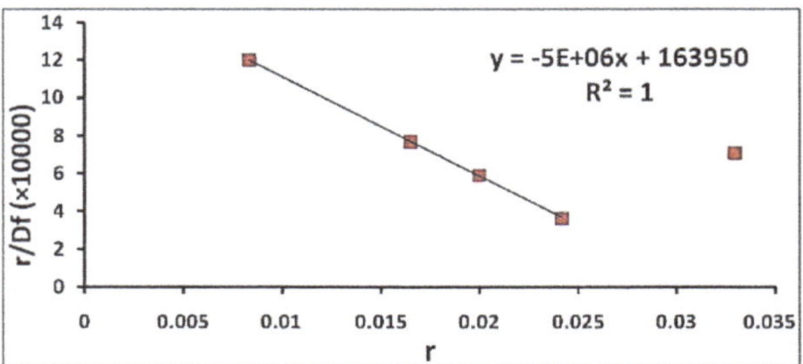

Figure 3. Scatchard plot of erlotinib.

Acknowledgments

The authors would like to thank the authorities of Drug Applied Research Center, Tabriz University of Medical Sciences, for their financial support.

Conflict of Interest

The authors report no conflict of interest in this study.

References

1. Xu XH, Su J, Fu XY, Xue F, Huang Q, Li DJ, et al. Clinical effect of erlotinib as first-line treatment for asian elderly patients with advanced non-small-cell lung cancer. *Cancer Chemother Pharmacol* 2011;67(2):475-9.
2. Fan WC, Yu CJ, Tsai CM, Huang MS, Lai CL, Hsia TC, et al. Different efficacies of erlotinib and gefitinib in taiwanese patients with advanced non-small cell lung cancer: A retrospective multicenter study. *J Thorac Oncol* 2011;6(1):148-55.
3. Padmalatha M, Kulsum S, Rahul C, Thimma Reddy D, Vidyasagar G. Spectrophotometric methods for the determination of erlotinib in pure and pharmaceutical dosage forms. *Int J Pharm Res Dev* 2011;3(6):103-9.
4. Paez JG, Janne PA, Lee JC, Tracy S, Greulich H, Gabriel S, et al. EGFR mutations in lung cancer:

correlation with clinical response to gefitinib therapy. *Science* 2004;304(5676):1497-500.
5. Arora A, Scholar EM. Role of tyrosine kinase inhibitors in cancer therapy. *J Pharmacol Exp Ther* 2005;315(3):971-9.
6. Schaefer G, Shao L, Totpal K, Akita RW. Erlotinib directly inhibits HER2 kinase activation and downstream signaling events in intact cells lacking epidermal growth factor receptor expression. *Cancer Res* 2007;67(3):1228-38.
7. Barghi L, Aghanejad A, Valizadeh H, Barar J, Asgari D. Modified synthesis of erlotinib hydrochloride. *Adv Pharm Bull* 2012;2(1):119-22.
8. Australia Government. Tarceva. Roche Products Pty Ltd; 2010; Available from: http://www.tga.gov.au/pdf/auspar/auspar-tarceva.pdf.
9. Johnson JR, Cohen M, Sridhara R, Chen YF, Williams GM, Duan J, et al. Approval summary for erlotinib for treatment of patients with locally advanced or metastatic non-small cell lung cancer after failure of at least one prior chemotherapy regimen. *Clin Cancer Res* 2005;11(18):6414-21.
10. Cayman Chemical Company wcc. Product information:Erlotinib. *No10483* 2010.
11. Ling J, Johnson KA, Miao Z, Rakhit A, Pantze MP, Hamilton M, et al. Metabolism and excretion of erlotinib, a small molecule inhibitor of epidermal growth factor receptor tyrosine kinase, in healthy male volunteers. *Drug Metab Dispos* 2006;34(3):420-6.
12. Rudin CM, Liu W, Desai A, Karrison T, Jiang X, Janisch L, et al. Pharmacogenomic and pharmacokinetic determinants of erlotinib toxicity. *J Clin Oncol* 2008;26(7):1119-27.
13. Faivre L, Gomo C, Mir O, Taieb F, Schoemann-Thomas A, Ropert S, et al. A simple HPLC-UV method for the simultaneous quantification of gefitinib and erlotinib in human plasma. *J Chromatogr B Analyt Technol Biomed Life Sci* 2011;879(23):2345-50.
14. Karunakara C, Aparna U, Chandregowda V, Reddy CG. Separation and determination of process-related impurities of erlotinib using reverse-phase HPLC with a photo-diode array detector. *Anal Sci* 2012;28(3):305-8.
15. Masters AR, Sweeney CJ, Jones DR. The quantification of erlotinib (OSI-774) and OSI-420 in human plasma by liquid chromatography-tandem mass spectrometry. *J Chromatogr B Analyt Technol Biomed Life Sci* 2007;848(2):379-83.
16. Chahbouni A, Den Burger JC, Vos RM, Sinjewel A, Wilhelm AJ. Simultaneous quantification of erlotinib, gefitinib, and imatinib in human plasma by liquid chromatography tandem mass spectrometry. *Ther Drug Monit* 2009;31(6):683-7.
17. Lankheet NA, Hillebrand MJ, Rosing H, Schellens JH, Beijnen JH, Huitema AD. Method development and validation for the quantification of dasatinib, erlotinib, gefitinib, imatinib, lapatinib, nilotinib, sorafenib and sunitinib in human plasma by liquid chromatography coupled with tandem mass spectrometry. *Biomed Chromatogr* 2012.
18. Thappali SR, Varanasi K, Veeraraghavan S, Arla R, Chennupati S, Rajamanickam M, et al. Simultaneous determination of celecoxib, erlotinib, and its metabolite desmethyl-erlotinib (OSI-420) in rat plasma by liquid chromatography/tandem mass spectrometry with positive/negative ion-switching electrospray ionisation. *Sci Pharm* 2012;80(3):633-46.
19. Islambulchilar Z, Ghanbarzadeh S, Emami S, Valizadeh H, Zakeri-Milani P. Development and validation of an HPLC method for the analysis of sirolimus in drug products. *Adv Pharm Bull* 2012;2(2):135-9.
20. Chakravarthy VK, Sankar DG. Development and validation of RP-HPLC method for estimation of erlotinib in bulk and its pharmaceuticals formulations. *RASAYAN J Chem* 2011;4:393-9.
21. Islambulchilar Z, Valizadeh H, Zakeri-Milani P. Rapid hplc determination of pioglitazone in human plasma by protein precipitation and its application to pharmacokinetic studies. *J AOAC Int* 2010;93(3):876-81.
22. Holt DW, Lee T, Johnston A. Measurement of sirolimus in whole blood using high-performance liquid chromatography with ultraviolet detection. *Clin Ther* 2000;22 Suppl B:B38-48.
23. Zeitlinger M, Derendorf H, Mouton J, Cars O, Craig W, Andes D, et al. Protein binding: Do we ever learn? . *Antimicrob agents chemother* 2011;55(7):3067-74.

3

Protective Effect against Hydroxyl-induced DNA Damage and Antioxidant Activity of *Citri reticulatae* Pericarpium

Xican Li[1]*, Yanping Huang[1], Dongfeng Chen[2]

[1] *School of Chinese Herbal Medicine, Guangzhou University of Chinese Medicine, Waihuang East Road No.232, Guangzhou Higher Education Mega Center, 510006, Guangzhou, China.*

[2] *School of Basic Medical Science, Guangzhou University of Chinese Medicine, Guangzhou, 510006, China.*

ARTICLEINFO

Keywords:
Citri reticulatae pericarpium
Antioxidant activity
DNA oxidative damage
Chenpi
Hesperidin
Narirutin

ABSTRACT

Purpose: As a typical Chinese herbal medicine, *Citri reticulatae* pericarpium (CRP) possesses various pharmacological effects involved in antioxidant ability. However, its antioxidant effects have not been reported yet. The objective of this work was to investigate its antioxidant ability, then further discuss the antioxidant mechanism. ***Methods:*** CRP was extracted by ethanol to obtain ethanol extract of *Citri reticulatae* pericarpium (ECRP). ECRP was then measured by various antioxidant methods, including DNA damage assay, DPPH assay, ABTS assay, Fe^{3+}-reducing assay and Cu^{2+}-reducing assay. Finally, the content of total flavonoids was analyzed by spectrophotometric method. ***Results:*** Our results revealed that ECRP could effectively protect against hydroxyl-induced DNA damage (IC_{50} 944.47±147.74 μg/mL). In addition, it could also scavenge DPPH· radical (IC_{50}349.67±1.91 μg/mL) and $ABTS^{+}$• radical (IC_{50}11.33±0.10 μg/mL), reduce Fe^{3+} (IC_{50} 140.95±2.15 μg/mL) and Cu^{2+} (IC_{50} 70.46±1.77 μg/mL). Chemical analysis demonstrated that the content of total flavonoids in ECRP was 198.29±12.24 mg quercetin/g. ***Conclusion:*** *Citri reticulatae* pericarpium can effectively protect against hydroxyl-induced DNA damage. One mechanism of protective effect may be radical-scavenging which is via donating hydrogen atom (H·), donating electron (e). Its antioxidant ability can be mainly attributed to the flavonoids, especially hesperidin and narirutin.

Introduction

Reactive oxygen species (ROS) include hydroxyl radical (·OH), superoxide anion ($\cdot O_2^-$), hydrogen peroxide (H_2O_2), and nitric oxide (NO), with the ·OH being the most harmful. All macromolecules are sensitive to free radical damage. For example, DNA can be easily damaged by ·OH then lead to severe biological consequences including mutation, cell death, carcinogenesis, and aging.[1]

Therefore, it is vital to search for potential therapeutic agents for DNA oxidative damage. Over the last two decades, much attention has been focused on the antioxidant of medicinal plants especially Chinese medicinal herbals.

As a typical Chinese herbal medicine, *Citri reticulatae* pericarpium (CRP, 陈皮 in Chinese, Figure 1A) has been used in traditional Chinese medicine (TCM) for about 2000 years[2,3] CRP is the dried and ripe pericarpium of *Citri reticulatae* Blanco (Figure 1B). From the viewpoint of TCM, CRP can invigorate *spleen,* replenish *qi,* eliminate dampness and phlegm.[3] Modern medicine has demonstrated that CRP possessed various pharmacological effects. For example, the extract from CRP could induce the apoptosis on SNU-C4 (human colon cancer cells) via Bax-related caspase-3 activation.[4] Ou reported that the extract from CRP could protect rats against myocardial ischemia.[5] Fang pointed out that CRP had antibacterial action.[6] Fan indicated an insecticidal effect of CRP.[7] In addition, CRP was also proved to be of anti-ulcer and anti-inflammatory.[8] However, according to free radical biology & medicine,[9] all these pharmacological effects may be associated with antioxidant ability.

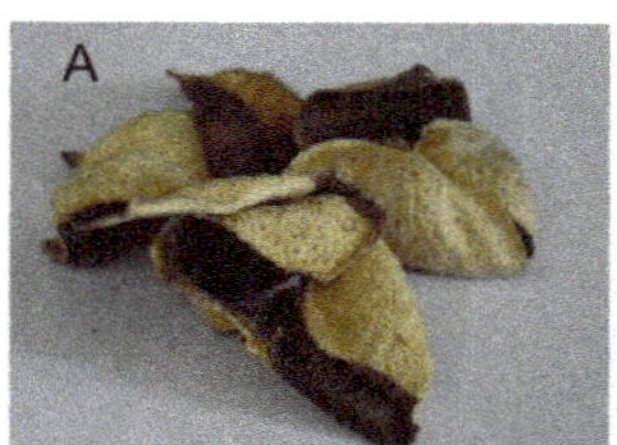

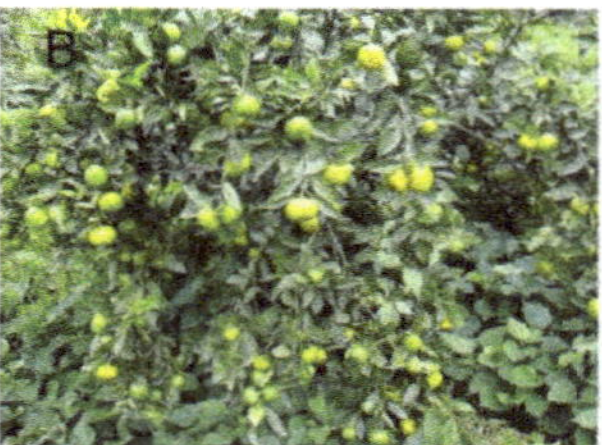

Figure 1. Dried *Citri reticulatae* pericarpium (A) and its plant *Citri reticulatae* Blanco (B)
Figure 1A was contributed by Weikang Chen, Figure 1B was contributed by www.plantphoto.cn

***Corresponding author:** Xican Li, School of Chinese Herbal Medicine, Guangzhou University of Chinese Medicine, Waihuang East Road No.232, Guangzhou Higher Education Mega Center, 510006, Guangzhou, China. Email: lixican@126.com

Until now, its antioxidant ability has not been reported. Therefore, the purpose of the study was to investigate the antioxidant ability, then further discuss the antioxidant mechanism.

Materials and Methods

Plant Material

Citri reticulatae pericarpium was purchased from Caizhilin pharmacy located in Guangzhou University of Chinese Medicine (Guangzhou, China), and authenticated by Professor Shuhui Tan. A voucher specimen was deposited in our laboratory.

Chemicals

DPPH• (1,1-diphenyl-2-picryl-hydrazl radical), ABTS [2,2′-azino-bis(3-ethylbenzo- thiazoline-6-sulfonic acid diammonium salt)], BHA (butylated hydroxyanisole), Trolox [(±)-6- hydroxyl-2,5,7,8-tetramethlychromane-2-carboxylic acid], DNA sodium salt (fish sperm), and neocuproine (2,9-dimethyl-1,10-phenanthroline) were purchased from Sigma Co. (Sigma-Aldrich Shanghai Trading Co., China). Other chemicals used in this study were of analytic grade.

Preparation of Extracts from Citri reticulatae Pericarpium

Citri reticulatae pericarpium was powdered then extracted by absolute ethanol using a Soxhlet extractor for 6 hr. The extract was filtered using a Buckner funnel and Whatman No 1 filter paper. The filtrate was then concentrated to dryness under reduced pressure to yield ECRP (ethanol extract of *Citri reticulatae* pericarpium). It was stored at 4°C for analysis.

Protective Effect against Hydroxyl-Induced DNA Damage

The experiment was conducted as described in previous report.[10] However, deoxyribose was replaced by DNA sodium. Briefly, sample was dissolved in methanol at 8 mg/mL. Various amounts (20-100 μL) of sample methanolic solutions were then separately taken into mini tubes. After evaporating the sample solutions in tubes to dryness, 400 μL of phosphate buffer (0.2 mol/L, pH 7.4) was added to the sample residue. Subsequently, 50 μL DNA sodium (10.0 mg/mL), 50 μL H_2O_2 (50 mmol/L), 50 μL $FeCl_3$ (3.2 mmol/L) and 50 μL Na_2EDTA (1 mmol/L) were added. The reaction was initiated by adding 50 μL ascorbic acid (18 mmol/L) and the total volume of the reaction mixture was adjusted to 800 μL with buffer. After incubation in a water bath at 55 °C for 20 min, the reaction was terminated by adding 250 μL trichloroacetic acid (10g/100mL water). The color was then developed by addition of 150 μL of TBA (2-thiobarbituric acid)(0.4 mol/L, in 1.25% NaOH aqueous solution) and heating in an oven at 105 °C for 15 min. The mixture was cooled and absorbance was measured at 530 nm against the buffer (as blank). The percent of protection against DNA damage is expressed as follows:

$$\text{Protective effect \%} = (1 - A/A_0)\times 100\%$$

Where A_0 is the absorbance of the mixture without sample, and A is the absorbance of the mixture with sample.

DPPH• Radical-Scavenging Assay

DPPH• radical-scavenging activity was determined as previously described by Li.[11] Briefly, 1 mL DPPH• ethanolic solution (0.1 mM) was mixed with 0.5 mL sample alcoholic solution (4.0 mg/mL). The mixture was kept at room temperature for 30 min, and then measured with a spectrophotometer (Unico 2100, Shanghai, China) at 519 nm. The DPPH• inhibition percentage was calculated as:

$$\text{Inhibition \%} = (1 - A/A_0)\times 100\%,$$

where A is the absorbance with sample, while A_0 is the absorbance without sample.

$ABTS^{+}$• Radical-Scavenging Assay

The $ABTS^{+}$• -scavenging activity was measured as described[12] with some modifications. The $ABTS^{+}$• was produced by mixing 0.35 mL ABTS diammonium salt (7.4 mmol/L) with potassium 0.35 mL persulfate (2.6 mmol/L). The mixture was kept in the dark at room temperature for 12 h to allow completion of radical generation, then diluted with 95% ethanol (about 1:50) so that its absorbance at 734 nm was 0.70 ± 0.02. To determine the scavenging activity, 1.2 mL aliquot of diluted $ABTS^{+}$• reagent was mixed with 0.3 mL of sample ethanolic solution (0.08-0.4 mg/mL). After incubation for 6 min, the absorbance at 734 nm was read on a spectrophotometer (Unico 2100, Shanghai, China). The percentage inhibition was calculated as:

$$\text{Inhibition \%} = (1 - A/A_0)\times 100\%$$

Here, A_0 is the absorbance of the mixture without sample, A is the absorbance of the mixture with sample.

Reducing Power (Fe^{3+}) Assay

Ferric (Fe^{3+}) reducing power was determined according to the method of Oyaizu.[13] In brief, sample solution x μL (2 mg/mL, x = 30, 60, 90, 120, and 150) was mixed with (350-x) μL Na_2HPO_4/KH_2PO_4 buffer (0.2 mol/L, pH 6.6) and 250 μL $K_3Fe(CN)_6$ aqueous solution (1 g/100 mL). After incubation at 50 °C for 20 min, the mixture was added by 250 μL of trichloroacetic acid (10 g/100 mL), then centrifuged at 3500 r/min for 10 min. As soon as 400 μL supernatant was aliquoted into 400 μL $FeCl_3$ (0.1 g/100 mL in distilled water), the timer was started. At 90 s, absorbance of the mixture was read at 700 nm (Unico 2100, Shanghai, China). Samples were analyzed in groups of three, and when the analysis of one group has finished, the next group of three samples was aliquoted into $FeCl_3$ to avoid oxidization by air. The relative reducing ability of the sample was calculated by using the formula:

$$\text{Relative reducing effect \%} = (A-A_{min})/(A_{max}-A_{min})\times 100\%$$

Here, A_{max} is the maximum absorbance and A_{min} is the minimum absorbance in the test. A is the absorbance of sample.

Cu^{2+}-Reducing Power Assay

The Cu^{2+}-reducing capacity was determined by the method,[14] with minor modifications. Briefly, 125 μL $CuSO_4$ aqueous solution (0.01 mol/L), 125 μL neocuproine ethanolic solution (7.5 mmol/L) and (750-*x*) μL CH_3COONH_4 buffer solution (0.1 mol/L, pH 7.5) were brought to test tubes. Then, different volumes of samples (2mg/mL, x = 40-120 μL) were added to the tubes. Then, the total volume was adjusted to 1000 μL with the buffer and mixed vigorously. Absorbance against a buffer blank was measured at 450 nm after 30 min (Unico 2100, Shanghai, China). The relative reducing power of the sample as compared with the maximum absorbance, was calculated by the formula:

$$\text{Relative reducing effect } \% = (A-A_{min})/(A_{max}-A_{min}) \times 100\%$$

where, A_{max} is the maximum absorbance at 450 nm and A_{min} is the minimum absorbance in the test. A is the absorbance of sample.

Determination of Total Flavonoids

The content of total flavonoids was measured using the $NaNO_2$ -Al $(NO_3)_3$ method.[15] In brief, 0.05mL sample methanolic solution (20 mg/mL) was mixed with 0.15 mL $NaNO_2$ aqueous solution (5%, w/w). The mixture stood for 6 min, followed by the addition of 0.15 mL Al $(NO_3)_3$ aqueous solution (10%, w/w). After incubation at ambient temperature for 6 min, 2 mL NaOH aqueous solution (4%, w/w) was added to the mixture which was then adjusted to 5 mL with distilled water. The absorbance was read at 508 nm on a spectrophotometer (Unico 2100, Shanghai, China). The standard curve was prepared using different concentrations of quercetin and the results were also expressed as quercetin in milligrams per gram extract.

Statistical Analysis

Data are given as the mean ± SD of three measurements. The IC_{50} values were calculated by linear regression analysis. All linear regression in this paper was analyzed by Origin 6.0 professional software. Significant differences were performed using the *T*-test ($p < 0.05$). The analysis was performed using SPSS software (v.12, SPSS, USA).

Results and Discussion

It is well known that hydroxyl radical (•OH) is generated in human body via Fenton reaction. Since •OH radical has extreme reactivity, it can easily damage DNA to produce malondialdehyde (MDA) and various oxidative lesions.[16,17] MDA combines TBA (2-thiobarbituric acid) to produce TBARS (thiobarbituric acid reactive substances) which present a maximum absorbance at 530 nm.[18] On the other hand, as the oxidative lesions mentioned above have no conjugative system in the molecules (Figure 2), they cannot be detected by a spectrophotometer at 530 nm. It means that these oxidative lesions can bring about no interference with the determination of MDA.

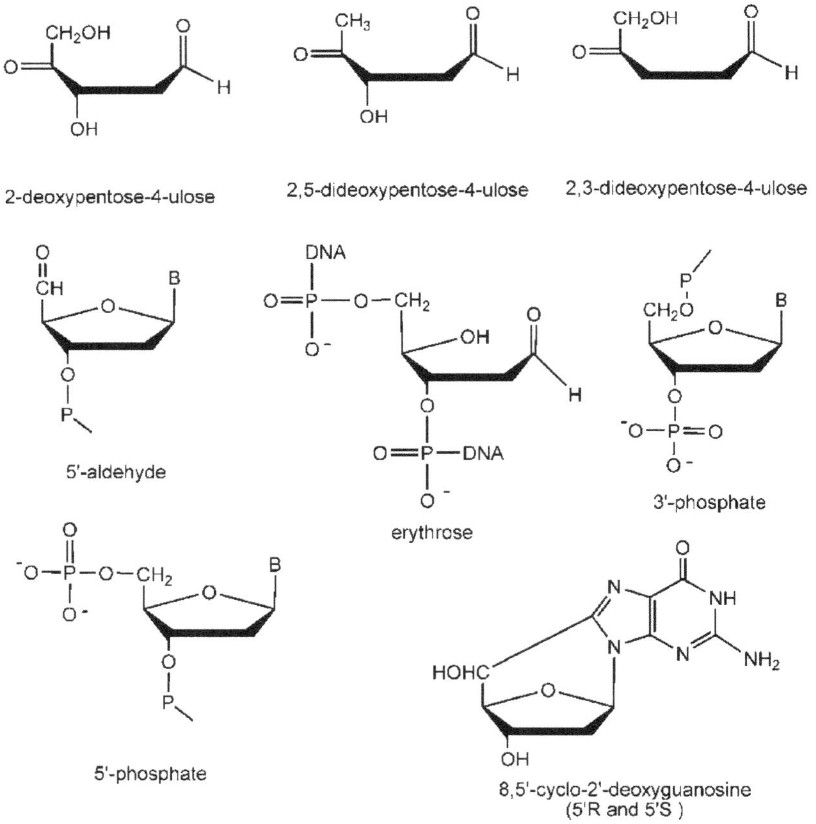

2-deoxypentose-4-ulose
2,5-dideoxypentose-4-ulose
2,3-dideoxypentose-4-ulose
5'-aldehyde
erythrose
3'-phosphate
5'-phosphate
8,5'-cyclo-2'-deoxyguanosine (5'R and 5'S)

Figure 2. The structures of some oxidative lesions.

Hence, the value of A_{532nm} can evaluate the amount of MDA, and ultimately reflect the extent of DNA damage. Based on the formula "protective effect % = $(1 - A/A_0) \times 100\%$", it can be deduced that the decrease of A_{530nm} value indicates a protective effect against DNA damage. As seen in Figure 3A, ECRP dose-dependently increased the protective effect against DNA damage from 0-1240 μg/mL and its IC_{50} value was 944.47±147.74 μg/mL (Table 1).

Previous works have shown that there were two approaches for natural antioxidant to protect DNA oxidative damage: one was to scavenge the •OH radicals then to reduce its attack; one was to fast repair the deoxynucleotide radical cations which were damaged by •OH radicals.[19] To further confirm whether the protective effect of ECRP was associated with its radical-scavenging ability, we determined the DPPH· and $ABTS^{+}\cdot$ radical-scavenging abilities.

The DPPH and ABTS assays have been widely used to determine the free radical-scavenging activity of various plants and pure compounds. Both DPPH• and $ABTS^{+}\cdot$ are stable free radicals which dissolve in methanol or ethanol, and their colors show characteristic absorptions at 519 nm or 734 nm, respectively. When an antioxidant scavenges the free radicals, the values of A_{519nm} or A_{734nm} will decrease. On this basis, the inhibition percentages were defined as: inhibition % = $(1 - A/A_0) \times 100\%$.

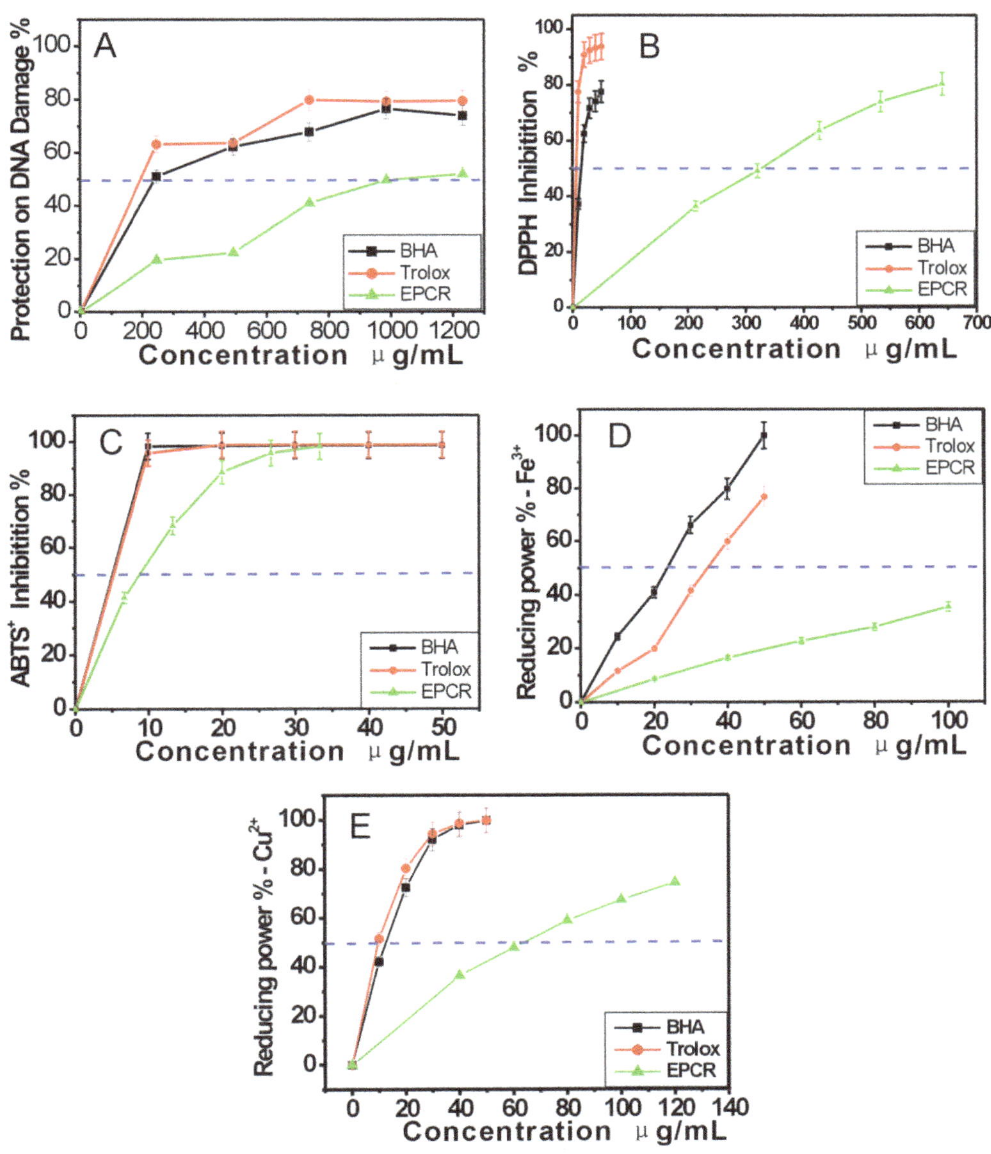

Figure 3. The dose response curves of ECRP in the antioxidant assays: (A) protective effect against DAN damage; (B)DPPH· scavenging; (C)$ABTS^{+}\cdot$ scavenging (D) Fe^{3+}-reducing; (E) Cu^{2+}-reducing.

ECRP, absolute ethanol extract of *Citri reticulatae* pericarpium. Trolox and BHA (butylated hydroxyanisole) were used as the positive controls. Each value is expressed as Mean±SD (*n*=3).

Table 1. The IC_{50} values of ethanol extract from *Citri reticulatae* pericarpium (ECRP) (μg/mL)

	ECRP	Positive controls	
		Trolox	BHA
Protecting DNA damage	944.47±147.74 ^{c}	306.13±26.11 ^{a}	344.89±30.28 ^{b}
DPPH· scavenging	349.67±1.91 ^{c}	9.75±0.06 ^{a}	22.35±0.58 ^{b}
$ABTS^{+}$· scavenging	11.33±0.10 ^{b}	5.09±0.02 ^{a}	5.21±0.25 ^{a}
Fe^{3+}-reducing	140.95±2.15 ^{c}	34.58±1.45 ^{b}	22.88±1.03 ^{a}
Cu^{2+}-reducing	70.46±1.77 ^{c}	13.82±0.30 ^{a}	16.09±0.47 ^{b}

IC_{50} value is defined as the concentration of 50% effect percentage and expressed as Mean±SD (n=3). Means values with different superscripts in the same row are significantly different (p<0.05), while with same superscripts are not signifiacntly different (p<0.05). BHA , butylated hydroxyanisole.

As can be seen in Figure 3B, ECRP can effectively inhibit DPPH• radical from 0-648 μg/mL and its IC_{50} was 349.67±1.91 μg/mL (Table 1). The previous study suggested that DPPH· may be scavenged by an antioxidant through donation of hydrogen atom (H·) to form a stable DPPH-H molecule.[20] For example, hesperidin which occurred in *Citri reticulatae* pericarpium,[21] may scavenge DPPH• via the following proposed reaction[22,23] (Figure 4).

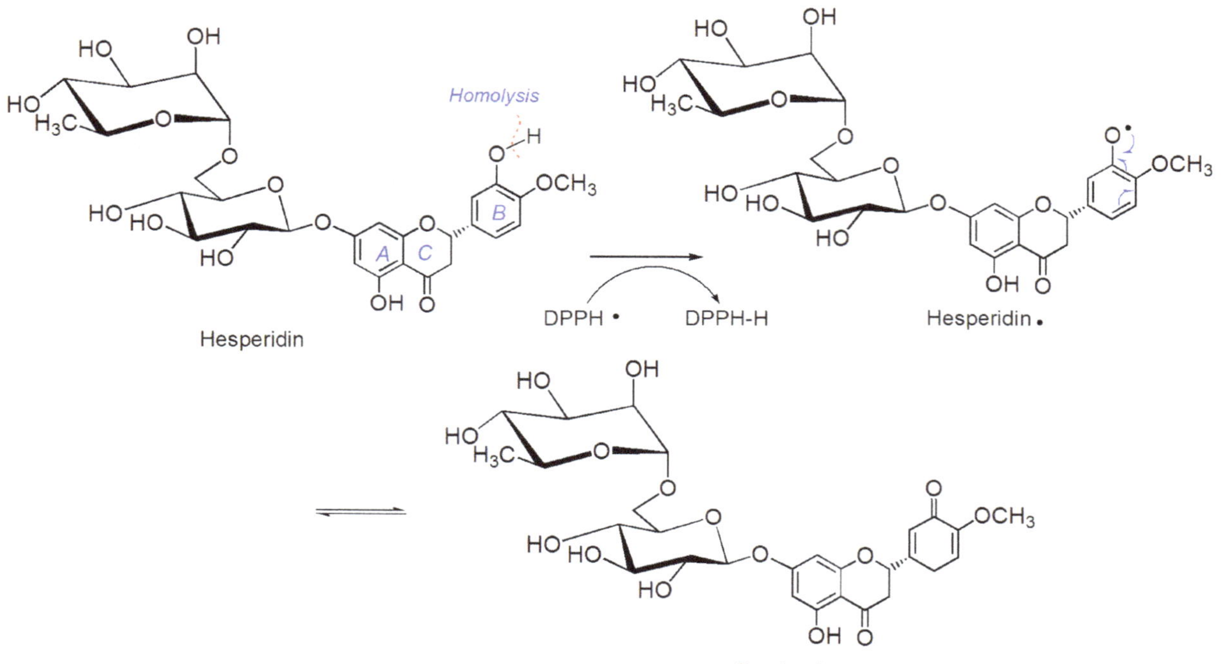

Figure 4. The proposed reaction of hesperidin with DPPH•.

The data in Figure 3C indicated that ECRP could also scavenge $ABTS^{+}$· in a dose-dependent manner (0-35μg/mL) and its IC_{50} was 11.33±0.10μg/mL (Table 1). However, $ABTS·^{+}$ scavenging is regarded as an electron (e) transfer reaction.[24]

The fact that ECRP can effectively scavenge both DPPH· and $ABTS^{+}$·radicals, suggests that: (1) the protective effect of ECRP against DNA oxidative damage was associated with its radical-scavenging ability; (2) ECRP exerted its radical-scavenging action by donating hydrogen atom (H·) and electron (e).

Although a reductant is not necessarily an antioxidant, an antioxidant is commonly a reductant.[25] The reducing power of an antioxidant may therefore serve as a significant indicator of its potential antioxidant activity.[26] Figure 3D&3E showed that ECRP exhibited its reducing powers on Fe^{3+} and Cu^{2+} in a concentration dependent manner. The IC_{50} values were 140.95±2.15 μg/mL & 70.46±1.77 μg/mL, respectively for Fe^{3+}-reducing and Cu^{2+}-reducing) (Table 1). Obviously, these data further support the findings mentioned above.

Previous studies have shown that flavonoids can be responsible for the antioxidant ability in plants, we then determined the content of total flavonoids in ECRP. Our results indicated a high amount of total flavonoids (198.29±12.24 mg quercetin/g) in ECRP. In fact, at least 9 flavonoids have been isolated from *Citri reticulatae* pericarpium until now, including hesperidin,[27] narirutin,[27] nobiletin,[27] tangeretin,[27] natsudaidain,[21] 3,5,6,7,8,3', 4'-heptamethoxylflavones,[27] 5-hydroxyl-6,7,8,3',4'–pentamethoxylflavone,[28] 5,6,7,8, 4'–pentamethoxylflavone,[28] and 5,6,7,8,3',4'–hexamethoxylflavone (Figure 5).[28] Among them, hesperidin and narirutin presented much higher content that the others in CRP.[27] Therefore, hesperidin and narirutin were regarded as two main active components of antioxidant in CRP.

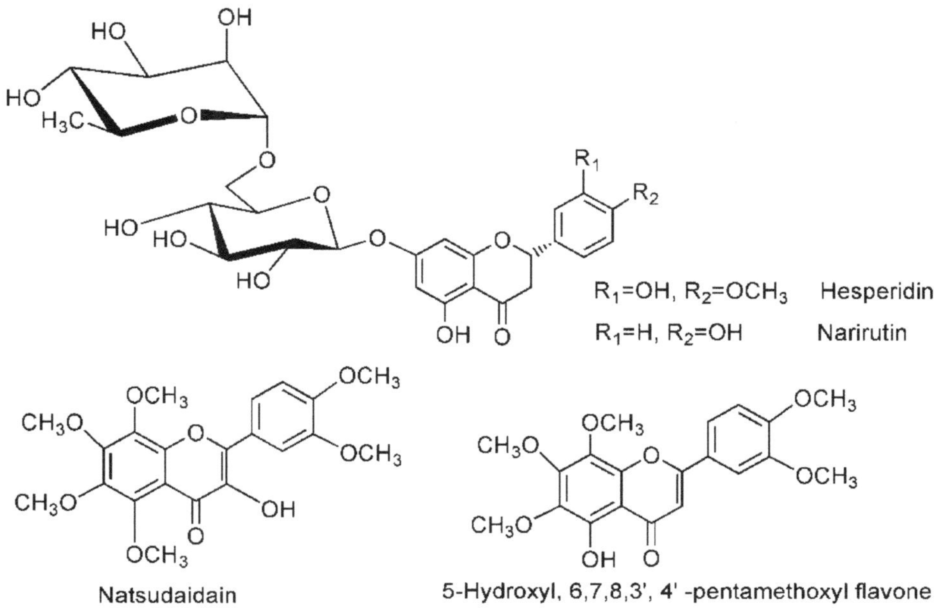

R_1=OH, R_2=OCH_3 Hesperidin

R_1=H, R_2=OH Narirutin

Natsudaidain

5-Hydroxyl, 6,7,8,3', 4' -pentamethoxyl flavone

Figure 5. The structures of some flavonoids in *Citri reticulatae* pericarpium.

Conclusion

As a typical Chinese herbal medicine, *Citri reticulatae* pericarpium can effectively protect against hydroxyl-induced DNA damage. One mechanism of protective effect may be radical-scavenging which is via donating hydrogen atom (H·), donating electron (e). Its antioxidant ability can be mainly attributed to flavonoids (especially hesperidin and narirutin).

Conflict of Interest

The authors declare there is no Conflict of interest in the content of this study.

References

1. Bhattacharjee S, Deterding LJ, Chatterjee S, Jiang J, Ehrenshaft M, Lardinois O, et al. Site-specific radical formation in DNA induced by cu(ii)-h_2o_2 oxidizing system, using esr, immuno-spin trapping, lc-ms, and ms/ms. *Free Radic Biol Med* 2011;50(11):1536-45.
2. Luan YJ, Hou WS. The Divine Farmer's Materia Medica. China: People's Medical Press; 2010.
3. China pharmacopoeia committee. Pharmacopoeia of the people's republic of China. China: Chemical Industry Press; 2005.
4. Kang SA, Park HJ, Kim MJ, Lee SY, Han SW, Leem KH. Citri reticulatae Viride Pericarpium extract induced apoptosis in SNU-C4, human colon cancer cells. *J Ethnopharmacol* 2005;97(2):231-5.
5. Ou LJ, Sun XP, Liu QD, Mi SQ, Wang NS. Effects of rhizoma zingiberis and pericarpium citri reticulatae extracts on myocardial ischemia in rats. *Zhong Yao Cai* 2009;32(11):1723-6.
6. Fang YF, Wei YP, Ding XA. Tangerine peel on the the superficial fungal test tube the antibacterial experiments and clinical efficacy observed. *Chin J Dermatol Venereol* 1997;11(5):275.
7. Fan J, Ding ZM. The tangerine peel several citrus bark extract on aphids, mites, worms insecticidal activity preliminary study. *Tradit Chin Med* 1995;20(7):397-8.
8. Yu H, Li CX, Gan QX. Pharmacological effects of Citrus. *Biomagnetism* 2005;5:44-5.
9. Zheng RL, Huang ZY. Free radical biology. 3rd Ed. China: Higher Education Press; 2007.
10. Wang X, Li X, Chen D. Evaluation of antioxdiant activity of isoferulic acid in vitro. *Nat Prod Commun* 2011;6:1285-8.
11. Li X, Chen C. Systematic Evaluation on Antioxidant of Magnolol in vitro. *Int Res J Pure Appl Chem* 2012;2(1):68-76.
12. Gao Y, Hu Q, Li X. Chemical composition and antioxidant activity of essential oil from Syzygium samarangense (BL.) Merr.et Perry flower-bud. *Spatula DD* 2012;2(1):23-33.
13. Oyaizu M. Studies on product of browning reaction prepared from glucoseamine. *Jpn J Nutr* 1986;44:307-15.

14. Li X, Wang X, Chen D, Chen S: Antioxidant activity and mechanism of protocatechuic acid *in vitro*. *Funct Foods Health Dis* 2011;7:232-44.
15. Li XC, Chen D, Mai Y, Wen B, Wang X. Concordance between antioxidant activities in vitro and chemical components of *Radix Astragali* (Huangqi). *Nat prod Res* 2012;26(11):1050-3.
16. Dizdaroglu M, Jaruga P, Birincioglu M, Rodriguez H. Free radical-induced damage to DNA: Mechanisms and measurement. *Free Radic Biol Med* 2002;32(11):1102-15.
17. Jaruga P, Rozalski R, Jawien A, Migdalski A, Olinski R, Dizdaroglu M. DNA damage products (5'r)- and (5's)-8,5'-cyclo-2'-deoxyadenosines as potential biomarkers in human urine for atherosclerosis. *Biochemistry* 2012;51(9):1822-4.
18. Cheeseman KH, Beavis A, Esterbauer H. Hydroxyl-radical-induced iron-catalysed degradation of 2-deoxyribose. Quantitative determination of malondialdehyde. *Biochem J* 1988;252(3):649-53.
19. Fang Y, Zheng R. Theory and application of free radical biology. China: Science Press; 2002.
20. Bondet V, Brand-Williams W, Berset C. Kinetics and mechanisms of antioxidant activity using the DPPH• free radical method. *LWT-Food Sci Technol* 1997;30(6):609-15.
21. Qian SH, Chen L. Tangerine peel flavonoids in the study. *Chin Herb Med* 1998,6:57-9.
22. Tsimogiannis DI, Oreopoulou V. The contribution of flavonoid C-ring on the DPPH free radical scavenging efficiency. A kinetic approach for the 3′,4′-hydroxy substituted members. *Innov Food Sci Emerg Technol* 2006;7(1-2):140-6.
23. Khanduja KL, Bhardwaj A. Stable free radical scavenging and antiperoxidative properties of resveratrol compared in vitro with some other bioflavonoids. *Indian J Biochem Biophys* 2003;40(6):416-22.
24. Aliaga C, Lissi EA. Reaction of 2, 2′-azinobis (3-ethylbenzothiazoline-6-sulfonic acid (ABTS) derived radicals with hydroperoxides: Kinetics and mechanism. *Int J Chem Kinet* 1998;30:565-70.
25. Prior RL, Cao G. In vivo total antioxidant capacity: Comparison of different analytical methods. *Free Radic Biol Med* 1999;27(11-12):1173-81.
26. Jung MJ, Heo SI, Wang MH. Free radical scavenging and total phenolic contents from methanolic extracts of Ulmus davidiana. *Food Chem* 2008;108(2):482-7.
27. Feng YF, Zhang HW, Zou ZM, Sun CH. HPLC simultaneous determination of contents of five flavonoids in Pericarpium Citri Reticulatae. *Pharm Anal mag* 2009;20:47-8.
28. Zhang ZH, Wang CY, Yang TM, Zhou JB, Huang YB. The tangerine peel chemical composition and pharmacological research. *Northwest Pharm J* 2005;29:10-5.

Combination Studies of *Oreganum Vulgare* Extract Fractions and Volatile Oil along with Ciprofloxacin and Fluconazole against Common Fish Pathogens

Veni Bharti[1], Neeru Vasudeva[1]*, Joginder Singh Dhuhan[2]

[1] *Department of Pharmaceutical Sciences, Guru Jambheshwer University of Science and Technology, Hisar, Haryana, India.*

[2] *Department of Biotechnology, Chaudhary Devilal University, Sirsa, Haryana, India.*

ARTICLEINFO

Keywords:
Antibiotics
Antimicrobial resistance
Aquaculture
Fish pathogens
Minimum Inhibitory Concentration
Oreganum vulgure

ABSTRACT

Purpose: The study is aimed at finding new antibiotic therapy for aquaculture due to potential of bacteria to develop resistance to the existing therapies. Use of large quantities of synthetic antibiotics in aquaculture thus has the potential to be detrimental to fish health, to the environment and wildlife and to human health. ***Methods:*** Antimicrobial potential of volatile oil and fractions of chloroform extract of *Oreganum vulgare* was evaluated alone and in the presence of standard antimicrobials against common fish pathogens by disc-diffusion, agar well assay and two fold microdilution method by nanodrop spectrophotometric method. ***Results:*** The best results were represented by volatile oil followed by phenolic fraction by disc-diffusion, agar well and microdilution assays (Minimum inhibitory concentration). By the interaction studies, it was observed that the volatile oil and phenolic fraction were able to inhibit the pathogens at very low concentration compared to standard drugs. The fractional inhibitory concentration index (FICI) was calculated and volatile oil and phenolic fractions were found to be synergistic against *Pseudomonas fluorescens* and *Candida albicans*. ***Conclusion:*** The experimental data suggests the use of volatile oil and phenolic fraction in combination with standard antimicrobials to maintain healthy aquaculture with lesser adverse effects as compared to synthetic antibiotic therapy.

Introduction

Seafood has always been important for human being since time immortal as it is nutrient- rich and plays an important role in reducing health risks like cardiovascular complications. Consumption of seafood provides many benefits like neurological development during gestation and infancy.[1-4] Along with benefits, seafood may prove harmful if it is contaminated with pathogens, heavy metals and marine toxins. Bacteria are a major group of pathogens, which infects fishes all over world.[5] The infection may be transmitted to humans by exposure to infected organisms by any means. Major group of bacteria associated with pathogenicity of fish are Aeromonads, Pesudomonads and Edwardsiella tarda.[6,7] *Pseudomonas fluorescens* causes Red Skin Disease in fish.[8] *Pseudomonas aeruginosa* are opportunistic human pathogens that are one of the main causes of human infections. *Aeromonas* infection in human being causes several gastrointestinal syndromes like bloody mucoid stools, vomiting, abdominal pain and acute and self-limiting diarrhea. Not only bacteria, but also fungi are infectious agents in marine environment. *Candida albicans* is one of pathogenic fungi affecting killer whales. Control of fish disease is not only necessary for management of aquaculture but also for welfare of human being which can be possible due to chemotherapy.[9] Various marketed formulations available to control fish disease are chemicals like Malachite green, piperazine, formalin, copper sulfate, organic compounds like napthaquinones, tea tree oil and antibiotics naladixic acid, ciprofloxacin, triple sulfa etc. Although there is wide range of synthetic and semi-synthetic antibiotics and antifungal compounds present in market, none of them is completely effective and there is emergence of resistance. Moreover, if organic compounds obtained from natural sources exhibiting antimicrobial activities are given along with synthetic antibiotics, not only antibiotic resistance in humans but also in fishes can also be solved to a great extent.

The main objective of this study was to determine the interaction effect studies of isolated phenolic and non-phenolic fractions of chloroform extract of *Oreganum vulgare* Linn. (Lamiaceae) against common fish pathogenic strains *Pseudomonas fluorescens*, *Aeromonas hydophila, Candida albicans* along with ciprofloxacin and fluconazole for bacterial and fungal

***Corresponding author:** Neeru Vasudeva, Department of Pharmaceutical Sciences, Guru Jambheshwer University of Science and Technology, Hisar-125001, Haryana, India. Email: neeruvasudeva@gmail.com

strains respectively. Antimicrobial interaction studies were performed by using disc diffusion method, agar well assay, minimum inhibitory concentration (MIC) by microdilution method, fractional inhibitory index (FICI) determination.

Materials and Methods

Plant Material and preparation of extracts

The freeze dried leaves of *Oreganum vulgare* Linn. were procured from Aum Agreefresh pvt. Ltd., Vadodara, Gujarat and were identified by the same company. The voucher specimen (Pcog 1101) was deposited in Department of Pharmaceutical sciences, Guru Jambheshwar University of Science and Technology for future references.

Crude drug (500 g) was placed in a closed flask with chloroform and after 24 h, filtered and concentrated in rotary vacuum to yield 12.5 g of paste like extract.[10] In order to separate the phenolic from non-phenolic fraction of the chloroform extract, a liquid-liquid extraction was done. In a seperating funnel, 2 g of the extract was diluted in 40 ml of chloroform and washed three times with 120 ml of 0.1 N sodium hydroxide. The chloroform phase was separated and was concentrated to obtain the crude non- phenolic fraction. To further purify this fraction, 0.3 g of it were diluted in ethanol and centrifuged at 3600×g at 10°C for 15 min. Ethanol was concentrated from the supernatant to obtain purified non- phenolic fraction. The basic aqueous phase was acidified with 6N HCl to pH 3.0 and 40 ml of chloroform was added to extract the phenolic fraction. The phenolic fraction was dissolved in chloroform and separated by preparative thin layer chromatography (TLC) on silica gel-G eluting with benzene- methanol 95:5.[10]

Extraction of volatile oil

Volatile oil was extracted from freeze dried leaves (1000 g) by hydro-distillation method by using clevenger's apparatus. The yellowish oil (16.6 ml, yield= 1.66 % v/w) obtained was separated from aqueous phase and dried over anhydrous sodium sulphate and stored at 4°C until used.

GC-MS analysis of Volatile oil

The oil sample was diluted with hexane in ratio of 1:100 and used for the further analysis. The quantitative analysis was done with the help of chromatographer in gas phase (Agilent 7890A GC system) equipped with MS detector (5975C inert XL EI/CI MSD), HP-5MS capillary column (Agilent 19091S-433: 1548.52849 HP-5MS 5% Phenyl Methyl Silox) having dimensions 30 m x 250 μm x 0.25 μm. The column temperature was programmed from initial 80°C upto 300°C. The temperature of the injector was fixed to 270°C. The debit of gas (helium) vector was fixed to 1ml/min and split injection with split ratio 50:1. The volume of injected sample was 2 μL of diluted oil in hexane (10%). The components were identified based on comparison of their relative retention time and mass spectra with those of standards, W9N08.L library data of the GC-MS system and literature data.

Bacterial strains and antibiotics

The microorganisms used for antimicrobial studies of volatile oil and extract were procured from Microbial Type Culture Collection (MTCC), Institute of Microbial Technology, Chandigarh. The bacterial strains used were *P.fluorescens* MTCC 7200 and *A.hydrophila* and fungal strain used was *C.albicans* MTCC 854. *A.hydrophila* was procured from slant cultures of Department of Biotechnology, CDLU, Sirsa. The media used for the growth and maintenance of microorganisms were nutrient agar (NA), for bacteria, potato dextrose agar (PDA) for fungi (Hi-media). The organic solvents used for extraction and fractionation of plant metabolites were of analytical grade.

Antimicrobial Screening

Disc Diffusion Assay

Antimicrobial activity of volatile oil was investigated along with ciprofloxacin and fluconazole using the standard method of diffusion disc plates on agar taking ciprofloxacin and fluconazole as positive control for bacterial and fungal strains respectively and DMSO as negative control.[11,12] For interaction effect studies, 0.25 mg ml^{-1} ciprofloxacin in DMSO was mixed with volatile oil in 1:1 concentration for antibacterial activity determination and 1:1 combination of 0.25 mg ml^{-1} of fluconazole dissolved in DMSO for the determination of antifungal activity. In this method 60 μl of 24 hr. old culture of test organism was inoculated on the agar plates and spread on to the surface of the agar with the help of sterilized glass spreader. After five minutes of inoculation of test organism, sterile paper discs (5mm diameter) were placed in each agar plate disc dipped in volatile oil and solution of volatile oil along with ciprofloxacin and fluconazole respectively. The bacterial cultures were incubated at 37°C for 18-24 h and fungal cultures at room temperature for 48 h. Zones of inhibition were measured. All the tests were done in triplicate.

Agar well assay

The preliminary investigation of the antibacterial activity of phenolic and non-phenolic fractions as well as interaction effect studies with that of synthetic antibiotics, ciprofloxacin and fluconazole was performed for bacterial and fungal strains respectively.[13] In this method 60 μl of 24 h old culture of test organism was inoculated on the agar plates and spread on to the surface of the agar with the help of sterilized glass spreader. After five minutes of inoculation of test organism, wells (2.5 mm diameter) were prepared with the help of sterilized steel cork borer.

Two wells of each plate were loaded with 60 μl of phenolic and non-phenolic fractions respectively. One well loaded well was loaded with 60 μl standard antibiotics viz. ciprofloxacin for bacterial strains and fluconazole for fungal strains were used as positive controls. One well was loaded with DMSO was used as a negative control. The bacterial cultures were incubated at 37°C for 18-24 h and fungal culture at room temperature for 48 h. For interaction effect studies, phenolic and non-phenolic fractions were mixed with 0.25 mg ml^{-1} of ciprofloxacin dissolved in DMSO in 1:1 combination and fluconazole dissolved in DMSO in 1:1 combination for bacterial and fungal strains respectively. Zones of inhibition were measured. Antimicrobial activity was determined by measuring zone of inhibition and compared with the growth inhibition results, obtained from standard microbial. The diameter (in mm) of zone inhibition was measured at cross-angles and the mean of two reading was taken. All the tests were done in triplicate.

Minimum Inhibitory Concentration (MIC) determination and comparison of MIC determination by spectrophotometric and visual methods and growth curve

MIC was determined by modified microdilution method.[14,15] The concentration of stock solutions of phenolic and non-phenolic fractions were 10 mg ml^{-1} and that of ciprofloxacin and fluconazole were 0.25 mg ml^{-1} in DMSO respectively for bacterial and fungal strains. Phenolic and non- phenolic fractions and volatile oil (0.5 ml each) were mixed with 0.5 ml of ciprofloxacin respectively. MIC of phenolic, non-phenolic fraction, volatile oil and ciprofloxacin was determined using two fold serial dilution method. For determination of interaction effect of phenolic, non-phenolic fractions and volatile oil, 0.5 ml of respective test sample were mixed with 0.5 ml of ciprofloxacin stock solution and 0.5 ml of fluconazole for bacterial and fungal strains respectively. MIC was determined using two fold serial dilution method. Tubes containing only bacterial suspensions and nutrient broth were used as positive control and negative control were the tubes with only nutrient broth.

Optical Densities (ODs) were measured for at 35°C using Thermo Scientific 2000/2000 C nanodrop spectrophotometer at 405 nm. OD of each replicate at before incubation (T_0) was subtracted from OD after incubation at 37° C (T_{24}) for bacterial cultures and at room temperature for fungal strains respectively. The adjusted OD of each control tube was then assigned a value of 100% growth. The percent inhibition of growth was thus determined using the formula:

Percent Inhibition = 1- (OD of tube containing test solution/OD of corresponding control tube) × 100.

The MIC is reported as the lowest concentration of test material which results in 100% inhibition of growth of the test organism. Visual MIC was determined by noting down the concentration of that first tube in which there is no appearance of turbidity after incubation of 24 h and it was compared with that of MIC determined by spectrophotometric method.

Fractional Inhibitory Concentration (FIC) Index Determination

The FIC index (FICI) was calculated by dividing the MIC of the combination of phenolic fraction, non-phenolic fraction, volatile oil and reference antibiotic respectively.[16]

FIC of vol. oil= MIC of vol. oil in combination with antibiotic drug/MIC of vol. oil

FIC of Phenolic Fraction= MIC of Phenolic Fraction in combination with antibiotic drug/ MIC of Phenolic Fraction

FIC of Non-Phenolic Fraction= MIC of Non-Phenolic Fraction in combination with antibiotic drug/ MIC of Non-Phenolic Fraction

FIC of antibiotic drug= MIC of antibiotic drug with particular fraction/MIC of drug

FICI (Vol. Oil) = FIC of Vol. oil+ FIC of antibiotic drug

FICI (Phenolic Fraction) = FIC of Phenolic Fraction+ FIC of antibiotic drug

FICI (Non-Phenolic Fraction) = FIC of Non-Phenolic Fraction+ FIC of antibiotic drug

Results and Discussion

GC-MS of volatile oil, Disc-diffusion and agar well assay

GC-MS analysis of volatile oil characterized and quantified total 35 compounds (Table 1). The major component of volatile oil *Oreganum vulgare* is carvacrol (86.5%), followed by p-cymene (7.2%), γ-Terpinene (0.6%), 3-Cyclohexen-1-ol (0.5%), δ-Cadinene (0.4%), β- Bisabolene (0.4%). The diameters of zones of inhibition of volatile oil, phenolic and non-phenolic fractions are shown in Table 2 against *P.fuorescens, A.hydrophila* and *C.albicans.* Non-phenolic fraction in terms of zone of inhibition was only effective against *A.hydrophila* while phenolic fraction and volatile oil showed antimicrobial activity against all the three tested strains.

MIC determination by spectrophotometric method and growth curve

Minimum inhibitory concentration is that concentration at which absorbance at time initiation time (T0) and after 24 h incubation, (T24) becomes equal. The MIC of non-phenolic fraction, phenolic fraction, volatile oil, combination of non-phenolic fraction, phenolic fraction and volatile oil respectively and ciprofloxacin in 1:1 ratio are shown in Table 2 and 3 were at 0.625, 0.01953, 0.00061, 0.156, 0.00122, 0.00030 mg ml^{-1} as compared to MIC of ciprofloxacin at 0.03900 mg ml^{-1} against *P.fluorescens* while against *A.hydrophila,* MIC of non-phenolic fraction, phenolic fraction, volatile oil, combination of non-phenolic fraction, phenolic fraction and volatile oil respectively and ciprofloxacin in 1:1

ratio was found to be 0.625, 0.156, 0.00030, 0.625, 0.00122, 0.00015 mg ml^{-1} as compared to MIC of ciprofloxacin at 0.00122 mg ml^{-1} (Table 3, 4). MIC exhibited by non-phenolic fraction, phenolic fraction, volatile oil, combination of non-phenolic fraction, phenolic fraction, volatile oil and fluconazole and fluconazole respectively was 5, 1.25, 0.01953, 0.07800, 0.00970, 0.00244 and 0.03900 mg ml^{-1} (Table 3, 4). A growth curve (% inhibition in concentration in mg ml^{-1}) was prepared for *P.fluorescens, A.hydrophila* and *C.albicans* in the presence of phenolic, non-phenolic fractions of chloroform extract and volatile oil respectively (Figure 1A, 1B and 1C respectively). The growth curve (Figure 1A) shows % inhibition of bacteria *P.fluorescens* at increasing concentrations (from 0.00015 mg ml^{-1} upto 10 mg ml^{-1}). The curve and Table 3 vividly indicates that at the concentration of 0.00015 mg ml^{-1} for non-phenolic fraction, combination of non-phenolic fraction and ciprofloxacin, phenolic fraction, combination of phenolic fraction and ciprofloxacin, volatile oil, combination of volatile oil and ciprofloxacin and ciprofloxacin, the % inhibition of *P.fluorescens* was found to be approximately 14%, 25%, 53%, 78%, 87% and 27% respectively. The % of inhibition of growth was found to be higher as the concentrations increased. The 100% inhibition of growth of bacteria was observed at 0.625, 0.156, 0.01953, 0.00122, 0.0006, 0.00030 and 0.03900 mg ml^{-1} for non-phenolic fraction, combination of non-phenolic fraction and ciprofloxacin, phenolic fraction, combination of phenolic fraction-ciprofloxacin, volatile oil, combination of volatile oil-ciprofloxacin and ciprofloxacin respectively. The curve indicates the superiority of phenolic fraction, combination of phenolic fraction and ciprofloxacin, volatile oil and volatile oil along with ciprofloxacin over ciprofloxacin alone against *P.fluorescens.* The growth curve (Figure 1B) and Table 3 depicts that at the lowest concentration chosen (0.00015mg ml^{-1}) non-phenolic fraction, non-phenolic fraction and ciprofloxacin, phenolic fraction, phenolic fraction in combination with ciprofloxacin, volatile oil, volatile oil and ciprofloxacin and ciprofloxacin the % inhibition of *A.hydrophila* was found to be 10, 25.7, 12.8, 78.5, 95.7, 100% respectively. The 100% inhibition concentration was 0.625, 0.625, 0.156, 0.00122, 0.00030 and 0.00015 mg/ml respectively. The curve indicates that volatile oil, volatile oil in combination with ciprofloxacin and phenolic fraction in combination with ciprofloxacin are more potent than ciprofloxacin against *A.hydrophila.* Figure 1C and Table 4 represents that at 0.00015 mg ml^{-1} concentration non-phenolic fraction showed least inhibition against *C.albicans* (2%) followed by phenolic fraction (8%), fluconazole (20%), non-phenolic fraction along with fluconazole (34%), phenolic fraction in combination with fluconazole (50%), volatile oil (48%) and volatile oil in combination with fluconazole (66.8%) respectively. Volatile oil, combination of volatile oil and fluconazole, phenolic fraction and fluconazole were found to have 100% inhibitory effect at less concentration (0.01953, 0.00244, 0.00970 mg ml^{-1} respectively) than that of fluconazole alone (0.03900 mg ml^{-1}).

Table 1. Gc-MS analysis of volatile oil of Oreganum vulgare Linn.

Chemical constituent	Retention Time	% of Chemical constituent
α-Thujene	3.482	0.076
α- Pinene	3.609	0.341
Camphene	3.851	0.114
1-Octen-3-ol	4.226	0.091
2-β- Pinene	4.300	0.060
3-Octanone	4.359	0.046
β- Myrcene	4.435	0.143
1-Phellandrene	4.756	0.029
α-Terpinene	4.989	0.333
Þ-cymene	5.153	7.249
Dl- limonene	5.240	0.179
1,8- Cineole	5.333	0.064
γ-Terpinene	5.883	0.642
Cis- Sabinenehydrate	6.116	0.058
α-Terpinolene	6.604	0.062
β-Linalool	6.840	0.154
3-Cyclohexen-1-ol	9.013	0.565
Benzenemethanol	9.2449	0.068
α-Terpineol	9.402	0.126
2-cyclohexen-1-one	11.039	0.053
m-Thymophenol	12.457	0.254
Carvacrol	12.857	86.586
Carvol	13.322	0.489
Eugenol	15.886	0.106
Caryophyllene	16.305	0.373
Aromadendrene	16.889	0.045
α- Humulene	17.332	0.063
Viridiflorene	18.582	0.037
β- Bisabolene	18.958	0.400
γ-Cadinene	19.142	0.152
δ- Cadinene	19.416	0.421
Caryophyllene oxide	21.186	0.271
Virdiflorol	22.820	0.094

It was reported that phenolic components of essential oil have the strongest antimicrobial activity, followed by aldehydes, ketones and alcohols.[17] In other research, the antimicrobial effect of volatile oil of *O. vulgare* on several Gram-positive and Gram-negative bacteria and saprophytic or foodborne pathogenic bacteria was investigated; results showed that this volatile oil has a strong antimicrobial activity. Polyphenols are well documented to have microbicide activities against a large number of pathogenic bacteria and fungal species.[18,19] The mechanisms responsible for phenolic toxicity to microorganisms include: adsorption and disruption of microbial membranes, interaction with enzymes and metal ion deprivation.[20,21]

Table 2. Measurement of zone of inhibition in mm of volatile oil, phenolic and non-phenolic fractions of chloroform extract of *Oreganum vulgare* against fish pathogenic strains.

Strain	NP	P	O	S
P.fuorescens	<10	12.34± 0.12	27.71± 1.31	32.60± 0.98
A.hydrophila	21.66± 1.31	22.28± 0.33	22.30± 1.11	26.57± 0.18
C.albicans	<10	<10	20.33± 0.64	16.43± 0.37

Note: The data are expressed as mean±error of mean (n=3). NP= non-phenolic fraction, P= phenolic fraction, O= volatile oil, S= standard drug (ciprofloxacin for bacterial strains and fluconazole for fungal strains).

Table 3. MIC and percent growth inhibition of volatile oil, phenolic, non-phenolic fractions of chloroform extract alone and in combination with ciprofloxacin against *P.fluorescens* and *A.hydrophila* by microdilution method.

	P.fluorescens							*A.hydrophila*						
Conc. (mg/ml)	**NP**	**NP+C**	**P**	**P+C**	**O**	**O+C**	**C**	**NP**	**NP+C**	**P**	**P+C**	**O**	**O+C**	**C**
0.00015	13.3	25	53	78	95	86.6	26.6	10	25.7	12.8	78.5	95.7	100	76.2
0.00030	23.3	33	58.3	88.3	96.6	100	33.3	22.8	34.2	27.1	85.7	100	>100	81.4
0.00061	30	42.3	63.3	92.3	100	>100	40	31.4	42.8	35.7	94.2	>100	>100	92.8
0.00122	40.6	55	66.7	100	>100	>100	53.3	40	51.4	44.2	100	>100	>100	100
0.00244	51.6	61.6	75	>100	>100	>100	61.6	50	52.8	54.2	>100	>100	>100	>100
0.00488	53.3	63.3	85	>100	>100	>100	73.3	61	64.2	67.1	>100	>100	>100	>100
0.00970	60	74.3	91.6	>100	>100	>100	80	62.8	65.7	77.1	>100	>100	>100	>100
0.01953	71.6	77	100	>100	>100	>100	93.3	71.4	72.8	85.1	>100	>100	>100	>100
0.03900	72.3	83.3	>100	>100	>100	>100	100	74.2	75.7	87.1	>100	>100	>100	>100
0.07800	81.6	93	>100	>100	>100	>100	>100	81.4	83.7	91.4	>100	>100	>100	>100
0.15600	87	100	>100	>100	>100	>100	>100	82.8	84.2	100	>100	>100	>100	>100
0.31200	91	>100	>100	>100	>100	>100	>100	90	92.8	>100	>100	>100	>100	>100
0.62500	100	>100	>100	>100	>100	>100	-	100	100	>100	>100	>100	>100	-
1.25000	>100	>100	>100	>100	-	-	-	>100	>100	>100	>100	-	-	-
2.50000	>100	>100	>100	>100	-	-	-	>100	>100	>100	>100	-	-	-
5.00000	>100	>100	>100	>100	-	-	-	>100	>100	>100	>100	-	-	-
10.0000	>100	-	>100	-	-	-	-	>100	-	>100	-	-	-	-

NP= non-phenolic fraction, P= phenolic fraction, O= volatile oil, S= standard drug ciprofloxacin, % in= inhibition, MIC= minimum inhibitory concentration, - = Dilution was not made in this concentration range for the given sample.

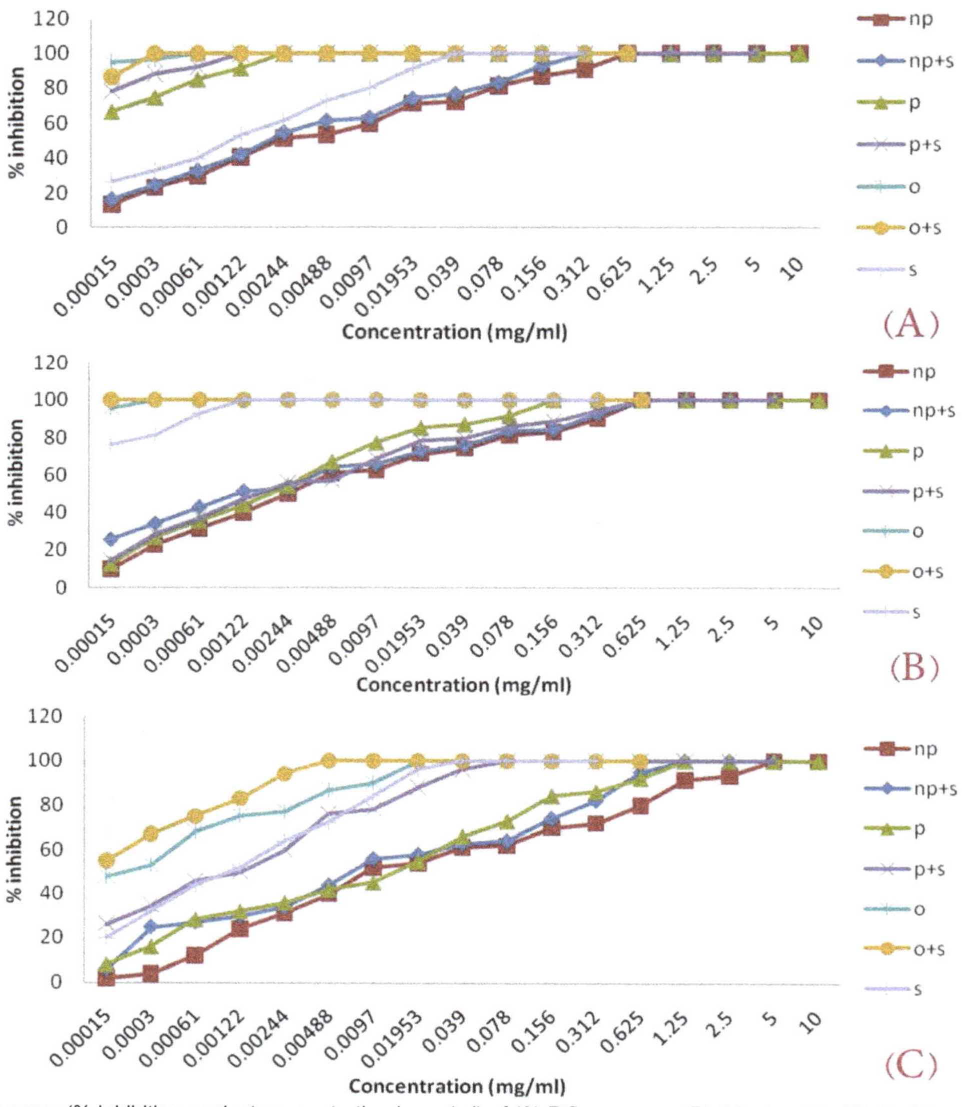

Figure 1. Growth curve (% inhibition against concentration in mg/ml) of (A) P.fluorescens (B) A.hydrophila (C) C.albicans in presence of phenolic, non-phenolic fractions and volatile oil alone and in combination with ciprofloxacin and fluconazole.

Fractional Inhibitory Concentration Index

Fractional inhibitory concentration was calculated to calculate FIC index which is an indicator of degree of interaction between standard drugs ciprofloxacin and fluconazole along with volatile oil, phenolic and non-phenolic fractions respectively for bacterial and fungal strains. FIC for volatile oil was found to be 0.491, 0.500 and 0.124 and that of phenolic fraction was found to be 0.062, 0.007 and 0.007 respectively against *P.fluorescens, A.hydrophila* and *C.albicans* (Table 5). Synergy is defined as an FIC index of ≤0.5. Indifference was defined as an FIC index of ≥0.5 but of ≤4.0. Antagonism was defined as an FIC index of >4.0.[22] Synergism was shown by volatile oil with a FICI of 0.498 and phenolic fraction with FICI of 0.093 respectively against *P.fluorescens* and 0.186 and 0.255 respectively against *C.albicans*. Indifference was exhibited by volatile oil phenolic fraction with FICI of 0.622 and 1.007 respectively against *A.hydrophila* and by non-phenolic fraction with FICI of 2.015 against *C.albicans.* Antagoistic interaction effect was observed for non-phenolic fraction with FICI of 4.249 and 513.295 against *P.fluorescence* and *A.hydrophila* (Table 5). The literature studies reveal that essential oil of *Oreganum vulgare* is effective against various strains of *Candida albicans* (13 to 15 mm diameter of zone of inhibition) and synergism is exhibited along with amphotericin B (16 to 23 mm diameter of zone of inhibition) and along with nystatin (17 to 20.1 mm) shown by disc-diffusion assay.[23,24] Very scanty information is available on this plant for the interaction studies with synthetic antibiotics as well as with other natural products. Synergism was shown by *Oreganum vulgare* and *Rosmarinus officinalis* combination against *S.aureus, L.monocytogens, Aeromonas hydrophila, Yersinia enterocolitica, P.fluorescens.*[25] Extracts of *Origanum vulgare* and *Vaccinium macrocarpon* presented a combined antimicrobial effect potentialized against *Vibrio parahaemolyticus*, an effect which is even more marked in the presence of lactic acid, suggesting that these may be viable alternatives for extending the preservation time of foods.[26] The same extracts combined were also active and synergic against *Helicobacter pylori*, and it is suggested to manage this bacteria with a diet containing these juices.[27] The results reviewed by above referred literature support to present studies results when compared.

Table 4. MIC and percent growth inhibition of volatile oil, phenolic, non-phenolic fractions of chloroform extract alone and in combination with ciprofloxacin against *C.albicans* by microdilution method.

Concentration (mg/ml)	NP	NP+C	P	P+C	O	O+C	C
0.00015	2	34	8	50	48	66.8	20
0.00030	4	44	16	60	53.2	74.8	32
0.00061	12	56	28	76	68	82.8	44
0.00122	24	58	32	78	75.2	94	52
0.00244	31.2	62.8	36	88	77.2	100	64
0.00488	40	64	42	96	86.8	>100	72
0.00970	52	74	45.2	100	90	>100	84
0.01953	54	82	54.8	>100	100	>100	96
0.03900	61.2	94.8	66	>100	>100	>100	100
0.07800	62	100	72.8	>100	>100	>100	>100
0.15600	70	>100	84	>100	>100	>100	>100
0.31200	72	>100	86	>100	>100	>100	>100
0.62500	80	>100	92	>100	>100	>100	-
1.25000	91.2	>100	100	>100	-	-	-
2.50000	93.2	>100	>100	>100	-	-	-
5.00000	100	>100	>100	>100	-	-	-
10.0000	>100	-	>100	-	-	-	-

NP= non-phenolic fraction, P= phenolic fraction, O= volatile oil, S= standard drug ciprofloxacin, % in= inhibition, - = Dilution was not made in this concentration range for the given sample, MIC= Minimum inhibitory concentration.

Table 5. FIC determination of volatile oil, phenolic, non-phenolic fractions of chloroform extract and standard antibiotic/antifungal drug and FICI determination.

strain	FIC		FIC		FIC		FICI		
	O	S	P	S	NP	S	O	P	NP
P.fluorescens	0.491	0.007	0.062	0.031	0.249	4.000	0.498	0.093	4.249
A.hydrophila	0.500	0.122	0.007	1.000	1.000	512.295	0.622	1.007	513.295
C.albicans	0.124	0.062	0.007	0.248	0.015	2.000	0.186	0.255	2.015

O= volatile oil, P= phenolic fraction, NP= non-phenolic fraction, S= standard (ciprofloxacin for bacterial strain and fluconazole for fungal strain), FIC= Fractional inhibitory concentration, FICI= Fractional inhibitory concentration index.

Conclusion

The experimental data suggests the use of volatile oil and phenolic fraction of the chloroform extract to be used against common fish pathogens *P.fluorescence, A.hydrophila* and *C.albicans* in combination with ciprofloxacin and fluconazole respectively to maintain healthy aquaculture and that of the people consuming seafood. The problem of emerging resistance of the micro-organisms against established antibiotics and toxicity can be solved by using these combinations.

Conflict of interest

The authors report no conflicts of interest.

References

1. Daviglus ML, Stamler J, Orencia AJ, Dyer AR, Liu K, Greenland P, et al. Fish consumption and the 30-year risk of fatal myocardial infarction. *N Engl J Med* 1997;336(15):1046-53.
2. Kris-Etherton PM, Harris WS, Appel LJ, American Heart Association. Nutrition C. Fish consumption, fish oil, omega-3 fatty acids, and cardiovascular disease. *Circulation* 2002;106(21):2747-57.
3. Kromhout D, Bosschieter EB, de Lezenne Coulander C. The inverse relation between fish consumption and 20-year mortality from coronary heart disease. *N Engl J Med* 1985; 312(19): 1205-9.
4. Mozaffarian D, Rimm EB. Fish intake, contaminants, and human health: evaluating the risks and the benefits. *JAMA* 2006;296(15):1885-99.
5. Roberts RJ. Fish Pathology. 2nd ed. London: Bailliene Tindall; 1989.
6. Banu GR. Studies on the bacteria Aeromonas spp in farmed fish and water in Mymensingh region [MS Dissertation]. Mymensingh, Bangladesh: Faculty of Fisheries, Bangladesh Agricultural University; 1996.
7. Islam MS. Studies on the bacteria Pseudomonas spp in farmed fishes and in water around Mymensingh [MS Dissertation]. Mymensingh, Bangladesh: Faculty of Fisheries, Bangladesh Agricultural University; 1996.
8. Zhang WW, Hu YH, Wang HL, Sun L. Identification and characterization of a virulence-associated protease from a pathogenic *Pseudomonas fluorescens* strain. *Vet Microbiol* 2009;139(1-2):183-8.
9. Roberts RJ. Aquatic Animal Health Towards. In: Shariff M, Arthur JR, Subasinghe RP, Editors. *Diseases in Asian Aquaculture II*. Philippines: Asian Fisheries Society; 1995. P. 3-7.
10. Avila-Sosa R, Gastelum-Franco MG, Camacho-Davila A, Torres-Munoz JV, Nevarez-Moorillon GV. Extracts of Mexican oregano (*Lippia berlandieri* Schauer) with antioxidant and antimicrobial activity. *Food Bioprocess Technol* 2010; 3(3): 434-40.
11. Rajeshwar Y, Gupta M, Mazumder UK. In Vitro Lipid Peroxidation and Antimicrobial Activity of *Mucuna pruriens* Seeds. *Iran J Pharmacol Therapeut* 2005; 4(1): 32-5.
12. Abou Z, Abou-Zeid A, Youssef S. 13-anti diabetic effect and flanonoids of Grewia asiatica L. leaves. *Indian J Pharmacol* 1969; 31: 72-8.
13. Salar RK, Suchitra. Evaluation of antimicrobial potential of different extracts of *Solanum xanthocarpum* Schrad. and Wendl. *Afr J Microbiol Res* 2009; 3(3): 97-100.
14. Kaya E, Ozbilge H. Determination of the effect of fluconazole against *Candida albicans* and *Candida glabrata* by using microbroth kinetic assay. *Turk J Med Sci* 2012; 42(2): 325-8.
15. Eloff JN. A sensitive and quick microplate method to determine the minimal inhibitory concentration of plant extracts for bacteria. *Planta Med* 1998;64(8):711-3.
16. Saad A, Fadli M, Bouaziz M, Benharref A, Mezrioui NE, Hassani L. Anticandidal activity of the essential oils of Thymus maroccanus and Thymus broussonetii and their synergism with amphotericin B and fluconazol. *Phytomedicine* 2010;17(13):1057-60.
17. Ozcan M, Erkmen O. Antimicrobial activity of the essential oils of Turkish plant spices. *Eur Food Res Technol* 2001; 212(6): 658-60.
18. Scalbert A. Antimicrobial properties of tannins. *Phytochemistry* 1991; 30: 3875-83.
19. Cowan MM. Plants products as antimicrobial agents. *J Clin Microbiol* 1999; 12(4): 564-82.
20. Fattouch S, Caboni P, Coroneo V, Tuberoso CI, Angioni A, Dessi S, et al. Antimicrobial activity of Tunisian quince (Cydonia oblonga Miller) pulp and peel polyphenolic extracts. *J Agric Food Chem* 2007;55(3):963-9.
21. Xia D, Wu X, Shi J, Yang Q, Zhang Y. Phenolic compounds from the edible seeds extract of Chinese Mei (*Prunus mume* Sieb. et Zucc) and their antimicrobial activity. *LWT-Food Sci Technol* 2011; 44(1): 347-9.
22. Agrawal A, Jain N, Jain A. Synergistic effect of cefixime and cloxacillin combination against common bacterial pathogens causing community acquired pneumonia. *Indian J Pharmacol* 2007; 39(5): 251-2.
23. Rosato A, Vitali C, Gallo D, Balenzano L, Mallamaci R. The inhibition of Candida species by selected essential oils and their synergism with amphotericin B. *Phytomedicine* 2008;15(8):635-8.
24. Rosato A, Vitali C, Piarulli M, Mazzotta M, Argentieri MP, Mallamaci R. In vitro synergic efficacy of the combination of Nystatin with the essential oils of Origanum vulgare and Pelargonium graveolens against some Candida species. *Phytomedicine* 2009;16(10):972-5.
25. Azeredo GA, Stamford TLM, Nunes PC, Neto NJG, de Oliveira MEG, de Souza EL. Combined application of essential oils from *Origanum vulgare* L. and *Rosmarinus officinalis* L. to inhibit bacteria and autochthonous microflora associated with minimally processed vegetables. *Food Res Int* 2011; 44(5): 1541-8.
26. Lin YT, Labbe RG, Shetty K. Inhibition of *Vibrio parahaemolyticus* in seafood systems using oregano and cranberry phytochemical synergies and lactic acid. *Innov Food Sci Emerg Technol* 2005; 6(4): 453-58.
27. Vattem DA, Lin YT, Ghaedi R, Shetty K. Cranberry synergies for dietary management of *Helicobacter pylori* infections. *Process Biochem* 2005; 40(5): 1583-92.

5

Anti-Inflammatory Effects of *Zingiber Officinale* in Type 2 Diabetic Patients

Sepide Mahluji[1], Alireza Ostadrahimi[2]*, Majid Mobasseri[3], Vahide Ebrahimzade Attari[1], Laleh Payahoo[1]

[1] *Student Research Committee, Tabriz University of Medical Science, Tabriz, Iran.*

2 Nutrition Research Center, Tabriz University of Medical Sciences, Tabriz, Iran.

[3] *Endocrinology and Metabolism Section, Department of Medicine, Imam Reza Hospital, Tabriz, Iran.*

ARTICLEINFO

Keywords:
Ginger
Inflammation
TNF-α
Diabetes

ABSTRACT

Purpose: Low-grade inflammation, a common feature in type 2 diabetes (DM2), causes some chronic complications in these patients. The present study was aimed to evaluate the effects of ginger (*Zingiber officinale*) on pro-inflammatory cytokines (IL-6 and TNF-α) and the acute phase protein hs-CRP in DM2 patients as a randomized double-blind placebo controlled trial. ***Methods:*** A total of 64 DM2 patients randomly were assigned to ginger or placebo groups and received 2 tablets/day of each for 2 months. The concentrations of IL-6, TNF-α and hs-CRP in blood samples were analyzed before and after the intervention. ***Results:*** Ginger supplementation significantly reduced the levels of TNF-α ($P = 0.006$), IL-6 ($P = 0.02$) and hs-CRP ($P = 0.012$) in ginger group in comparison to baseline. Moreover, the analysis of covariance showed that the group received ginger supplementation significantly lowered TNF- α (15.3 ± 4.6 vs. 19.6 ± 5.2; $P = 0.005$) and hs-CRP (2.42 ± 1.7 vs. 2.56 ± 2.18; $P = .016$) concentrations in comparison to control group. While there were no significant changes in IL-6 (7.9 ± 2.1 vs. 7.8 ± 2.9; $P > .05$). ***Conclusion:*** In conclusion, ginger supplementation in oral administration reduced inflammation in type 2 diabetic patients. So it may be a good remedy to diminish the risk of some chronic complications of diabetes.

Introduction

Ginger (*Zingiber officina*le) has been cultivated for thousands of years as a flavoring agent and cooking spice. In addition, it has been used in traditional systems of medicine for a wide range of ailments including pain, muscholar aches, fever, sore throats, indigestion and vomiting.[1] On the other hand, recent studies showed some benefits of ginger to treat musculoskeletal disorder,[2] nausea and vomiting,[3] inflammation or inflammatory states[4] such as osteoarthritis,[4,5] migraine,[6] cancer[7], hyperlipidemia and hyperglycemia.[1,8]

According to the results of some in vitro studies, rhizome of ginger and its main components, gingerols and shogaols, can inhibit synthesis of several pro-inflammatory cytokines including IL-1, TNF-α and IL-8 along with inhibiting prostaglandin (PG) and leukotriene (LT) synthesis enzymes.[9]

More recently, investigations showed that ginger has an effect on several genes encoding cytokines, chemokines and the inducible enzyme cyclo-oxygenase-2 (COX-2).[10] Besides, it has been shown that the components of ginger are more effective than conventional non-steroidal anti-inflammatory drugs (NSAIDs) with fewer side effects.[11]

Therefore, there is a hypothesis that ginger may have useful effects on diabetes with a chronic low-grade inflammation. Chronic hyperglycemia increases circulating levels of inflammatory biomarkers such as IL-6 (IL6), tumor necrosis factor-α (TNF-α) and C-reactive protein (CRP). TNF-α and IL-6, as the major cytokines, initiate inflammatory responses and cause the production of CRP as an acute-phase reactant.[12] Moreover, lots of evidences showed that low-grade inflammation, a common feature in type 2 diabetes mellitus (DM2), play a major role in pathogenesis of its secondary complications such as atherothrombosis.[13]

Although, ginger has hypoglycemic and anti-inflammatory effects, just a few studies have reported its anti-inflammatory activity during diabetes.[14] An animal study on the anti-inflammatory effects of ginger extract on diabetic rats reported the reduced level of TNF-α consequent to ginger extract treatment.[15] Therefore, the present study was planned to evaluate the effect of ginger powder supplementation on pro-inflammatory cytokines (IL-6, TNF-α) and hs-CRP in DM2 patients.

***Corresponding author:** Alireza Ostadrahimi, Tabriz University of Medical Sciences, Tabriz, Iran.
Email: ostadrahimi@tbzmed.ac.ir

Materials and Methods

Study Design

This study was a randomized, double blind, placebo controlled trial performed on type 2 diabetic patients with at least 2 years experience. Subjects were recruited from diabetes association in Tabriz, Iran. The study was approved by Medical Ethical Committee of the Tabriz University of medical science under the number of 5/4/3832. Exclusion criteria were insulin therapy at baseline or during the study, smoking, presence of pregnancy and breastfeeding, consumption of ginger or other botanical supplements, any acute illnesses and presence of some chronic diseases including kidney, liver, cardiovascular, and gastrointestinal diseases. 64 eligible patients with the age group of 38-65 yrs of either sex fulfilled consent paper prior to inclusion in the study.

Sample size was determined based on data from previous study[16] by considering α= 0.05 with power of 80%. The sample size was computed as 25 per group. Regarding a possible loss to follow-up, a safety margin of 30% was determined, and therefore 32 patients were allocated in each group.

Treatment

All patients were randomly assigned to two groups of 32 subjects in each to receive either ginger or placebo one tablet twice a day immediately after lunch and dinner for 8 weeks. The patients were instructed to maintain their diet and physical activity during the intervention. All subjects were permitted to consume their usual medications according to their physicians' recommendation. The three-day food record was taken from all patients at the beginning and end of intervention to be confidant of constant dietary intake.

Tablets Preparation

Fresh rhizomes of zingiber officinale were purchased from local market and were ground as a fine particle after drying. The powder was delivered to a pharmaceutical lab (Tabriz university of medical science, Iran) to prepare tablets containing 1 gram ginger in each. Starch was also used to make placebo. The tablets were placed in the identical bottles by a third person not directly involved in this study. This person labeled the bottles with 2 cods which retained unknown for researchers until the end of intervention. To evaluate the compliance of patients, bottles containing ginger (or placebo) tablets were given monthly.

Anthropometric and Biochemical Assessments

Anthropometric parameters including height and weight were measured at the beginning and end of the intervention to calculate body mass index (BMI) as the formula (Wt/Ht2). Body weight was measured without shoes and light clothing by using a Seca scale (Seca, Hamburg, Germany). Heights were also measured using a statiometer (Seca) without shoes.

Blood samples (5ml) were taken in a 12-14 hrs fasting state (water permitted) at the beginning and after two months of intervention. The serum was obtained by high speed centrifugation and was frozen immediately at −70 °C until assay. The concentration of hs-CRP was measured by spectrophotometer method using parsazmun kit. IL-6 and TNF-α were also assayed using ELISA kits according to the manufacturer's instruction.

Statistical Analysis

The data were analyzed by SPSS software (version 17; SPSS Inc., Chicago, IL) and the results were expressed as mean ± standard error. The normality of the distribution of variables was determined by the Kolmogorov-Smirnov test. The background characteristics and baseline experimental data in the 2 groups were compared using independent sample *t*-tests and chi-squared test. Analysis of covariance (ANCOVA) was used to identify any differences between 2 groups after intervention, adjusting for baseline measurements and covariates including age and hypoglycemic drugs. The changes of anthropometric measurements and the concentration of IL-6, TNF-α and hs-CRP were assessed by paired sample *t*-tests in each group. Differences with $P < 0.05$ were considered to be statistically significant.[17]

Results

Of 64 patients initially recruited, 6 persons were excluded during the study. In ginger group 2 persons did not consume tablets according to plan, one person traveled and one person needed to change his medication during the intervention. In placebo group also one people did not consume tablets according to plan and one person traveled.

Participants represented good compliance with the ginger consumption and no serious adverse side effects or symptoms were reported except for two patients with slight heart burn in the beginning of intervention. Despite the differences in consumed hypoglycemic drugs, it remained constant for all participants during the study.

Table 1 shows baseline anthropometric parameters and the levels of IL-6, TNF-α and hs-CRP in two groups. There were no statistically significant differences between the ginger and placebo groups ($P > 0.05$).

Table 1. Baseline characteristics of study participants[a]

Item	Intervention (ginger)	placebo
Age (yr)	49.27±5.18	53.14±7.9
Sex[b] (M:F)	14:12	16:12
Weight (kg)	79.38±11.87	76.89±14.59
BMI (kg/m2)	29.2±4.07	29.8±5.05
TNF-α (Pg/ml)	16.7±4.4	18.9±5.3
IL-6 (Pg/ml)	8.6±2.7	7.6±3.0
Hs-CRP (Pg/ml)	3.37±2.8	2.23±2.3

[a] Data are presented as means ± standard error
[b] Frequency

Table 2 shows the concentrations of IL-6, TNF-α and hs-CRP before and after intervention in both groups. Ginger supplementation significantly reduced the levels of TNF-α (P=0.006), IL-6 (P=0.02) and hs-CRP (P=0.012) in ginger group in comparison to baseline. These parameters remained unchanged in placebo group during the study.

Table 2. Effects of ginger or placebo consumption on some parameters in diabetic patients[1]

Item	Intervention (ginger)		placebo		P
	Before	after	before	after	
TNF-α (Pg/ml)	16.7±4.4	15.3±4.6*	18.9±5.3	19.6±5.2	0.005
IL-6 (Pg/ml)	8.6±2.7	7.9±2.1*	7.6±3.0	7.8±2.9	0.11
Hs-CRP (Pg/ml)	3.37±2.8	2.42±1.7*	2.23±2.3	2.56±2.18	0.016

1 Data are presented as means ± SD
*P < 0.05 significantly different from baseline according to paired sample t

On the other hand, results of analysis of covariance showed significant differences in TNF-α (P=0.005) and hs-CRP (P=0.016) levels between two groups at the end of study, that were in accordance with the type of consumed hypoglycemic drug, age and baseline values. While no statistically significant differences were observed for IL-6 (P > 0.05) between 2 groups (Table 2).

Discussion

Recent studies have reported that ginger has anti-inflammatory effects[7] which can decline pain associated with rheumatoid and osteoarthritis.[8] On the other hand, the role of inflammation on diabetes has been reported in numerous studies.[18] Cytokines are associated with the pathogenesis of both type 1 and type 2 diabetes through accelerating beta-cell apoptosis and death. Besides, evidence have shows that insulin resistance as a pro-inflammatory status may have existed for years before the occurrence of type 2 diabetes.[19] Moreover, increased CRP, IL-6 and TNF-α are associated with nephropathy, retinopathy and cardiovascular disease in both types of diabetes.[20]

The present study was performed with the aim of assessing the effects of ginger powder on inflammation under diabetic condition. The results showed that ginger supplementation alleviated the inflammation by reduced levels of TNF-α and hs-CRP without any significant effects on IL-6 levels. In consistent with our study Morakinyo et al.[15] indicated that treatment with aqueous and ethanol extracts of ginger in diabetic rats significantly decreased the levels of TNF-α. Besides, Fatehi-Hassanabad et al.[14] reported the anti-inflammatory effects of the aqueous extract of ginger in diabetic mice.

A large body of evidence indicated that the major pharmacological activity of ginger is due to gingerols and shogaols. These compounds reduce prostaglandin synthesis through suppression of cyclooxygenase- 1 and cyclooxygenase-2. It also has been reported that ginger suppresses leukotriene biosynthesis by inhibiting 5-lipoxygenase.[21] In addition, ginger extract was found to inhibit beta-amyloid peptide-induced cytokine and chemokine expression in cell line of human monocytes.[10]

Conclusion

In conclusion, during the present study oral ginger supplementation ameliorated inflammation through reduction in levels of TNF-α and hs-CRP concentrations in blood samples of the patients with type 2 diabetes mellitus. Regarding negligible side effects of ginger, it may be a good remedy for diabetic patients to diminish the risk of some secondary chronic complications.

Acknowledgements

This study was supported by a grant from Research Vice-Chancellor of Tabriz University of Medical Sciences (Tabriz, Iran). The authors thank Tabriz association of diabetes for helping in recruiting patients.

Conflict of Interest

The authors have no conflict of interest.

References

1. Ali BH, Blunden G, Tanira MO, Nemmar A. Some phytochemical, pharmacological and toxicological properties of ginger (Zingiber officinale Roscoe): a review of recent research. *Food Chem Toxicol* 2008;46(2):409-20.
2. Srivastava KC, Mustafa T. Ginger (zingiber officinale) in rheumatism and musculoskeletal disorders. *Med Hypotheses* 1992;39(4):342-8.
3. Bryer E. A literature review of the effectiveness of ginger in alleviating mild-to-moderate nausea and vomiting of pregnancy. *J Midwifery Womens Health* 2005;50(1):e1-3.
4. Leach MJ, Kumar S. The clinical effectiveness of ginger (zingiber officinale) in adults with osteoarthritis. *Int J Evid Based Healthc* 2008;6(3):311-20.
5. Altman RD, Marcussen KC. Effects of a ginger extract on knee pain in patients with osteoarthritis. *Arthritis Rheum* 2001;44(11):2531-8.

6. Mustafa T, Srivastava KC. Ginger (Zingiber officinale) in migraine headache. *J Ethnopharmacol* 1990;29(3):267-73.
7. Shukla Y, Singh M. Cancer preventive properties of ginger: A brief review. *Food Chem Toxicol* 2007;45(5):683-90.
8. White B. Ginger: An overview. *Am Fam Physician* 2007;75(11):1689-91.
9. Grzanna R, Lindmark L, Frondoza CG. Ginger-an herbal medicinal product with broad anti-inflammatory actions. *J Med Food* 2005;8(2):125-32.
10. Grzanna R, Phan P, Polotsky A, Lindmark L, Frondoza CG. Ginger extract inhibits β-amyloid peptide-induced cytokine and chemokine expression in cultured thp-1 monocytes. *J Altern Complement Med* 2004;10(6):1009-1013.
11. Charlier C, Michaux C. Dual inhibition of cyclooxygenase-2 (cox-2) and 5-lipoxygenase (5-lox) as a new strategy to provide safer non-steroidal anti-inflammatory drugs. *Eur J Med Chem* 2003;38(7-8):645-59.
12. Spranger J, Kroke A, Mohlig M, Hoffmann K, Bergmann MM, Ristow M, et al. Inflammatory cytokines and the risk to develop type 2 diabetes: Results of the prospective population-based european prospective investigation into cancer and nutrition (epic)-potsdam study. *Diabetes* 2003;52(3):812-7.
13. Ray A, Huisman MV, Tamsma JT, van Asten J, Bingen BO, Broeders EA, et al. The role of inflammation on atherosclerosis, intermediate and clinical cardiovascular endpoints in type 2 diabetes mellitus. *Eur J Intern Med* 2009;20(3):253-60.
14. Fatehi-Hassanabad Z, Gholamnezhad Z, Jafarzadeh M, Fatehi M. The anti-inflammatory effects of aqueous extract of ginger root in diabetic mice. *DARU J Pharm Sci* 2005;13(2):70-3.
15. Morakinyo OA, Akindele AJJ, Ahmned Z. Modulation of antioxidant enzymes and inflammatory cytokines: possible mechanism of antidiabetic effect of ginger extracts. *Afr J Biomed Res* 2011;14(3):195-202.
16. Alizadeh-Navaei R, Roozbeh F, Saravi M, Pouramir M, Jalali F, Moghadamnia AA. Investigation of the effect of ginger on the lipid levels: A double blind controlled clinical trial. *Saudi Med J* 2008;29(9):1280-4.
17. Zar JH. Biostatistical analysis. 4th ed. New Jersey: Prentice Hall;1999.
18. Pradhan AD, Manson JE, Rifai N, Buring JE, Ridker PM. C-reactive protein, interleukin 6, and risk of developing type 2 diabetes mellitus. *JAMA* 2001;286(3):327-34.
19. Festa A, D'Agostino R, Jr., Howard G, Mykkanen L, Tracy RP, Haffner SM. Chronic subclinical inflammation as part of the insulin resistance syndrome: The insulin resistance atherosclerosis study (iras). *Circulation* 2000;102(1):42-7.
20. Goldberg RB. Cytokine and cytokine-like inflammation markers, endothelial dysfunction, and imbalanced coagulation in development of diabetes and its complications. *J Clin Endocrinol Metab* 2009;94(9):3171-82
21. Ramadan G, Al-Kahtani MA, El-Sayed WM. Anti-inflammatory and anti-oxidant properties of curcuma longa (turmeric) versus zingiber officinale (ginger) rhizomes in rat adjuvant-induced arthritis. *Inflammation* 2011;34(4):291-301.

6

Phytochemical Screening and Anti-nociceptive Properties of the Ethanolic Leaf Extract of *Trema Cannabina* Lour

Hossain Hemayet[1]*, Ismet Ara Jahan[1], Howlader Sariful Islam[2], Dey Shubhra Kanti[3], Hira Arpona[3], Ahmed Arif[3]

[1] *BCSIR Laboratories, Dhaka, Bangladesh Council of Scientific and Industrial Research, Dhaka-1205, Bangladesh.*

[2] *Department of Pharmacy, World University of Bangladesh, Dhaka-1205, Bangladesh.*

[3] *Pharmacy Discipline, Life Science School, Khulna University, Khulna-9208, Bangladesh.*

ARTICLE INFO

Keywords:
Trema cannabina
Anti-nociceptive
Hot plate test
Tail immersion test
Acetic acid induced writhing test

ABSTRACT

Purpose: The present study was designed to investigate the anti-nociceptive activity of ethanolic leaf extract of *Trema cannabina* Lour (family: Cannabaceae) in experimental animal models. ***Methods:*** The anti-nociceptive action was carried out against two types of noxious stimuli, thermal (hot plate and tail immersion tests) and chemical (acetic acid-induced writhing) in mice. ***Results:*** Phytochemical analysis of crude extract indicated the presence of reducing sugar, tannins, steroid and alkaloid types of secondary metabolites. Crude extract of *T. cannabina* (500 mg/kg dose) showed maximum time needed for the response against thermal stimuli (6.79±0.15 seconds) which is comparable to diclofenac sodium (8.26±0.14 seconds) in the hot plate test. Hot tail immersion test also showed similar results as in hot plate test. At the dose of 250 and 500 mg/kg body weight, the extract showed significantly and in a dose-dependent ($p<0.001$) reduction in acetic acid induced writhing in mice with a maximum effect of 47.56% reduction at 500 mg/kg dose comparable to that of diclofenac sodium (67.07%) at 25 mg/kg. ***Conclusion:*** The obtained results tend to suggest the Anti-nociceptive activity of ethanolic leaf extract of *Trema cannabina* and thus provide the scientific basis for the traditional uses of this plant part as a remedy for pain.

Introduction

Bangladesh possesses rich floristic wealth and diversified genetic resources of medicinal plants. It has a widely ranging tropical and the agro climatic conditions, which are conducive for introducing and domesticating new and exotic plant varieties. The use of plant extracts and pure compounds isolated from natural sources provided the foundation to modern pharmaceutical compounds. *Trema cannabina* is one of the common medicinal plants grown in India and almost all districts of Bangladesh.

Trema cannabina (*T. cannabina*) is a tree of Cannabaceae family. The plant is used in traditional folk remedy by the rural people and shows various pharmacological activities.[1] The root of the plant is used in the treatment of asthma, diarrhoea and passing of blood in urine; the bark is used as poultice in muscular pain; the roots, barks and leaves are used in epilepsy.[1,2] In Africa, this plant is used in various diseases including, hypertension and dysentery.[3] The leaves are used to treat cough and sore throats and bark are used to make cough syrups in traditional medicine. It has been also reported to be used in bronchitis, gonorrhea, malaria, yellow fever, toothache and intestinal worms.[1,4]

Since no literature is currently available to substantiate Anti-nociceptive property from ethanolic extract of *T. cannabina*, therefore the present study was designed to provide scientific evidence for its use as a traditional folk remedy by investigating the Anti-nociceptive activity that also confirms its use as pain killer.

Materials and Methods

Collection and Identification of Plant Materials

The plant selected for present work was the leaves of *T. cannabina*, which were collected from Khulna, Bangladesh in March, 2011 at the daytime. The leaves were collected from the fresh plants. The samples were identified by Sarder Nasir Uddin, Senior Scientific Officer, Bangladesh National Herbarium, Mirpur, Dhaka, Bangladesh. A voucher specimen (DACB: 35921) has been deposited in the Herbarium for further reference.

Preparation of Ethanolic Extract

The leaves of *T. cannabina* were freed from any of the foreign materials. Then the leaves were air-dried under shed temperature followed by drying in an electric oven at 40 °C. The dried plant materials were then ground

***Corresponding author:** Hossain Hemayet, Chemical Research Division, BCSIR Laboratories, Council of Scientific and Industrial Research (BCSIR), Dhaka-1205, Bangladesh. E-mail: hemayethossain02@yahoo.com

into powder. About 200 g of powdered material was taken in a clean, flat-bottomed glass container and soaked in 800 ml of 95% ethanol. The container with its contents was sealed and kept for a period of 7 days accompanying occasional shaking and stirring. The whole mixture then underwent a coarse filtration by a piece of clean, white cotton material. Then it was filtered through whatman filter paper (Bibby RE200, Sterilin Ltd., UK) which was concentrated with rotary evaporator at bath temperature not exceeding 40 °C to have gummy concentrate of extract (yield approx. 5.77%).

Chemicals

Gallic acid, Folin-ciocalteu phenol reagent and atropine were obtained from Sigma Chemical Co. [(St. Louis, MO, USA)]. Bromocresol green, Phosphate buffer, Sodium hydroxide, hydrochloric acid, sodium carbonate, ethanol and chloroform were of analytical grade and purchased from Merck (Darmstadt, Germany).

Test Animals and Drug

Swiss albino mice of either sex and male rats of Wister strain weighing between 20-25 g and 175-202 g respectively were used for in-vivo pharmacological screening. The mice and rats were collected from the animal research branch of the International Center for Diarrhoeal Disease and Research, Bangladesh (ICDDR, B). The animals were housed under standard laboratory (at Pharmacology Laboratory of BCSIR, Chittagong) conditions maintained at 25±1 °C and under 12/12 h light/dark cycle and feed with Balanced Trusty Chunts and water ad libitum (Chatterjee 1993) during acclimatization period. The animals were acclimatized to this laboratory condition for a period of 14 days prior to performing the experiments. The animals were fasted overnight before the experiments. All the experimental animals were treated following the Ethical Principles and Guidelines for Scientific Experiments on Animals (1995) formulated by The Swiss Academy of Medical Sciences and the Swiss Academy of Sciences. All experimental protocols were approved by the BCSIR Ethics Committee.
The standard drug diclofenac Na used for this study and purchased from Square Pharmaceuticals Ltd, Bangladesh.

Phytochemical Screening

The freshly prepared crude extract was qualitatively tested for the presence of chemical constituents, by using the following reagents and chemicals, for example, alkaloids were identified by the Dragendorff's reagent, flavonoids with the use of Mg and HCl, tannins with ferric chloride and potassium dichromate solutions, steroids with Libermann-Burchard reagent and reducing sugars with Benedict's reagent.[5-7]

Quantification of Total Phenolic Content

The total phenolic content of the extract was determined by the modified Folin-Ciocaltu method.[8] 1.0 ml of extract (1 mg/ml) was mixed with 5 ml of Folin-Ciocaltu reagent (1:10 v/v distilled water) and 4 ml (75 g/l) of sodium carbonate solution. The mixture was then allowed to stand for 30 min at 40 °C for color development .The absorbance was read at 765 nm against blank using a double beam UV/Visible spectrophotometer (Analykjena, Model 205, Jena, Germany). Total phenolic content was determined as mg/g of gallic acid equivalent using the equation obtained from a standard gallic acid calibration curve $y=6.2548x - 0.0925$, $R^2=0.9962$.

Quantification of Total Alkaloid Content

Total alkaloid content was determined by the Fazel et al., method.[9] The plant extract (1mg/ml) was dissolved in 2 N HCl and then filtered. The pH of phosphate buffer solution was adjusted to neutral with 0.1 N NaOH. One ml of this solution was transferred to a separating funnel and then 5 ml of bromocresol green solution along with 5 ml of phosphate buffer were added. The mixture was shaken and the complex formed was extracted with chloroform by vigorous shaking. The extracts were collected in a 10 ml volumetric flask and diluted to volume with chloroform. The absorbance of the complex in chloroform was measured at 470 nm. Atropine was used as reference standard for this study. All experiments were performed thrice; the results were averaged and reported in the form of mean ± S.E.M.

Anti-nociceptive Activity

Hot Plate Test

Albino mice were placed in aluminum hot plate kept at a temperature of 55±0.5 °C for a maximum time of 10 second.[10] The animals were divided into control, positive control and test groups with five mice in each group. The animals of test groups received test substance at the dose of 250 and 500 mg/kg body weight. Positive control group was administered with diclofenac Na (standard drug) at the dose of 25 mg/kg body weight and vehicle control group was treated with 1% tween 80 in water at the dose of 10 ml/kg body weight. Reaction time was recorded when animals licked their forepaws and jumped at before and at 0, 15, 30 and 45 min followed by oral administration of control and crude extract. Diclofenac sodium (25 mg/kg) was administered intra-peritoneally.

Tail Immersion Test

Anti-nociceptive effect of the test substances was determined by the tail immersion test method described by Sewell and Spencer.[11] Mice were treated with diclofenac sodium (25 mg/kg) and two doses of the crude extract (250 and 500 mg/kg). One to two centimeter of the tail of mice was immersed in warm water kept constant at 50 °C. The reaction time was the time taken by the mice to deflect their tails. The first reading is discarded and the reaction time was taken as a mean of the next two readings. The latent period of the tail-flick response was taken as the index of antinociception and was determined at 0, 30 and 60 min after the administration of drugs. The maximum reaction time was fixed at 10 seconds.

Acetic Acid-Induced Writhing Test

The Anti-nociceptive activity of the crude ethanolic leaf extract of *T. cannabina* was studied using acetic acid induced writhing model in mice.[12,13] The animals were divided into control, positive control and test groups with five mice in each group. The animals of test groups received test substance at the dose of 250 and 500 mg/kg body weight. Positive control group was administered with diclofenac Na (standard drug) at the dose of 25 mg/kg body weight and vehicle control group was treated with 1% tween 80 in water at the dose of 10 ml/kg body weight. Test samples, standard drug and control vehicle were administered orally 30 min before intra-peritoneal administration of 0.7% acetic acid. After an interval of 15 min, the mice were observed writhing (constriction of abdomen, turning of trunk and extension of hind legs) for 5 min.

Statistical analysis

The results are presented as mean±SEM. The statistical analysis of the results was performed using one way analysis of variance (ANOVA) followed by Dunnett's test using SPSS 11.5 software. Differences between groups were considered significant at a level of $p<0.05$.

Results

Chemical Group Test

Results of different chemical tests on the ethanolic extract of leaves of *T. cannabina* showed the presence of alkaloids, reducing sugars, tannins and steroids (Table 1).

Table 1. Results of different group tests of ethanolic extract of leaves of *T. cannabina*

Serial No.	Chemical Constituents	Test	Extract	Result
1.	Test for Reducing Sugar	Benedict's Test	Ethanolic	+
		Fehling's Test	Ethanolic	+
		Alpha Napthol Solution Test	Ethanolic	+
2.	Test for Tannins	Ferric Chloride Test	Ethanolic	++
		Potassium dichromate Test	Ethanolic	+
3.	Test for Flavonoids	Hydrochloric Acid Test	Ethanolic	-
4.	Test for Saponins	Foam Test	Ethanolic	-
5.	Test for Gums	Molisch Test	Ethanolic	-
6.	Test for Steroids	Libermann-Burchard Test	Ethanolic	+
		Sulphuric acid Test	Ethanolic	+
7.	Test for Alkaloids	Mayer's Test	Ethanolic	+
		Wagner's Test	Ethanolic	+
		Dragendroff's Test	Ethanolic	+
		Hager's Test	Ethanolic	+

+: Positive result; - : Negative result; ++: significantly positive

Total Phenolic & Alkaloid Content

The amount of total phenolic content was calculated as quite high in the ethanolic crude extract of *T. cannabina* (152.37±1.32 mg/g of gallic acid equivalent). The alkaloid content was also found high in ethanolic extract (28.59±0.73 mg/gm) (Table 2).

Table 2. Total phenolicand alkaloid content of *T. cannabina* extracts.

Extract	Total phenolic content (mg/gm of gallic acid equivalent)	Total alkaloid content (mg/gm)
Ethanol extract of *T. cannabina*	152.37±1.32	28.59±0.73

The values are expressed as mean ± SEM (n=3)

Analgesic Activity

Hot Plate Test

Two doses of ethanolic extract of leaves of *T. cannabina* increased the reaction time in a dose dependent manner to the thermal stimulus which was summarized in Table 3. The highest nociceptive inhibition of thermal stimulus was exhibited at a higher dose 500 mg/kg of crude extract which has maximum time needed for the response against thermal stimuli (6.79±0.15 seconds) which is comparable to diclofenac sodium (8.26±0.14 seconds) and found statistically significant ($p<0.001$).

Tail Immersion Test

The Anti-nociceptive activity of *T. cannabina* and diclofenac Na demonstrated in tail immersion test are given in Table 4. *T. cannabina* at all two doses (250 and 500 mg/kg) significantly increased the latency period to hot-water induced thermal stimuli ($p<0.001$) in a dose-dependent manner. The highest nociceptive inhibition of thermal stimulus was exhibited at a higher dose 500 mg/kg of crude extract (8.14±0.11 seconds) comparable to diclofenac sodium (8.17±0.11 seconds) and was also statistically significant ($p<0.001$).

Table 3. Effect of ethanolic extract of leaves of *T. cannabina* on hot plate test in mice.

Treatment	Dose (mg/kg, p.o.)	Response Time (sec)			
		0 min (Latency)	15 min	30 min	45 min
Control (1% aq. Tween 80)	10 ml/ kg	1.80±0.08	2.56±0.25	2.96±0.21	3.13±0.16
Diclofenac-Na	25	2.08±0.06	5.84±0.31*	6.75±0.17*	8.26±0.14*
Et. of leaves of *T. cannabina*	250	1.96±0.04	3.92±0.16*	4.11±0.10*	4.90±0.28*
	500	2.02±0.09	5.19±0.21*	6.20±0.21*	6.79±0.15*

Values are expressed as mean±SEM (Standard Error Mean); Et.:Ethanolic; *indicates P < 0.001; one-way ANOVA followed by Dennett's test as compared to control; p.o.: per oral

Table 4. Effect of ethanolic leaf extract of *T. cannabina* on tail immersion test in mice

Treatment	Dose (mg/kg, p.o.)	Response Time (sec)		
		0 min	30 min	60 min
Control(1% aq. Tween 80)	10 ml/ kg	2.22±0.22	3.19±0.19	3.76±0.20
Diclofenac-Na	25	4.20±0.26*	7.89±0.16*	8.17±0.22*
Et. of leaves of *T. cannabina*	250	3.21±0.11*	4.89±0.17*	5.79±0.16*
	500	4.04±0.33*	7.07±0.35*	8.14±0.11*

Values are expressed as mean±SEM; Et.:Ethanolic; *indicates P < 0.001; one-way ANOVA followed by Dennett's test as compared to control; p.o.: per oral.

Acetic Acid-Induced Writhing Test

Table 5 showed the effect of the ethanolic extract of leaves of *T. cannabina* on acetic acid induced writhing in mice. At the dose of 250 mg/kg and 500 mg/kg of body weight, the extract produced 34.15% & 47.56 % writhing inhibition in test animals respectively. The results were statistically significant ($p <0.001$) and was comparable to the standard drug diclofenac Na, which showed 67.07% at a dose of 25 mg/kg weight.

Table 5. Effects of the ethanolic leaf extract of T. cannabina on acetic acid induced writhing of mice (n=5)

Group	Treatment and Dose	Number of writhes (% Writhing)	% Writhing Inhibition
Control	1% tween 80 solution 10 ml/kg, p.o.	16.4± 1.72 (100)	---
Positive Control	Diclofenac Na 25 mg/kg, p.o.	5.4 ± 0.68 * (32.93)	67.07
Test Group- 1	Et. Extract of *T. cannabina* 250 mg/kg, p.o.	10.80± 0.58 * (65.85)	34.15
Test group- 2	Et. Extract of *T. cannabina* 500 mg/kg, p.o.	8.60 ± 0.68 * (52.44)	47.56

Values are expressed as mean ± SEM; Et.:Ethanolic; * indicates P < 0.001; one-way ANOVA followed by Dennett's test as compared to control; n = Number of mice; p o.: per oral

Discussion

A number of natural products are used in various traditional medical systems to treat relief of symptoms from pain. The crude extracts of leaves of *T. cannabina* demonstrated significant anti-nociceptive activity at two different dose levels in various animal models of pain. Acetic acid-induced writhing response elucidated peripheral activity, while the hot plate tests, hot tail flick test investigated both peripheral and central activity.[14,15] Nociceptive reaction towards thermal stimuli in hot plate test and tail immersion in hot water test using mice is a well-validated model for the detection of opiate analgesic as well as several types of analgesic drugs from spinal origin.[11,16] Nociceptive pain inhibition was noticed highest in both the test at 45 minutes after administration of the extracts and the response time is increased from 2.02 seconds to 6.79 seconds in hot plate test at dose 500 mg/kg while it was also increased from 4.04 seconds to 8.14 seconds in tail flick test at the same dose level. Other doses used in this study also increases the latent period significantly with the time being in both tests. Acetic acid-induced writhing test has been used as a model of chemo-nociceptive induced pain, which increases PGE2 and PGF2a peripherally. The crude ethanolic extract of leaves of *T. cannabina* showed significant reduction of abdominal contraction in mice. Local peritoneal receptors were postulated to be partly involved in the abdominal constriction (writhing) response.[11,17] The method has been associated with prostanoids in general, i.e. increased levels of PGE2 and PGF2α in peritoneal fluids[17] as well as lipoxygenase products by some researchers.[15] In the present study, the reduction of the Anti-nociceptive process obtained within the first hour is probably related to reduction in the release of preformed inflammatory agents, rather than to a reduced synthesis of the inflammatory mediators by inhibition of cyclooxygenases and/or lipoxygenases (and other inflammatory mediators). Thus the anti-nociceptive activity shown by crude extracts of leaves of *T. cannabina* in hot plate, hot tail-flick and acetic acid induced writhing test indicate that ethanolic extract of the plant might possess centrally and peripherally mediated Anti-nociceptive properties.

Furthermore, phytochemical screening of the ethanol extract of *F. hispida* reveals the presence of steroid, reducing sugars, alkaloid and significant amount of phenolic compounds (tannins). Inhibition of pain is associating with presence of steroidal constituents.[18] Tannins also play a role in Anti-nociceptive and anti-inflammatory activities in some studies.[19] Because tannins inhibit prostaglandin synthesis by modifying the production of cyclooxygenase (cox-1 and cox-2) and lipooxygenase involved in the prostaglandin synthesis.[20,21] Besides, alkaloids are well known for their ability to inhibit pain perception.[22] So these phyto-constituents might be responsible for its Anti-nociceptive activity.

Conclusion

In conclusion, it can be revealed that the crude ethanolic leaf extract of *T. cannabina* plant possess significant Anti-nociceptive activity. The potential of the extract of *T. cannabina* as Anti-nociceptive agent may be due to the presence of phyto-constituents like tannins, alkaloids etc and might be responsible for its activity and justify its use as a traditional folk remedy. However, a more extensive study is necessary to determine the exact mechanism(s) of action of the extract and its active compound(s).

Acknowledgements

The authors are thankful to Prof. Dr. Samir Kumar Sadhu, Pharmacy Discipline, Khulna University; Dr. Jamil Ahmed Shilpi, Associate professor, Pharmacy Discipline, Khulna University; Dr. Mahiuddin Alamgir, Research Scientist, National Measurement institute (NMI), Australia, for their encouragement during the research time. All the informants of the study area are cordially acknowledged for their valuable cooperation.

Conflict of Interest

There is no conflict of interest in this study.

References

1. Uddin SN, Uddin KMA, Ahmed F. Analgesic and antidiarrhoeal activities of *Treamaorientalis* Linn. in mice. *Oriental Pharm and Exp Med* 2008;8(2):187-91.
2. Kirtikar KR, Basu BD. Indian Med Plants. 2nd ed. India: Singh B and Singh MP publishers; 1980.
3. Iwe MM. Handbook of african medicinal plants. Boca Raton: CRC Press; 1993.
4. Rulangaranga ZK. Conservation of medicinal and aromatic plants in Tanzania proceedings of a workshop on priority species for tree planting and afforestation in Tanzania. Tanzania: Morogoro; 1991.
5. Ghani A. Medicinal Plants of Bangladesh. 1st ed. Bangladesh: Dhaka; 1998.
6. Evans WC. Trease and Evan's Textbook of Pharmacognosy. 13th ed. London: Cambidge University Press; 1989.
7. Harborne JB. *Phytochemal methods* (A guide to modern techniques to plantanalysis). 3rd ed. London: Chapman and Hall; 1984.
8. Singleton V, Orthofer R, Lamuela-Raventos RM. Analysis of total phenols and other oxidation substrates and antioxidants by means of folin-ciocalteu reagent. *Methods Enzymol* 1999;99:152-58.
9. Shamsa F, Monsef H, Ghamooshi R, Verdian-rizi M. Spectrophotometric determination of total alkaloids in some Iranian medicinal plants. *Thai J Pharm Sci* 2008;32: 17-20.
10. Franzotti EM, Santos CV, Rodrigues HM, Mourao RH, Andrade MR, Antoniolli AR. Anti-inflammatory, analgesic activity and acute toxicity of sida cordifolia l. (malva-branca). *J Ethnopharmacol* 2000;72(1-2):273-7.
11. Sewell RDE, Spencer PSJ. Anti-nociceptive activity of narcotic agonist and partial agonist analgesics and other agents in the tail-immersion test in mice and rats. *Neuropharmacol* 1976; 15(11):683-8.
12. Whittle BA. The use of changes in capillary permeability in mice to distinguish between

narcotic and non-narcotic analgesics. *Br J Pharmacol Chemother* 1964; 22: 246-53.

13. Ahmed F, Selim MS, Das AK, Choudhuri MS. Anti-inflammatory and Anti-nociceptive activities of lippia nodiflora linn. *Pharmazie* 2004;59(4):329-30.
14. Starec M, Waitzova D, Elis J. evaluation of the analgesic effect of rg-tannin using the "hot plate" and "tail flick" method in mice. *Cesk Farm* 1988;37(7):319-21.
15. Ghule BV, Ghante MH, Upaganlawar AB, Yeole PG. Analgesic and Anti Inflammatory activities of *Lagenaria siceraria Stand.* Fruit juice extract in rats and mice. *Pharmacogn Mag* 2006; 2(8): 232-8.
16. D'Amour FE, Smith DL. A method for determining loss of pain sensation. *J Pharmacol Exper Therap*1941; 72: 74-9.
17. Adzu B, Amos S, Kapu SD, Gamaniel KS. Anti-inflammatory and Anti-nociceptive effects of Sphaeranthussene galensis. *J Ethnopharmacol* 2003;84:169-73.
18. Miguel OG, Calixto JB, Santos AR, Messana I, Ferrari F, Cechinel Filho V, et al. Chemical and preliminary analgesic evaluation of geraniin and furosin isolated from phyllanthus sellowianus. *Planta Med* 1996;62(2):146-9.
19. Ramprasath VR, Shanthi P, Sachdanandam P. Immunomodulatory and anti-inflammatory effects of semecarpus anacardium linn. Nut milk extract in experimental inflammatory conditions. *Biol Pharm Bull* 2006;29(4):693-700.
20. Sreejayan, Rao MN. Nitric oxide scavenging by curcuminoids. *J Pharm Pharmacol* 1997;49(1):105-7.
21. Yokozawa T, Chen CP, Dong E, Tanaka T, Nonaka GI, Nishioka I. Study on the inhibitory effect of tannins and flavonoids against the 1,1-diphenyl-2 picrylhydrazyl radical. *Biochem Pharmacol* 1998;56(2):213-22.
22. Uche FI, Aprioku JS. The phytochemical constituents, analgesic and anti-inflammatory effects of methanol extract of Jatrophacurcas leaves in mice and Wister albino rats. *J Applied Sci Environ Manage* 2008; 12(4): 99-102.

7

Cadmium-Induced Toxicity and the Hepatoprotective Potentials of Aqueous Extract of *Jessiaea Nervosa* Leaf

Ama Udu Ibiam[1], Emmanuel Ike Ugwuja[1,2]*, Christ Ejeogo[3], Okechukwu Ugwu[4]

[1] *Department of Biochemistry, Faculty of Biological Sciences, Ebonyi State University, PMB 053, Abakaliki, Nigeria.*

[2] *Department of Chemical Pathology, Faculty of Clinical Medicine, Ebonyi State University, PMB 053 Abakaliki, Nigeria.*

[3] *Department of Biochemistry, Institute of Management and Technology (IMT), Enugu, Nigeria.*

[4] *Department of Biotechnology, Faculty of Biological Sciences, Ebonyi State University, PMB 053, Abakaliki, Nigeria.*

ARTICLEINFO

Keywords:
Jussiaea nervosa
Cadmium toxicity
Biochemical parameters
Hepatoprotection

ABSTRACT

Purpose: Hepatoprotective potentials of *Jussiaea nervosa* leaf extract against Cadmium-induced hepatotoxicity were investigated. ***Methods***: Forty albino rats were randomly assigned into groups A-G with 4 rats in each of the groups A-F. Group A served as control and were given feed only while rats in groups B-F were orally exposed to varying concentrations of cadmium for six weeks. Effects of cadmium were most significant at 12 mg/Kg body weight (BW), and this dose was used for subsequent test involving oral administration of *Jussiaea nervosa* leaf extracts. In this segment, group G (n= 16) was sub-divided into four: G_1-G_4, with each sub-group containing four rats. Rats in sub-group G_1 were given cadmium and feed only and served as positive control. Rats in sub-groups G_2, G_3, and G_4 were given cadmium and 20, 50 and 100g/kg BW of *Jussiaea nervosa* extract, respectively, for six weeks. Blood and liver were analysed using standard laboratory techniques and methods. ***Results:*** Liver function parameters (ALT, AST, ALP, bilirubin) were significantly ($p<0.05$) elevated in exposed rats in comparison to the controls, except for total protein and albumin, which were significantly decreased. Histopathological assessment reveals renal pathology in exposed rats in sharp contrast with the controls. *Jussiaea nervosa* extract however lowered the values of liver function parameters with 100mg/Kg BW dose producing the highest ameliorative effects. Similarly, the serum albumin and total protein significantly ($p<0.05$) improved with normal liver architecture. ***Conclusion:*** The results show the hepatoprotective potentials of *Jussiaea nervosa* extract against Cd toxicity.

Introduction

Cadmium (Cd) is a naturally occurring metal that is widely distributed throughout the biosphere. It is found in soils, sediments, air and water,[1,2] foods, especially of vegetable origin.[3] In fact about 98% of the ingested Cd comes from terrestrial foods while 1% comes from aquatic foods and another 1% from drinking water.[4] Other natural sources of Cd in the atmosphere include volcanic activity, forest fires and wind-borne transport of soil particles.[5] Industrialization has made Cd almost ubiquitous in the environment,[6] thereby increasing its propensity of exposure to humans. Occupational exposures to cadmium are encountered in the manufacturing of batteries, pigments, plastic stabilizers, production and processing of Cd alloys, recycling of domestic wastes and non-ferrous smelters.[7]

Cigarette smoke is one of the most common sources of Cd exposure in the environment.[8] A study conducted by Ibiam and Uwakwe[9] revealed high content of Cd in different brands of cigarettes smoked in Nigeria, especially, the locally manufactured ones; no wonder smoking in public places has been banned in many developed countries of the World.

Cadmium toxicity in humans and other primates is no longer in doubt. For instance, exposure to Cd produces deleterious effects on the cellular architecture and metabolism in a variety of body tissues,[10] including testis,[11] liver and pancreas,[12] kidneys,[13,14] and bone.[14]

In recent times, the use of traditional medicine is increasingly gaining popularity in both developed and developing Worlds.[15] The therapeutic values of many plants have been identified and exploited for the management of many disease conditions. *Jussiaea nervosa* is one of the herbal plants used for treating various diseases. The plant has been classified by the Association of Scientific Identification, Conservation and Utilization of Medicinal Plants in Nigeria.[16] It belongs to the family of *Onagracea*. Its common local names include *arira mmili* (Igbo), *sha shatau* (Hausa),

***Corresponding author:** Emmanuel Ike Ugwuja, Department of Biochemistry, Faculty of Biological Sciences, Ebonyi State University, PMB 053, Abakaliki, Nigeria. Email: ugwuja@yahoo.com

and *ewuru odo* (Yoruba). The chemotherapeutic uses of *J. nervosa* include antidote to poison, alcoholic intoxication and in the treatment of diarrhoea, dysentery as well as vomiting.[16] To the best of our knowledge, there is no report on the phytochemical constituents of *Jussiaea nervosa* and its protective effects against metal intoxication in animals. Considering the ease with which humans are exposed to Cd, both at home (foods, drinking water, cigarette), work places and the abundance of *Jussiaea nervosa* in our environment, it is pertinent to scientifically evaluate whether the consumption of the extract can protect against Cd toxicity. Therefore, this study evaluated the hepatoprotective potentials of the leaf extract of *Jussiaea nervosa* on Cd-intoxicated rats.

Materials and Methods

Collection and Preparation of Plant Material

The leaves of *Jussiaea nervosa* was collected from a farm in a swampy area of phase 6, Trans-Ekulu, Enugu East Local Government Area of Enugu State Nigeria. The plant was identified and authenticated by Prof. J.C. Okafor, Consultant Agro forester and Taxonomist, University of Nigeria, Nsukka.

The leaves were washed and sun dried for 3 days. The dried leaves were homogenized using a manual grinder. The resultant powder was soaked in distilled water and boiled on slow heat for about two hours. The preparation was then suction-filtered. Soaking and filtration was repeated until all the soluble compounds had been extracted. This was adjudged by loss of colour of the filtrate. The extract was concentrated to dryness at 60 °C using electric oven. It was carefully evaporated to dryness on water bath at 40 °C.[17] The extract was kept in a refrigerator until used.

Animals

Male Wister albino rats (n=40), weighing 145-165 g purchased from animal house of the Department of Pharmacy, University of Nigeria, Nsukka were kept in standard cages at 25 °C and 12h light/dark condition in the animal room of the Department of Biochemistry, Ebonyi State University, Abakaliki. The animals were fed on commercial rats' feeds and were given water *ad libitum* for a period of two week to allow them acclimatize. All the rats received human care in accordance with the National Institute of Health guidelines for the care and use of laboratory animals.

Experimental Design

The rats were randomly divided into seven groups (A, B, C, D, E, F and G). There were four (4) rats in each of the groups A-F. Rats in group A were given feed only and served as negative control while rats in groups B, C, D, E and F were orally exposed to varying concentrations (1, 2, 4, 8, 12mg/Kg body weight, respectively) of cadmium (cadmium chloride) for six weeks. Effects of cadmium were most significant at 12 mg/Kg body weight. This informed the use of cadmium at 12 mg/Kg body weight for the subsequent test, which involved oral administration of *Jussiaea nervosa* leaf extract. In this segment, group G (n=16 rats) was sub-divided into four: G_1, G_2, G_3 and G_4, with each sub-group containing four (4) rats.

Rats in sub-group G_1 were given cadmium and feed only and served as positive control. However, rats in sub-groups G_2 , G_3 and G_4 were in addition to cadmium, administered 20, 50 and 100g/kg body weight of *Jussiaea nervosa* leaf extract, respectively. The experiment lasted for six (6) weeks. Both the control and experimental animals were allowed free access to water. At the end of the experiment, the rats were sacrificed. Blood samples were collected for biochemical analysis while the livers were excised for histopathological examinations.

Phytochemical, Biochemical and Histochemical Analysis

The phytochemical analyses of *Jussiaea Nervosa* leaf extractwas done using A.O.A.C[18] and A.O.A.C,[19] while the levels of Alanine transaminase (ALT), Aspartate transminases (AST), alkaline phosphatase (ALP), serum bilirubin and albumin were determined using test kits (Randox Laboratories, UK) in accordance with manufacturer's instructions.

Statistical Analysis

All the tested parameters were subjected to statistical analysis. Statistical analysis was done by One-way Analysis of Variance (ANOVA) and means were compared by Dunnettes comparison.[20]

Results and Discussion

The results of the proximate composition of *Jussiaea nervosa* leaf extract are presented in Table 1. Carbohydrate recorded the highest value of 50.90±0. 96 % while protein was the lowest with a value of 3.60±0.58%. The plant is edible and the proximate analysis is important because it provides information of its nutritional worth and other beneficial effects on humans.[21]

Table 1. Proximate composition of *Jussiaea nervosa* aqueous extract.

Parameter	Mean ± S.D (%)
Moisture	10.00 ± 0.00
Ash	15.5 ± 0.86
Fat	5.5 ± 0.00
Protein	3.6 ± 0.58
Fibre	15.5 ± 1.54
Carbohydrate	50.9 ± 0.96

Data represent means ± SD of three measurements.

The results of the phytochemicals analysis as presented in Table 2 showed the presence of saponins, flavonoids, alkaloids and tannins. Steroids glycosides and phenols were absent. Comparatively, flavonoids had the highest value (30.33+0.64%) while tannins were the least with a mean value of 1.24+0.10%. These values are consistent with phytochemical analysis reports on some other medicinal plants found in Nigeria and West African sub region.[17]

Table 2. Phytochemical Analysis of *Jussiaea nervosa* aqueous leaf extract.

Parameter	Concentration (mg/l)
Steriod	ND
Glycosides	ND
Saponins	1.85 ± 0.50
Flavonoids	30.33 ± 0.64
Phenols	ND
Alkaloid	11.20 ± 0.99
Tannins	1.24 ± 0.10

Table 3 shows the effects of Cd exposure on some liver functions biomarkers. Exposure to cadmium was observed to cause impairment of hepatocyte functions in dose-dependent manner, with higher doses having more severe effects. For instance, the values of serum ALT, AST, ALP, total bilirubin and conjugated bilirubin increased significantly ($p<0.05$), while total protein and albumin decreased significantly ($p<0.05$). The values of ALT, AST, ALP, total bilirubin and conjugated bilirubin were observed to increase by up to 327, 160, 286, 154 and 208%, respectively, at Cd dose of 12 mg/Kg body weight. Total protein and albumin levels decreased by 67 and 61 %, respectively at the same cadmium dosage.

Table 3. Effects of cadmium exposure on some liver function biomarkers in albino rats.

Experimental groups	Proteins (g/dl)		Liver enzymes (U/L)			Bilirubin (µmol/l)	
	Total	Albumin	AST	ALT	ALP	Total	Conjugated
A	6.0±0.5^{a}	3.6±0.2^{a}	18.7±0.2^{a}	38.4±0.3^{a}	52.1±0.7^{a}	9.7±0.9^{a}	2.4±0.7^{a}
B	4.6±0.4^{b}	2.9±0.3^{b}	37.8±0.3^{b}	56.5±0.4^{b}	77.3±0.3^{b}	21.4±0.4^{b}	4.8±0.2^{b}
C	3.6.±0.1^{b}	2.4±0.1^{b}	45.0±0.0^{b}	58.8±0.2^{b}	82.4±1.2^{b}	22.8±0.5^{b}	5.70±0.2^{b}
D	3.3±0.1^{b}	2.0±0.1^{c}	47.1±0.4^{b}	68.0±0.1^{b}	99.1±0.1^{b}	23.2±0.3^{b}	5.9±0.6^{b}
E	2.9±0.1^{c}	1.6±0.1^{d}	63.0±0.1^{c}	94.5±0.4^{c}	198.4±0.7^{c}	23.8±0.6^{b}	6.7±1.1^{c}
F	2.0±0.9^{d}	1.4±0.1^{d}	79.8±1.0^{c}	100.1±1.2^{c}	209.2±1.1^{c}	24.5±0.6^{b}	7.4±0.8^{c}

Values represent means ±S.D. Values with different superscript in the same column are significantly different ($p<0.05$).

These results were corroborated by the results of the histopathological assessment of the liver which revealed extensive cells turnover, fibrosis, infiltration of inflammatory cells, extensive distortion of the hepatocytes, hepatitis and hepatic necrosis (Figure 1), which are in sharp contrast with the results from the control rats (Figure 2). These are indicative of the liver inflammation due to exposure of the rats to Cd. Cd is a known toxic metal and may have elicited some injuries to the hepatocytes.[22]

Figure 1. Micrograph of a section of the liver of normal albino rat (control). Section shows normal liver architecture with preserved hepatic vessels.

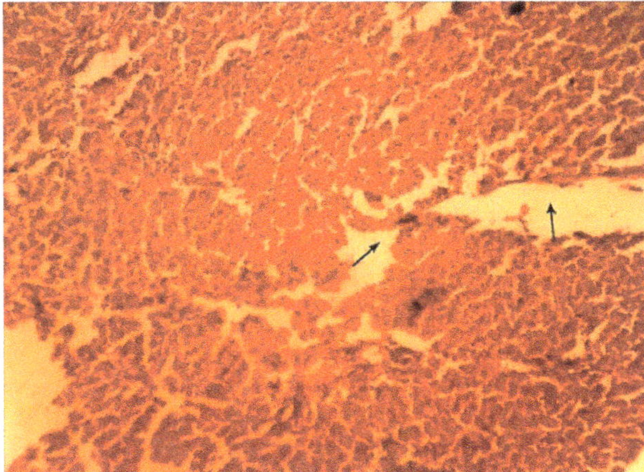

Figure 2. Micrograph of a section of the liver of albino rat exposed to 12 mg of Cd//Kg body weight. Arrows show extensive necrosis with inflammatory cells infiltrating into hepatocytes resulting in hepatisis.

Increased bilirubin levels may have been caused by breakdown of erythrocytes and other haem containing proteins, myoglobin and cytochromes. The haem (from porphrin) of the haemoglobin molecule is separated from the globin and haem is converted mainly in the spleen to bilverdin which is reduced to bilirubin.[23] This is also in tandem with the observed decrease in haemoglobin and packed cell volume levels due to exposure to Cd as previously reported.[24] Another possible explanation is that Cd exposure is known to induce generation of reactive oxygen species (ROS) in organisms[25] which have the potential to elicit oxidative damage to cells, tissues and organs and even death.

For rats which were exposed to 12 mg/kg Cd and co-treated with various concentrations of *Jussiaea nervosa* leaf extract, the results were different: The values of AST, ALT, ALP, bilirubin and conjugated bilirubin were significantly ($P<0.05$) lower than those found in rats that were exposed to Cd only (Table 4) and comparable to levels found in unexposed rats (negative control). The serum albumin and total protein levels significantly ($p<0.05$) improved in animals co-treated with *Jussaiea nervosa* leaf extract. For instance, ALT, AST, ALP, total bilirubin and conjugated bilirubin which were elevated in the untreated rats almost returned to the values found in the unexposed (negative control) rats on administration of aqueous extract of *J. nervosa* leaves at higher doses with only 97, 83, 245, 62, and 72 % elevation, respectively, and thus causing 233, 94, 23, 147, and 191% improvement, respectively, in the treated rats. Similarly, the values of total protein and albumin, which decreased by 67 and 61%, respectively, in the untreated rats, only decreased by 3 and 17%, respectively, in the *Jussiaea nervosa* treated rats, and thus causing 1811 and 267% improvement, respectively.

Table 4. Effects of *Jussiaea nervosa* extract on liver biochemical parameters of Cd- exposed rats

Experimental groups	Proteins (g/dl)		Liver enzymes (U/L)			Bilirubin (µml/l)	
	Total	Albumin	AST	ALT	ALP	Total	Conjugated
A	6.0±0.48^a	3.6±0.2^a	18.7±0.2^a	38.4±0.3^a	52.1±0.7^a	9.7±0.9^a	2.4±0.7^a
G_1	2.0±0.87^b	1.4±0.1^b	78.8±1.0^b	100.2±1.2^b	209.2±1.1^b	24.5±0.6^b	7.4±0.9^b
G_2	3.2±0.11^b	2.4±0.2^b	60.4±0.9^b	92.8±0.3$_b$	207.9±4.1^b	20.5±0.9^b	6.1±1.0^b
G_3	4.8±0.01^c	2.6±0.1^a	52.4±1.2^b	90.4±0.5^b	189.9±5.4^b	18.8±1.1^b	5.4±0.6^b
G_4	5.8±0.17^a	3.0±0.4^a	36.5±0.4^c	70.3±0.1^c	180.1±0.6^b	15.7±1.2^c	4.1±0.9^c

Values represent means ± S.D. Values with different superscript in the same column are statistically different ($p<0.05$).

The observed results are corroborated by histopathological examination of the liver (Figure 3) which showed minimal damage to the liver architecture and even normal integrity of the liver. The liver architecture was well preserved with moderate central fatty changes. The observed results could be attributed to the protective effects of *Jussiaea nervosa* leaf extract, which contains various bioactive chemical with established known therapeutic/antioxidant properties. The presence of the active principles could have caused chelation of the metals and prevented the adverse effects seen in animals exposed to Cd only.

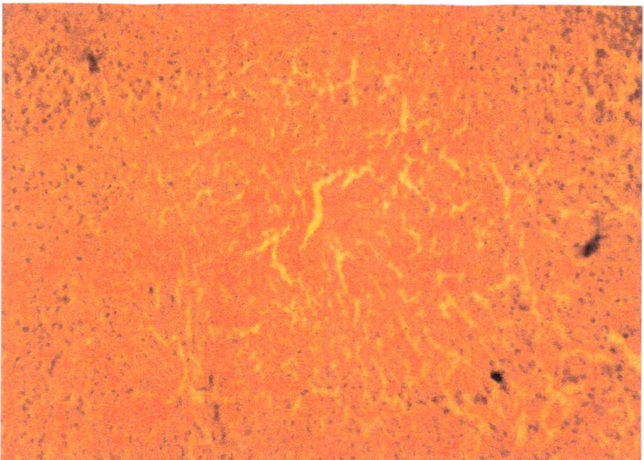

Figure 3. Micrograph of a section of the liver of albino rat exposed to 12 mg/Kg of Cd and treated with aqueous extract of *Jussiaea nervosa* leaf. Section shows normal integrity of liver architecture when compared with control, indicative of the extract protection.

It is therefore reasonable to state that *Jussiaea nervosa* leaf extract contain some phytochemicals which could protect against Cd intoxication, though the mechanism of its action is yet to be established. We can however speculate that the antioxidant properties of the phytochemicals present in *Jussiaea nervosa* leaf extract could have exerted its actions by scavenging ROS produced due to Cd exposure, and therefore, prevented the attendant damage on the liver and macromolecules.[26] It is also possible that some bioactive principles in *Jussiaea nervosa* leaf extract may have induced synthesis of small sulphur rich polypeptides termed phytochelatin which formed complexes with Cd^{2+} and neutralized its toxic effects.[27]

The present results suggest that *Jussiaea nervosa* leaf extract possess hepatoprotective properties against Cd-induced toxicity. Considering the ubiquity of Cd in the environment and the ease with which humans, especially children are exposed; it is recommended that *Jussiaea nervosa* leaf be included in the daily menu to ameliorate Cd toxicity.

Conflict of Interest

There is no conflict of interest to be reported.

References

1. WHO. Environmental Health Criteria. Geneva: World Health Organisation; 1992.
2. Waisberg M, Joseph P, Hale B, Beyersmann D. Molecular and cellular mechanism of cadmium carcinogenesis. Toxicology 2003;192(2-3):95-117.

3. Kiestin PG. Lactational transfer of cadmium in rodents, central nervous system: Effects in the offspring. *Agric Sci Vet* 2003;150:10-1.
4. Van-Assche FJ. A stepwise model to quantify the relative contribution of different environment sources to human cadmium exposure. *Toxicol*ogy1998;98:21-2.
5. Irwin RJ, Van-Mouwerik M, Stevend L, Seese MD, Rasham W. Environmental Contaminates Encyclopedia. 1st ed. Fort Collins, Colorado: National Park Service Water Resources Division; 2003.
6. Margeli A, Theocharis S, Skaltsas S, Skopelitou A, Mykoniatis M. Effect of cadmium pretreatment on liver regeneration after partial hepatectomy in rats. *Environ Health Perspect* 1994;102(Suppl 3):273-6.
7. Cook ME, and Morrow H. Anthropogenic sources of cadmium in Canada. *J Pharmacol* 1992; 60:20-5.
8. Bem EM, Piotrowski JK, Turzynska E. Cadmium, zinc, and copper levels in the kidneys and liver of the inhabitants of north-eastern Poland. *Pol J Occup Med Environ Health* 1993;6(2):133-41.
9. Uwakwe AA, Ibiam UA. Levels of cadmium in different brands of cigerettes sold in Abakaliki metropolis of Nigeria. *Afr J Biochem Res* 2009;3(8):317-20.
10. Al-Motabagani MAH. Effect of cadmium on the morphology of Adrenal Gland in Mice. *J Anat Soc India* 2002;51(2):212-6.
11. Martynowicz H, Skoczyńska A, Karczmarek-Wdowiak B, Andrzejak R. Effect of cadmium on testis function. *Med Pr* 2005;56(2):167-74.
12. Rastogi RB, Singhal RL. Effect of chronic cadmium treatment on rat adrenal catecholamines. *Endocr Res Commun* 1975;2(1):87-94.
13. Axelsson B, Piscator M. Renal damage after prolonged exposure to cadmium. An experimental study. *Arch Environ Health* 1966;12(3):360-73.
14. Jarup L, Alfven T. Low level cadmium exposure, renal and bone effects--the OSCAR study. *Biometals* 2004;17(5):505-9.
15. Jia W, Zhang H. Challenges and opportunities in the Chinese Herbal Drug Industry. 2nd ed. New Delhi: Eastern Publishers; 2005.
16. Sadiq D, Ezi-Ashi T, Onuaguluchi G. Checklist of medicinal plants of Nigeria and their uses. 1st ed. Enugu-Nigeria: Asicumptipn; 2003.
17. Sofowora A. The State of Medicinal Plants 1st ed. Enugu-Nigeria: University of Ibadan;1997.
18. AOAC. Official Methods of Analysis. 15th ed. Washington DC, USA: Association of Official Analytical Chemists; 1990.
19. AOAC. Official Methods of Analysis. 16th ed. Washington DC, USA: Association of Official Analytical Chemists; 1999.
20. William GC, Snedecor GW. Statistical Methods, 8th ed. New York: Lowa State University Press; 1994.
21. Pandey M, Abidi AB, Singh S, Sing RP. Nutritional Evaluation of Leafy Vegetable Paratha. *J Hum Ecol* 2006;19(2):155-6.
22. Suzuki Y, Morita I, Yamane Y, Murota S. Cadmium stimulates prostaglandin E2 production and bone resorption in cultured fetal mouse calvaria. *Biochem Biophys Res Commun* 1989;158(2):508-13.
23. Doumas BT, Perry BW, Sasse EA, Straumfjord JV, Jr. Standardization in bilirubin assays: evaluation of selected methods and stability of bilirubin solutions. *Clin Chem* 1973;19(9):984-93.
24. Ibiam UA, Ugwuj EI, Ejeogo C, Aja PM, Afiukwa C, Oji OU, et al. Hemoprotective and nephroprotective potentials of aqueous extract of *Jussiaea nervosa* leaf in cadmium exposed albino rats. *IOSR J Pharm Biol Sci* 2012;4(1):48-53.
25. Price DJ, Joshi JG. Ferritin. Binding of beryllium and other divalent metal ions. J Biol Chem 1983;258(18):10873-80.
26. Valko M, Izakoric M, Mazur M, Rhodes CJ, Telser J. Role of oxygen radicals in DNA damage and cancer incidence. *Mol Cell Biochem* 2004;266(1-2):37-56.
27. Ming Ho Yu. Environmental Toxicology, 1st ed. Washington DC, USA: Lewis Publishers;2000.

8

NPY Receptors Blockade Prevents Anticonvulsant Action of Ghrelin in the Hippocampus of Rat

Mina Ghahramanian Golzar[1], Shirin Babri[1,2], Zohre Ataie[1], Hadi Ebrahimi[1], Fariba Mirzaie[1], Gisou Mohaddes[1,2]*

[1] *Neuroscience Research Centre (NSRC), Tabriz University of Medical Sciences, Tabriz, Iran.*
[2] *Neuroscience Research Centre, Shahid Beheshti Universiy of Medical Sciences, Tehran, Iran.*

ARTICLEINFO

Keywords:
Ghrelin
Seizure
NPY
GR231118
BIIE0246
CGP71683

ABSTRACT

Purpose: Ghrelin has been shown to have antiepileptic function. However, the underlying mechanisms by which, ghrelin exerts its antiepileptic effects are still unclear. In the present study, we investigated whether neuropeptide Y (NPY) mediates ghrelin anticonvulsant effect in the brain through its Y_1, Y_2 or Y_5 receptors. ***Methods:*** Male Wistar rats were bilaterally microinjected with ghrelin 0.3 nmol/µl/side and NPY antagonists; GR231118 (Y_1 receptor antagonist), BIIE0246 (Y_2 receptor antagonist), CGP71683 (Y_5 receptor antagonist) or solvents (Saline, DMSO) into the dorsal hippocampus 20 minutes before ghrelin administration. Thirty minutes after ghrelin microinjection, a single convulsive dose of pentylenetetrazole (PTZ) (50 mg/kg) was injected intraperitoneally (ip). Afterwards, duration of seizure and total seizure score (TSS) were assessed for 30 minutes in all animals. ***Results:*** Intrahippocampal injection of 0.3 nmol/µl/side ghrelin decreased duration of seizure and TSS induced by PTZ. The suppression of both duration ($p< 0.001$) and TSS ($p< 0.001$) induced by ghrelin in hippocampus were significantly blocked by GR231118 (10 µg/µl/side), BIIE0246 (400 pmol/µl/side) and CGP 71683A (5 nmol/µl/side). ***Conclusion:*** Our findings suggest that NPY Y1, Y2 and Y5 receptors in the hippocampus may somehow mediate the anticonvulsive action of ghrelin. Therefore, it is possible to speculate that ghrelin acts in the hippocampus to modulate seizures via NPY.

Introduction

Ghrelin is a brain-gut peptide, which is mainly produced by stomach.[1,2] However, expression of the peptide has also been demonstrated in peripheral organs such as testis, ovary, placenta, kidney, pituitary, small intestine, pancreas, lymphocytes and brain.[3] Central tissues that express ghrelin include hippocampus, ependymal layer of third ventricle, pituitary and different hypothalamic nuclei such as arcuate, ventromedial, dorsomedial and paraventricular nuclei.[4] Two major forms of ghrelin are found in tissues and plasma: n-octanoyl-modified and des-acyl ghrelin and both cross the blood-brain barrier.[5,6] Ghrelin receptor, growth hormone secretagogue receptor (GHSR), has been detected in many brain regions such as hypothalamus-pituitary unit, CA1, CA2, CA3 and dentate gyrus of hippocampal formation.[7-9]

Ghrelin has many physiological functions but growth hormone release and stimulation of feeding are the most known functions for ghrelin.[4,10,11] Recently, it has been shown that there is a relationship between seizure and ghrelin. On the one hand, PTZ-induced seizure decreased acylated ghrelin of plasma.[12] On the other hand, intraperitoneal and intrahippocampal administration of ghrelin attenuated the intensity of PTZ-induced seizures in rats.[13,14] Electrophysiological evidence also showed that the intracerebroventricular injection of ghrelin has an inhibitory effect against epileptiform activity in the penicillin model of epilepsy.[15] Therefore, previous studies show that ghrelin has an attenuating effect on the severity of seizures, but the mechanism by which ghrelin shows its effect is unclear.

Neuropeptide Y, a potent inhibitory neurotransmitter expressed in the central neurons, is capable of inhibiting epileptiform discharge and its expression, and release is significantly upregulated in hippocampal neurons following an epileptic seizure.[16-18] Six NPY receptor subtypes have been reported (Y_1–Y_6) all of which belong to the G-protein coupled receptor superfamily. In the central nervous system, and specifically in hippocampus (an epileptogenic brain region), expression of Y_1, Y_2 and Y_5 are most prominent.[18]

The possible involvement of NPY in the several ghrelin-mediated effects has been shown in different functions. Ghrelin affects feeding behavior), energy

***Corresponding author:** Gisou Mohaddes, Neuroscience Research Centre, Tabriz University of Medical Sciences, Tabriz, Iran.
E-mail address: gmohades@yahoo.com, mohaddesg@tbzmed.ac.ir

balance, growth hormone secretion and gastrointestinal motility through regulating NPY system.[19-24]
To further substantiate the role of NPY as mediator of ghrelin's antiepileptic actions, intrahippocampal administration of ghrelin was done and the role of Y_1, Y_2 and Y_5 receptors investigated in PTZ-induced seizures in rats.

Materials and Methods

Chemicals and Drugs

Rat ghrelin, GR231118 (Y_1 receptor antagonist), BIIE0246 (Y_2 receptor antagonist), CGP71683 (Y_5 receptor antagonist), and PTZ were purchased from Tocris Bioscience, (Bristol, UK) and DMSO Sigma, (Germany). Ghrelin was dissolved in saline (1mg/100µl), and stocked at -20 °C. Immediately before intrahippocampal microinjection, ghrelin was diluted with 0.9% saline to give a final concentration of 0.3 nmol/ µl. The control group received equal amounts of saline (1µl). Both GR231118 and BIIE0246 were dissolved in saline and CGP71683 was dissolved in DMSO.

Animals and Treatments

The Regional Ethics Committee of Tabriz University of Medical Sciences approved all experimental procedures. Every effort was made to minimize the number of used animals and their suffering. Animals were obtained from the colony of Tabriz university of Medical Sciences. The experiments were performed in adult male Wistar rats weighting 220-250 g at the beginning of experiments. They were housed in a temperature (22±2 °C) and humidity-controlled room. The animals were maintained under a 12:12 h light/ dark cycle, with lights off at 8:00 p.m. Food and water provided ad libitum except for the periods of behavioral testing. The behavioral testing was done during the light phase.

Surgery

For surgical procedures, rats were anesthetized with i.p. injection of ketamine (60 mg/kg) and xylazine (12 mg/kg).[25] Animals were positioned in a stereotaxic apparatus. Then trepanation of the skull cap was performed according to coordinates obtained from Paxinos and Watson brain atlas (mm from bregma: AP= -3.8; ML= ± 2.2; DV= -2.7).[26] According to these coordinates, two 22-gauge guide cannulae were implanted bilaterally into the dorsal hippocampus. The guide cannulae were anchored to the skull using stainless steel screws and acrylic cement. After cannulae implantation, animals were individually housed and allowed 7 days recovery before the behavioral test.

Intrahippocampal Microinjection Procedure

All microinjections were done slowly (1µl/2 min) using a 5µl Hamilton syringe connected by Pe-20 polyethylene tube. The stainless steel injection needle (30 G) were cut to protrude 0.5 mm beyond the tips of the guide cannulae. The conscious animals were gently restrained by hand, the injection needle was inserted through the guide cannulae, and vehicles (1 µl saline or DMSO) or NPY receptor antagonists (GR231118 10 µg/µl; BIIE0246 400 pmol/µl; CGP71683 5 nmol/µl) and ghrelin (0.3 nmol/µl), were sequentially injected. A twenty min interval between i.h. injection of receptor antagonist or vehicles and ghrelin was considered. The injection needle was left in place for 1 min after injection to allow diffusion of the solution and to prevent back flow. Thirty minutes after the last microinjection, a single convulsive dose of PTZ (50 mg/kg) was administered intraperitoneally. The doses of antagonists and administration schedule were chosen based on previous studies demonstrating block of the relevant receptor subtype at the selected dose.[27-29] Effective dose of ghrelin to attenuate seizure intensity obtained from our previous study.[14] Microinjections were done between 9:00 and 12:00 a.m. to prevent variations determined by circadian rhythms.

Seizure Assessment

The rats were housed in Plexiglas cages (50 cm × 50 cm × 40 cm) after PTZ injection and their behavior was observed and videotaped for 30 min. The duration and severity of seizures were monitored in all animals. Then videotapes were reviewed, and detected seizures were scored based on Racine's scale as following: (0) normal, non epileptic activity; (1) mouth and facial movements, hyperactivity, grooming, sniffing, scratching, wet dog shakes; (2) head nodding, staring, tremor; (3) forelimb clonus, forelimb extension; (4) rearing, salivating, tonic clonic activity; (5) falling, status epilepticus.[30] Rats were assigned the score of the most severe seizure observed as seizure score (SS) for each 5 min interval over the course of the 30 min session.[31] Then a mean SS was calculated for the entire 30 min session for each rat and referred as total seizure score (TSS).[32]

Experimental Design

After 7 days of recovery seventy rats were randomly divided into six groups (n=10) as follows:
Group (saline): 1µl/side saline i.h.
Group (ghrelin): 0.3 nmol/µl/side ghrelin i.h.
Group (Saline + ghrelin): 1µl/side saline, 20 min before 0.3 nmol/µl/side ghrelin i.h.
Group (DMSO + ghrelin): 1µl/side DMSO, 20 min before 0.3 nmol/µl/side ghrelin i.h.
Group (GR231118+ ghrelin): 10 µg/µl/side GR231118, 20 min before 0.3 nmol/µl/side ghrelin i.h.
Group (BIIE0246 + ghrelin): 400 pmol/µl/side BIIE 0246, 20 min before 0.3 nmol/µl/side ghrelin i.h.
Group (CGP71683 + ghrelin): 5nmol/µl/side CGP71683, 20 min before 0.3 nmol/µl/side ghrelin i.h.
In all experimental groups, PTZ (50 mg/kg) was injected intraperitoneally 30 min after the administration of ghrelin.

On completion of each experiment, the rats were sacrificed, their brains were removed, fixed in formalin, and injection sides were verified in coronal sections. Only animals with the correct injection sides were taken for a further analysis.

Statistical Analysis

Data are expressed, as means ± SEM. The statistical analysis of the data was carried out by one-way ANOVA-followed by Tukey's test. In all comparisons, $P < 0.05$ was considered significant.

Results

Effect of Intrahippocampal Microinjection of Y_1 Antagonist on Seizure

Figure 1 shows the effects of GR231118 (Y_1 receptor antagonist) (10 µg/µl, i.h.), on the anticonvulsive activity of ghrelin in PTZ-induced seizure. Administration of GR231118, 20 min before the effective dose of ghrelin (0.3 nmol/µl), significantly ($P < 0.001$) prolonged duration of the seizures (Figure 1A) and increased total seizure score ($P < 0.001$) (Figure 1B.) in rats.

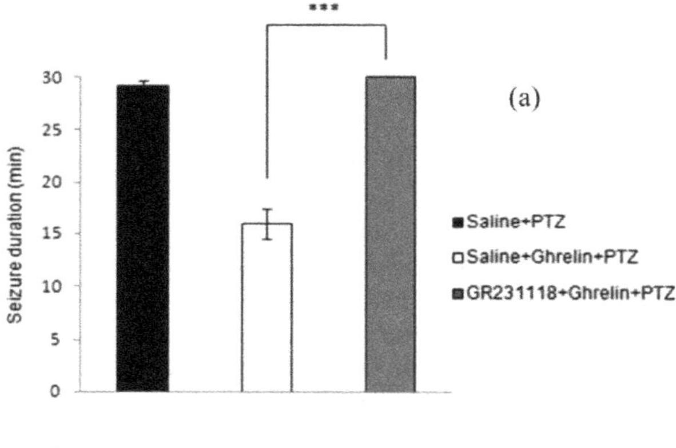

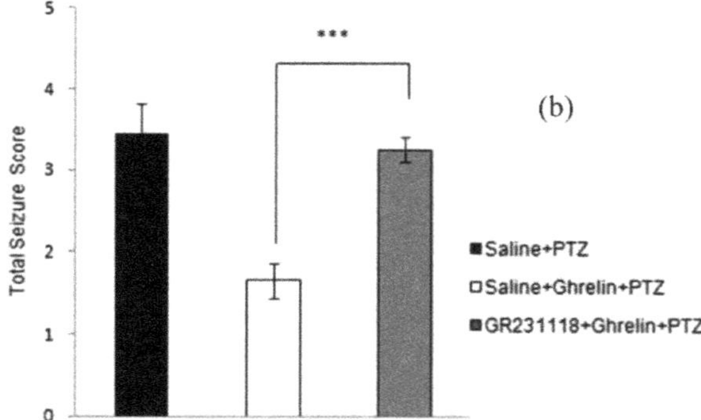

Figure 1. Effect of intrahippocampal injection of ghrelin preceded by GR231118 (Y1-receptor subtype antagonist) or saline on the duration of seizures (a) and total seizure score (b) during the 30-min post-PTZ behavior assessment. Data were analyzed by one-way ANOVA followed by Tukey's test. Results are expressed as mean ± SEM, n=10 animals per group; *** P < 0.001

Effect of Intrahippocampal Microinjection of Y_2 Antagonist on Seizure

As shown in Figure 2, pre-treatment with BIIE0246 (Y_2 receptor antagonist) in dorsal hippocampus, 20 min prior to ghrelin administration (0.3 nmol/µl i.h.) reversed the anticonvulsant effects of ghrelin. BIIE0246 (400 pmol/µl, i.h.) administration significantly prolonged duration of seizure ($p < 0.001$) (Figure 2A) and intensified total seizure score ($p < 0.001$) (Figure 2B).

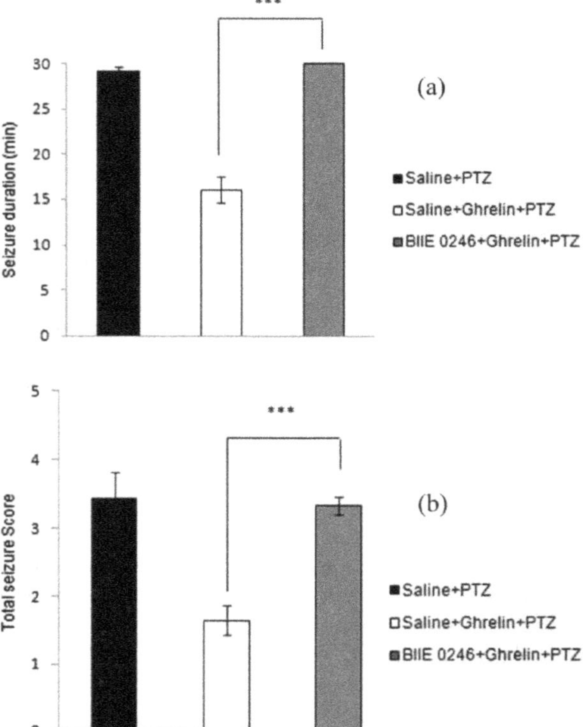

Figure 2. Effect of intrahippocampal injection of ghrelin preceded by BIIE 0246 (selective Y2-receptor subtype antagonist) or saline on the duration of seizures (a) and total seizure score (b) during the 30-min post-PTZ behavior assessment. Data were analyzed by one-way ANOVA followed by Tukey's test. Results are expressed as mean ± SEM, n=10 animals per group; *** P < 0.001

Effect of Intrahippocampal Microinjection of Y_5 Antagonist on Seizure

The effect of ghrelin in dorsal hippocampus of rats was reduced by GR231118 (Y_5 receptor antagonist) at a dose of 1 µg/µl. Data analysis showed that duration of seizure was increased significantly ($p < 0.001$) after GR231118 administration as shown in Figure 3A. In addition, injection of CGP71683 prior to ghrelin administration significantly intensified total seizure scores ($p < 0.001$) (Figure 3B.) in PTZ-induced seizure in rats.

None of the antagonists induced seizure when administered intrahippocampally alone (in the absence of PTZ) and there were no significant differences between saline or vehicle and ghrelin treated groups with ghrelin alone group in seizure duration and TSS.

Discussion

In the present study, in vivo PTZ model of epilepsy was used to determine one possible mechanism of action for anticonvulsant effect of ghrelin. We assessed the response to ghrelin and different antagonists of NPY receptors in area CA1 of hippocampus in rats. Our findings demonstrated that the NPY type 1, 2, 5 receptors are primarily involved in the anticonvulsive action of ghrelin. Our evidences have been obtained using GR231118 (potent Y_1 receptor antagonist), BIIE0246 (a specificY2 receptor antagonist) or CGP71683 (a potent and highly selective non-peptide antagonist).[27,28,33]

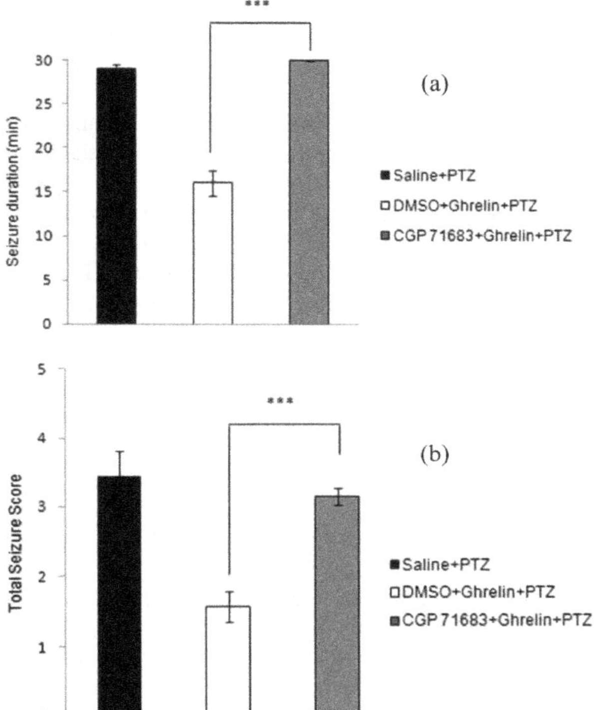

Figure 3. Effect of intrahippocampal injection of ghrelin preceded by CGP 71683 (Y5-receptor subtype antagonist) or DMSO on the duration of seizures (a) and total seizure score (b) during the 30-min post-PTZ behavior assessment. Data were analyzed by one-way ANOVA followed by Tukey's test. Results are expressed as mean ± SEM, n=10 animals per group; *** $P < 0.001$

Ghrelin is a 28 amino acid peptide with growth hormone-releasing and appetite-inducing activities.[1,2] Ghrelin is involved in many more processes than was initially postulated, and its endocrine, paracrine and autocrine effects play a role in its physiological and pathophysiological functions.[1] Recently, it has been shown that ghrelin has an antiepileptic effect and simultaneous treatment of animals with the ghrelin receptor antagonist significantly attenuates the neuroprotective effect of ghrelin against KA-induced excitotoxicity.[13,15,34,35]

Circulating ghrelin enter the hippocampus, where specially has been shown to be a critical region for temporal lobe epilepsy, and binds to the hippocampal neurons.[7,36] Ghrelin may exert modulator effects on neurotransmission.[21] It enhances NPY and GABA-ergic activity in the brain.[21] A number of studies show the possible involvement of NPY in the ghrelin-mediated effects.[20,21,37]

Neuropeptide Y is a 36 amino acid peptide which has been suggested to act as an endogenous anticonvulsant.[18,38,39] NPY is a powerful endogenous modulator of limbic seizure activity.[18] It has potent inhibitory effects on excitatory synaptic transmission from stratum radiatum to CA1 pyramidal cells and in both area CA1 and CA3 of hippocampus.[40,41] Mice lacking NPY had an enhanced susceptibility to PTZ-induced seizures suggesting that the peptide is an important modulator of excitability in the CNS.[42]

Six different NPY receptor subtypes have been reported (Y_1–Y_6). In the central nervous system, and specifically in hippocampus (an epileptogenic brain region), expression of Y_1, Y_2 and Y_5 are most prominent.[18] All three subtype receptors have been shown to influence epileptic activity.[43]

Our results showed that pretreatment with GR231118, BIIE 0246 or CGP 71683 reverse anticonvulsant effect of intrahippocampal ghrelin. All these three NPY receptor antagonists increased the duration and TSS of PTZ-induced generalized seizures that had been attenuated by intrahippocampal administration of ghrelin.

NPY could theoretically be acting to suppress generalized seizures via postsynaptic Y_1 or Y_5 receptors enhancing GABAergic inhibition within the nucleus reticularis thalami or cortex, or presynaptically via Y_2 receptors inhibiting GABA release from nRT axon terminals projecting onto VB neurons (and therefore reducing hyperpolarization-mediated T-channel de-inactivation).[44] Y_1, Y_2 and Y_5 receptors have all been shown to influence epileptic activity and their receptor agonists reduced seizure-like activity in hippocampal cultures.[43] Silva also suggested that selective Y_1, Y_2 or Y_5 receptor activation significantly inhibits glutamate (principal brain excitatory neurotransmitter) release in rat dentate gyrus of the epileptic hippocampus induced by kainite.[45]

The functional involvement of Y_1 receptors in seizures has been demonstrated by several researchers with either anticonvulsant or proconvulsant effects.[42,44,46] It has been reported that the Y_1 receptor subtype predominantly mediates the antiepileptic activity of NPY in the frontal cortex.[46] Conversely, Y1 receptors may mediate a facilitator role on seizure susceptibility and suggest that NPY Y_1 receptors have a permissive role in seizures.[18,42,47]

In accordance with these studies, our results suggest that Y_1 receptors mediate an attenuating action of ghrelin on seizures induced by PTZ.[44,46] Thus, we suggest that these receptors may play a role in ghrelin effects on PTZ-induced seizure. The controversial results about Y_1 receptors role may depend on several experimental difficulties such as the selection of the brain region, epilepsy model, the type and dosage of the used convulsant and the applied Y_1 receptor antagonists.

Y_2-like receptor is highly expressed in the hippocampal formation. Y_5 receptors are also expressed in high levels in the hippocampus.[48] Several studies showed that antiepileptic actions of NPY require activation of hippocampal Y_2 or Y_5 receptor subtypes.[17,39,43,49,50] There are strong evidences from in vitro and in vivo studies that the effect of NPY to suppress hippocampal seizures and absence seizures was mediated by the Y_2 receptors.[39,41,44] Some studies have also suggested that in rat CA1 neurons, Y_5 agonists reduce excitatory postsynaptic currents and the Y_5 antagonist CGP71683A as well the Y_2 antagonist BIIE0246 both block the inhibitory effect of NPY on glutamate release.[51,52] Taken together, these data suggest that both Y_2 and Y_5 receptors regulate hippocampal seizures.[53] Our results confirmed these findings and it seems that Y_2 and Y_5 receptors may play a critical role in modulating ghrelin induced hippocampal anticonvulsant effect.

In conclusion, intrahippocampal microinjection of ghrelin reduced the TSS and shortened the duration of epileptic activity in PTZ-induced seizures of rats and central administration of the $NPY_{1,\ 2,\ 5}$ receptor antagonists, prior to ghrelin antagonize the ghrelin anticonvulsant effects. Therefore, it is possible to speculate that ghrelin acts in the central nervous system to modulate seizures via NPY receptor dependent mechanisms. It will be beneficial to measure NPY levels after ghrelin administration to find out whether it acts through NPY release to control seizures in the hippocampus.

Acknowledgments
The Neuroscience Research Centre of Tabriz University of Medical Sciences and Neuroscience Research Centre of Shahid Beheshti University of Medical Sciences supported this study. The article is based on the MSc thesis of Mrs. Mina Ghahramanain Golzar entitled "Evaluation of the mechanism of antiepileptic effect of intrahippocampal injection of ghrelin through neuropeptide $Y_{1,2,5}$ receptors in pentylenetetrazole-induced seizure".

Conflict of Interest
The authors report no conflicts of interest in this work.

References

1. Leontiou CA, Franchi G, Korbonits M. Ghrelin in neuroendocrine organs and tumors. *Pituitary* 2007; 10(3):213-25.
2. Kojima M, Kangawa K. Ghrelin: structure and function. *Physiol Rev* 2005;85(2):495-522.
3. Ferrini F, Salio C, Lossi L, Merighi A. Ghrelin in central neurons. *Curr Neuropharmacol* 2009;7(1):37-49.
4. Korbonits M, Goldstone AP, Gueorguiev M, Grossman AB. Ghrelin a hormone with multiple functions. *Front Neuroendocrinol* 2004;25(1):27-68.
5. Hosoda H, Kojima M, Matsuo H, Kangawa K. Ghrelin and des-acyl ghrelin: two major forms of rat ghrelin peptide in gastrointestinal tissue. *Biochem Biophys Res Commun* 2000; 279(3):909-13.
6. Banks WA, Tschöp M, Robinson SM, Heiman ML. Extent and direction of ghrelin transport across the blood-brain barrier is determined by its unique primary structure. *J Pharmacol Exp Ther* 2002;302(2):822-7.
7. Diano S, Farr SA, Benoit SC, McNay EC, da Silva I, Horvath B, et al. Ghrelin controls hippocampal spine synapse density and memory performance. *Nat Neurosci* 2006;9(3):381-8.
8. Bennett PA, Thomas GB, Howard AD, Feighner SD, van der Ploeg LH, Smith RG, et al. Hypothalamic growth hormone secretagogue-receptor (ghs-r) expression is regulated by growth hormone in the rat. *Endocrinology* 1997;138(11):4552-7.
9. Van der Lely AJ, Tschop M, Heiman ML, Ghigo E. Biological, physiological, pathophysiological, and pharmacological aspects of ghrelin. *Endocr Rev* 2004; 25(3):426-57.
10. Carlini VP, Monzón ME, Varas MM, Cragnolini AB, Schioth HB, Scimonelli TN, et al. Ghrelin increases anxiety-like behavior and memory retention in rats. *Biochem Biophys Res Commun* 2002;299(5):739-43.
11. Nakazato M, Murakami N, Date Y, Kojima M, Matsuo H, Kangawa K, Matsukura S. A role for ghrelin in the central regulation of feeding. *Nature* 2001; 409(6817):194-8.
12. Ataie Z, Golzar MG, Babri Sh, Ebrahimi H, Mohaddes G. Does ghrelin level change after epileptic seizure in rats? *Seizure* 2011;20(4):347-9.
13. Obay BD, Tasdemir E, Tumer C, Bilgin HM, Sermet A. Antiepileptic effects of ghrelin on pentylenetetrazole-induced seizures in rats. *Peptides* 2007; 28(6):1214-9.
14. Ghahramanian Golzar M, Ataei Z, Babri Sh, Ebrahimi H, Mirzaie F, Mohaddes G. Effect of acute and chronic intrahippocampal microinjection of ghrelin on pentylenetetrazole-induced seizures in rats. *Pharmaceut Sci* 2011;17(1):11-8.
15. Aslan A, Yildirim M, Ayyildiz M, Guven A, Agar E. The role of nitric oxide in the inhibitory effect of ghrelin against penicillin-induced epileptiform activity in rat. *Neuropeptides* 2009;43(4):295-302.
16. Michalkiewicz M, Zhao G, Jia Z, Michalkiewicz T, Racadio MJ. Central neuropeptide Y signaling ameliorates N(omega)-nitro-L-arginine methyl ester hypertension in the rat through a Y1 receptor mechanism. *Hypertension* 2005;45(4):780-5.
17. Baraban SC. Antiepileptic actions of neuropeptide Y in the mouse hippocampus require Y5 receptors. *Epilepsia* 2002;43 Suppl 5:9-13.
18. Baraban SC. Neuropeptide Y and epilepsy: recent progress, prospects and controversies. *Neuropeptides* 2004;38(4):261–5.

19. Gualillo O, Lago F, Gomez-Reino J, Casanueva FF, Dieguez C. Ghrelin, a widespread hormone: insights into molecular and cellular regulation of its expression and mechanism of action. *FEBS Lett* 2003;552(2-3):105-9.
20. Chen HY, Trumbauer ME, Chen AS, Weingarth DT, Adams JR, Frazier EG, et al. Orexigenic action of peripheral ghrelin is mediated by neuropeptide Y and agouti-related protein. *Endocrinology* 2004; 145(6):2607-12.
21. Cowley MA, Smith RG, Diano S, Tschop M, Pronchuk N, Grove KL, et al. The distribution and mechanism of action of ghrelin in the cns demonstrates a novel hypothalamic circuit regulating energy homeostasis. *Neuron* 2003;37(4):649-61.
22. Horvath TL, Diano S, Sotonyi P, Heiman M, Tschop M. Minireview: Ghrelin and the regulation of energy balance--a hypothalamic perspective. *Endocrinology* 2001;142(10):4163-9.
23. Wren AM, Small CJ, Fribbens CV, Neary NM, Ward HL, Seal LJ, et al. The hypothalamic mechanisms of the hypophysiotropic action of ghrelin. *Neuroendocrinology* 2002;76(5):316-24.
24. Fujimiya M, Asakawa A, Ataka K, Chen CY, Kato I, Inui A. Ghrelin, des-acyl ghrelin, and obestatin: Regulatory roles on the gastrointestinal motility. *Int J Pept* 2010;2010.
25. Mohaddes G, Rasi S, Naghdi N. Evaluation of the effect of intrahippocampal injection of leptin on spatial memory. *Afr J Pharm Pharmacol* 2009;3:443-8.
26. Paxinos G, Watson C. The Rat Brain in Stereotaxic Coordinates. Sydney:Academic press;2004.
27. Ishihara A, Tanaka T, Kanatani A, Fukami T, Ihara M, Fukuroda T. A potent neuropeptide Y antagonist, 1229U91, suppressed spontaneous food intake in Zucker fatty rats. *Am J Physiol* 1998;274(5 Pt 2):R1500-4.
28. Smialowska M, Wieronska JM, Domin H, Zieba B. The effect of intrahippocampal injection of group II and III metobotropic glutamate receptor agonists on anxiety; the role of neuropeptide Y. *Neuropsychopharmacology* 2007;32(6):1242-50.
29. Westfall TC, Naes L, Gardner A, Yang CL. Neuropeptide Y induced attenuation of catecholamine synthesis in the rat mesenteric arterial bed. *J Cardiovasc Pharmacol* 2006;47(6):723-8.
30. Meurs A, Clinckers R, Ebinger G, Michotte Y, Smolders I. Seizure activity and changes in hippocampal extracellular glutamate, GABA, dopamine and serotonin. *Epilepsy Res* 2008;78(1):50-9.
31. Toscano CD, Ueda Y, Tomita YA, Vicini S, Bosetti F. Altered GABAergic neurotransmission is associated with increased kainate-induced seizure in prostaglandin-endoperoxide synthase-2 deficient mice. *Brain Res Bull* 2008; 75:598-609.
32. Lian XY, Zhang ZZ, Stringer JL. Anticonvulsant activity of ginseng on seizures induced by chemical convulsants. *Epilepsia* 2005;46(1):15-22.
33. Della Zuana O, Sadlo M, Germain M, Feletou M, Chamorro S, Tisserand F, et al. Reduced food intake in response to cgp 71683a may be due to mechanisms other than npy y5 receptor blockade. *Int J Obes Relat Metab Disord* 2001;25(1):84-94.
34. Portelli J, Aourz N, Ver Donck L, Moechars D, Schallier A, Michotte Y, et al. Anticonvulsant effects of ghrelin receptor ligands against pilocarpine-induced limbic seizures. 13th International Conference on In Vivo Methods; 12 - 16 September; Brussels, Belgium 2010.
35. Lee J, Lim E, Kim Y, Li E, Park S. Ghrelin attenuates kainic acid-induced neuronal cell death in the mouse hippocampus. *J Endocrinol* 2010; 205(3):263-70.
36. Acharya MM, Hattiangady B, Shetty AK. Progress in neuroprotective strategies for preventing epilepsy. *Prog Neurobiol* 2008;84(4):363-404.
37. Shintani M, Ogawa Y, Ebihara K, Aizawa-Abe M, Miyanaga F, Takaya K, et al. Ghrelin, an endogenous growth hormone secretagogue, is a novel orexigenic peptide that antagonizes leptin action through the activation of hypothalamic neuropeptide Y/Y1 receptor pathway. *Diabetes* 2001;50(2):227-32.
38. Colmers WF, El Bahh B. Neuropeptide Y and Epilepsy. *Epilepsy Curr* 2003;3(2):53-8.
39. El Bahh B, Cao JQ, Beck-Sickinger AG, Colmers WF. Blockade of neuropeptide Y(2) receptors and suppression of NPY's anti-epileptic actions in the rat hippocampal slice by BIIE0246. *Br J Pharmacol* 2002;136(4):502-9.
40. Colmers WF, Lukowiak K, Pittman QJ. Presynaptic action of neuropeptide Y in area CA1 of the rat hippocampal slice. *J Physiol* 1987;383:285-99.
41. El Bahh B, Balosso S, Hamilton T, Herzog H, Beck-Sickinger AG, Sperk G, et al. The anti-epileptic actions of neuropeptide Y in the hippocampus are mediated by Y and not Y receptors. Eur J Neurosci 2005;22(6):1417-30.
42. Gariboldi M, Conti M, Cavaleri D, Samanin R, Vezzani A. Anticonvulsant properties of BIBP3226, a non-peptide selective antagonist at neuropeptide Y Y1 receptors. *Eur J Neurosci* 1998;10(2):757-9.
43. Reibel S, Nadi S, Benmaamar R, Larmet Y, Carnahan J, Marescaux C, et al. Neuropeptide Y and epilepsy: Varying effects according to seizure type and receptor activation. *Peptides* 2001;22(3):529-39.
44. Morris MJ, Gannan E, Stroud LM, Beck-Sickinger AG, O'Brien TJ. Neuropeptide Y suppresses absence seizures in a genetic rat model primarily through effects on Y receptors. *Eur J Neurosci* 2007;25(4):1136-43.
45. Silva AP, Xapelli S, Pinheiro PS, Ferreira R, Lourenço J, Cristovao A, et al. Up-regulation of

neuropeptide Y levels and modulation of glutamate release through neuropeptide Y receptors in the hippocampus of kainate-induced epileptic rats. *J Neurochem* 2005;93(1):163-70.
46. Bijak M. Neuropeptide Y suppresses epileptiform activity in rat frontal cortex and hippocampus in vitro via different NPY receptor subtypes. *Neurosci Lett* 1999;268(3):115-8.
47. Benmaamar R, Pham-Le BT, Marescaux C, Pedrazzini T, Depaulis A. Induced down-regulation of neuropeptide Y-Y1 receptors delays initiation of kindling. *Eur J Neurosci* 2003;18(4):768-74.
48. Dumont Y, St-Pierre JA, Quirion R. Comparative autoradiographic distribution of neuropeptide Y Y1 receptors visualized with the Y1 receptor agonist [125I][Leu31,Pro34]PYY and the non-peptide antagonist [3H]BIBP3226. *Neuroreport* 1996;7(4):901-4.
49. Furtinger S, Pirker S, Czech T, Baumgartner C, Ransmayr G, Sperk G. Plasticity of Y1 and Y2 receptors and neuropeptide Y fibers in patients with temporal lobe epilepsy. *J Neurosci* 2001;21(15):5804-12.
50. Benmaamar R, Richichi C, Gobbi M, Daniels AJ, Beck-Sickinger AG, Vezzani A. Neuropeptide Y Y5 receptors inhibit kindling acquisition in rats. *Regul Pept* 2005;125(1-3):79-83.
51. Ho MW, Beck-Sickinger AG, Colmers WF. Neuropeptide Y (5) receptors reduce synaptic excitation in proximal subiculum, but not epileptiform activity in rat hippocampal slices. *J Neurophysiol* 2000; 83(2):723-34.
52. Rodi D, Mazzuferi M, Bregola G, Dumont Y, Fournier A, Quirion R, et al. Changes in NPY-mediated modulation of hippocampal [3H]D-aspartate outflow in the kindling model of epilepsy. *Synapse* 2003;49(2):116-24.
53. Woldbye DP, Nanobashvili A, Sorensen AT, Husum H, Bolwig TG, Sorensen G, et al. Differential suppression of seizures via Y2 and Y5 neuropeptide Y receptors. *Neurobiol Dis* 2005;20(3):760-72.

In Vivo Assessment of Antihyperglycemic and Antioxidant Activity from Oil of Seeds of *Brassica Nigra* in Streptozotocin Induced Diabetic Rats

Manoj Kumar[1], Sunil Sharma[2]*, Neeru Vasudeva[3]

[1] *Department of Pharmaceutical Sciences, Guru Jambheshwar University of Science and Technology, Post Box: 38, Hisar-125001, India.*

[2] *Pharmacology Divisions, Department of Pharmaceutical Sciences,Guru Jambheshwar University of Science and Technology, Post Box: 38, Hisar-125001, India.*

[3] *Pharmacognosy Divisions, Department of Pharmaceutical Sciences,Guru Jambheshwar University of Science and Technology, Post Box: 38, Hisar-125001, India.*

ARTICLEINFO

Keywords:
Brassica nigra
Seeds
Streptozotocin
Essential oil
MDA

ABSTRACT

Purpose: This study was made to investigate the antihyperglycemic and antioxidant potential of oil of seeds of *Brassica nigra* (BNO) in streptozotocin -nicotinamide (STZ) induced type 2 diabetic rats. ***Methods:*** BNO was orally administered to diabetic rats to study its effect in both acute and chronic antihyperglycemic study. The body weight, oral glucose tolerance test and biochemical parameters viz. glucose level, insulin level, liver glycogen content, glycosylated hemoglobin and antioxidant parameters were estimated for all treated groups and compared against diabetic control group. ***Results:*** Administration of BNO at a dose 500 mg/kg and 1000 mg/kg body weight p.o. to STZ diabetic rats showed reduction in blood glucose level from 335 mg/dl to 280 mg/dl at 4th h and from 330 mg/dl to 265 mg/dl respectively which was found significant ($p<0.01$) as compared with diabetic control. BNO (500 mg/kg and 1000 mg/kg) and glibenclamide (0.6 mg/kg) in respective groups of diabetic animals administered for 28 days reduced the blood glucose level in streptozotocin-nicotinamide induced diabetic rats. There was significant increase in body weight, liver glycogen content, plasma insulin level and decrease in glycosylated hemoglobin in test groups as compared to control group. *In vivo* antioxidant studies on STZ-nicotinamide induced diabetic rat's revealed decreased malondialdehyde (MDA) and increased reduced glutathione (GSH). ***Conclusion:*** Thus the results showed that the oil of seeds of *Brassica nigra* has significant antihyperglycemic and antioxidant activity.

Introduction

Now a day herbal remedies have become the popular source of medicines due to lesser adverse reactions and various other reasons. There are thousands of plants used from last years for the treatment of various diseases, species of the genus Brassica is one of them among the important medicinal plants used in various systems of medicine.[1] The genus Brassica contains over 150 species that are cultivated worldwide as oil seed crops or vegetables. *Brassica nigra* (black mustard) is a winter annual herb (family Brassicaceae). Like other mustards, black mustard grows profusely and produces allelopathic chemicals that prevent germination of native plants. Brassica nigra is an annual growing to 1.2 m (4ft) by 0.6 m (2ft in). It is hardy to zone 7 and is not frost tender. It is in flower from Jun to August, and the seeds ripen from July to September. The flowers are hermaphrodite (have both male and female organs) and are pollinated by Bees, flies. The plant is self-fertile.[2] The plant prefers light (sandy), medium (loamy) and heavy (clay) soils and requires well-drained soil. The plant prefers acid, neutral and basic (alkaline) soils and can grow in very acid soils. It can grow in semi-shade (light woodland) or no shade. It requires moist soil. The plant can tolerate maritime exposure.[3]

Diabetes is growing with a high speed in India and has become a capital of the world which is affecting the all age group of people.[4] There were an estimated 40 million persons with diabetes in India in 2007 and this number is predicted to rise to almost 70 million people by 2025 according to Diabetes Atlas published by the International Diabetes Federation (IDF). The country with the largest number of diabetic people will be India by 2030. Due to these sheer numbers, the economic burden due to diabetes in India is amongst the highest in the world.[5] Diabetes is of mainly three type's viz., Type I, type II, and Gestational. Type II diabetes is the most common type, accounting for 90–95% of all diabetic cases. So the main concern for management of

***Corresponding author:** Sunil Sharma, Pharmacology Divisions, Department of Pharmaceutical Sciences, Guru Jambheshwar University of Science and Technology, Post Box: 38, Hisar-125001, India. Email: sharmask71@rediffmail.com

this type of diabetes is very essential. Some studies have suggested that essential oils may be useful in the treatment of type II diabetes mellitus and various oils have been used as therapeutic agents for years without any significant adverse health effects.[6]

The oil has been widely used in the food industries from centuries. As long as we know, the effect of oil on the blood profiles in diabetic models has not been studied. In light of these findings, we carried out this study for the evaluation of antihyperglycemic, and antioxidant potential of oil of seeds of *Brassica nigra*.

Materials and Methods

Drugs and chemicals

The drugs and chemicals used in the study were glibenclamide (Torrent Pharmaceutical, Ahmadabad), streptozotocin, heparin (SRL, India), EDTA (Hi-media Lab. Pvt Ltd., Mumbai, India), Ellman's reagent (5,5'-dithiobis-(2-nitro-benzoic acid); DTNB), sodium sulphate, methanol, pyridine, anthrone, thiourea, benzoic acid, sodium chloride (SD Fine Chem Ltd., Mumbai, India). All the chemicals used in the study were of analytical grade.

Isolation of oil

The dried seeds of *Brassica nigra* were purchased from Oil and seed section of Chaudhary Charan Singh Haryana Agriculture University, Hisar, India. The seeds were crushed and oil was extracted with the help of Clevenger apparatus. The percentage yield of light yellow colored oil was found to be 30%.

Experimental animals

Healthy albino wistar rats (150-250 g) were procured from Disease Free Small Animal House, Lala Lajpat Rai University of Veterinary & Animal Sciences, Hisar (Haryana). The rats were housed in (Polycarbonate cage size: 29×22×14 cm) under laboratory standard conditions (25±3 °C:35-60% humidity) with alternating light and dark cycle of 12 h each and were feed fed with a standard rat pellet diet (Hindustan Lever Ltd, Mumbai, India) and water *ad libitum*. The experimental protocol was approved by Institutional Animals Ethics Committee (IAEC) and animal care was taken as per the guidelines of Committee for the Purpose of Control and Supervision of Experiments on Animals (CPCSEA), Govt. of India (Registration No. 0436).

Induction of Diabetes

Type II diabetes mellitus (NIDDM) was induced in overnight fasted animals by a single intraperitoneal injection of 50 mg/kg STZ in 0.1 M citrate buffer (pH-4.5) in a volume of 1 ml/kg body weight 15 minute after the i.p. administration of 110 mg/kg nicotinamide. Diabetes was developed and stabilized over a period of 7 days. Diabetes was confirmed by the elevated blood glucose levels determined at 72 h and on 7th day after injection. Only rats confirmed with permanent NIDDM (Glucose level above 250 mg/dl) were used in the study. Blood was collected by intraocular route.[7]

Acute toxicity studies

Healthy adult albino wistar rats, starved overnight were divided in to six groups (n=6) and were orally fed with the oil of *Brassica nigra* in the increasing dose of 100, 200, 500, 1000, 2000, 5000 mg/kg body weight. The rats were observed continuously for 4 h for behavioral changes and after 24 and 72 h for any lethality.

Oral Glucose Tolerance Test

In this test 2 g/kg of body weight of glucose was administered to the animals and then the blood samples were collected at the time interval of 30, 60, 90, 120 min and 24 h and glucose level was estimated.

Experimental design

Rats were divided into the following groups comprising six rats in each group after the induction and confirmation of diabetes.

a) Acute antihyperglycemic model

In the acute antihyperglycemic models the study was carried out for 4 hours to check whether the plant have some effect or not.

Group 1 Normal group
Group 2 Diabetic control group
Group 3 Test group administered glibenclamide (0.6 mg/kg p.o)
Group 4 Test group administered orally 500 mg/kg of BNO
Group 5 Test group administered orally 1000 mg/kg of BNO

b) Chronic antihyperglycemic model

In the chronic antihyperglycemic models the study was carried out for 28 days to study the various parameters of the diabetes to confirm the antihyperglycemic activity of BNO in streptozotocin induced diabetes in rats.

Group 1 Normal rats
Group 2 Diabetic control
Group 3 Diabetic animals were administered glibenclamide (0.6 mg/kg p.o)
Group 4 Diabetic animal were administered orally 500 mg/kg of BNO
Group 5 Diabetic animal were administered orally 1000 mg/kg of BNO

Sample collection

The 24h fasted animals were sacrificed by cervical decapitation on 28th day of treatment. Trunk blood was collected in heparinized tubes and the plasma was obtained by centrifugation at 5000 rpm for 5 min. for the determination of biochemical parameters; glucose, insulin, cholesterol etc.

Estimation of plasma glucose and cholesterol

Plasma cholesterol and glucose level were measured by commercial supplied biological kit Erba Glucose Kit (GOD-POD Method) and Erba Cholesterol Kit (CHOD-PAP Method) respectively using Chem 5 Plus-V_2 Auto-analyser (Erba Mannhein Germany) in plasma sample prepared as above. Glucose and cholesterol values were calculated as mg/dl blood sample.

Estimation of glycosylated hemoglobin (Hb1Ac)

Glycosylated hemoglobin was measured using commercial supplied biological kit (Erba Diagnostic) in plasma sample prepared as above using Chem 5 Plus-V_2 Auto-analyser (Erba Mannhein Germany). Values are expressed as the percent of total hemoglobin.

Estimation of liver glycogen content

Liver glycogen estimation was done by the method as described by Seifter *et al* (1950).[8] Immediately after excision from the animal, 1 g of the liver was dropped into a previously weighed test tube containing 3 ml of 30% potassium hydroxide solution. The weight of the liver sample was determined. The tissue was then digested by heating the tube for 20 min in boiling water bath, and following this the digest was cooled, transferred quantitatively to a 50 ml volumetric flask, and diluted to the mark with water. The contents of the flask were then thoroughly mixed and a measured portion was then further diluted with water in a second volumetric flask so as to yield a solution of glycogen of 3-30 μg/ml. Five ml aliquots of the final dilution were then pipette into Evelyn tube and the determination with anthrone was carried out. The amount of glycogen in the aliquot used was then calculated using the following equation:

μg of glycogen in aliquot = 100 U/ 1.11S

U is the optical density of unknown solution. S is the optical density of the 100 μg glucose and 1.11 is the factor determined by Morris in 1948 for the conversion of the glucose to the glycogen.

In vivo antioxidant activity

Estimation of MDA level

Malondialdehyde (MDA), an index of free radical generation/lipid peroxidation, was determined as described by Okhawa *et al* 1979.[9] Briefly, the reaction mixture consisted of 0.2 ml of 8.1% sodium lauryl sulphate, 1.5 ml of 20% acetic acid (pH 3.5) and 1.5 ml of 0.8% aqueous solution of thiobarbituric acid added to 0.2 ml of blood plasma. The mixture was made up to 4.0 ml with distilled water and heated at 95 °C for 60 min. After cooling the contents under running tap water, 5.0 ml of n-butanol and pyridine (15:1 v/v) and 1.0 ml of distilled water was added. The contents were centrifuged at about 3000 rpm for 10 min. The organic layer was separated out and its absorbance was measured at 532 nm using double beam UV-Visible spectrophotometer (Systronics 2203, Bangalore, India) against a blank. MDA values were calculated using the extinction coefficient of MDA-thiobarbituric acid complex 1.56×10^5 l/mol×cm and expressed as nmol/ml.

Estimation of reduced glutathione level

The tissue sample (liver 200 mg) was homogenized in 8.0 mL of 0.02M EDTA in an ice bath. The homogenates were kept in the ice bath until used. Aliquots of 5.0 mL of the homogenates were mixed in 15.0 mL test tubes with 4.0mL distilled water and 1.0mL of 50 % trichloroacetic acid (TCA). The tubes were centrifuged for 15 min at approximately 3000 rpm, 2.0 mL of supernatant was mixed with 4.0 ml of 0.4M Tris buffer pH 8.9, 0.1mL Ellman's reagent [5,5-dithiobis-(2-nitro-benzoic acid)] (DTNB) added and the sample shaken. The absorbance was read within 5 min of the addition of DTNB at 412 nm against a reagent blank with no homogenate. Results are expressed as μmol GSH/g tissue.

Statistical analysis

The data for various biochemical parameters were evaluated by use of one-way ANOVA, followed by Dunnett's t-test using the software Sigma-Stat 3. In all the tests, the criterion for statistical significance was $p<0.05$.

Results

Acute toxicity study

The oral administration of graded dose of BNO to the rats in our acute toxicity study was found to be non lethal up to the dose of 5000 mg/kg body weight.

Oral glucose tolerance test

The effect of BNO on plasma glucose level after glucose loading of 2 g/kg body weight orally to the STZ diabetic rats is expressed in the Table 1. The blood glucose level rises to a maximum in 60 min after glucose loading. The oil (500 mg/kg and 1000 mg/kg body weight) treated groups showed a significant decrease in level of glucose as compared to control group. The oil treated group showed a marked fall in glucose level in 90 min to 120 min interval (Table 1).

Table 1. Effect of *Brassica nigra* oil in oral glucose tolerance test (OGTT).

Treatment	Dose	Mean blood glucose concentration (mg/dl) ± S.E.M				
		0 min.	30 min.	60 min.	90 min.	120 min.
Normal	----	80±2.6	87 ±2.8	90 ± 3.8	86 ± 2.5	83 ± 2.7
Diabetic control	----	290 ± 4.6	390 ±5.3	413.2 ± 4.3	360 ± 2.7	331 ± 2.8
BNO	500 mg/kg	250 ± 3.0	287 ±3.7	329 ± 3.0	301 ± 4.6**	277 ± 3.9**
BNO	1000 mg/kg	272 ± 4.6	295 ± 4.5	356 ± 4.1	284 ± 3.4**	242 ± 3.3**

Values are presented as mean ± S.E.M.; n = 6 in each group. One way ANOVA followed by *Dunnett's* test **p < 0.01 vs. diabetic control; BNO: Oil of seed of *Brassica nigra*

Effect of BNO on STZ diabetic rats in acute study

Administration of BNO at a dose 500 mg/kg body weight p.o. to STZ diabetic rats showed reduction in blood glucose level from 335 mg/dl to 280 mg/dl at 4th h. When the dose was increased as 1000 mg/kg then the blood glucose level decreased from 330 mg/dl to 265 mg/dl which was found significant (p< 0.01) when compared with diabetic control (Table 2).

Table 2. Effect of *Brassica nigra* oil in STZ induced diabetic rats in acute antihyperglycemic study.

Treatment	Dose	Mean blood glucose concentration (mg/dl) ± S.E.M)				
		0 h	1/2 h	1h	2h	4h
Normal	--	76 ± 4.2	80 ± 3.2	77 ± 2.5	82 ± 4.1	79 ± 5.3
Control	--	340.5 ±10.2	342 ± 11.3	346 ± 7.6	341.0 ± 6.7	332.0 ± 7.2
BNO	500 mg/kg p.o	335 ±5.7	332.1± 5.4	310 ± 4.5**	303 ± 3.4**	280 ± 3.6**
BNO	1000 mg/kg p.o	330 ±1.8	315 ± 1.8*	297 ± 3.3**	275 ± 3.4**	265 ± 5.5**

Values are presented as mean ± S.E.M.; n=6 in each group. One way ANOVA followed by *Dunnett's* test *p<0.05; **p<0.01 vs. diabetic control; BNO: Oil of seed of *Brassica nigra*

Effect of BNO on STZ diabetic rats in chronic study

In chronic study administration of BNO at the dose of 500 mg/kg body weight to STZ diabetic rats for 28 days showed a fall in plasma glucose level from 335 mg/dl to 190 mg/dl on 28th day when compared to 0 day value. BNO at the dose of 1000 mg/kg body weight showed a significant (p<0.01) fall in plasma glucose level from 330 mg/dl to 160 mg/dl on 28th day (Table 3).

Table 3. Effect of *Brassica nigra* oil in STZ induced diabetic rats in chronic antihyperglycemic study.

Treatment	Dose	Mean blood glucose concentration (mg/dl) ± S.E.M				
		0th Day	7th Day	14th Day	21st Day	28th
Normal	--	80 ± 4.2	79 ± 3.2	82 ± 2.5	85.5 ± 4.1	78 ± 2.1
Control	--	380 ±7.3	379 ±7.6	384 ±6.7	416 ±7.2	410 ± 5.4
BNO	500 mg/kg p.o	335 ±10.4	298 ±9.5**	276 ±6.2**	240 ±6.9**	190 ± 7.2**
BNO	1000 mg/kg p.o	330 ±5.2	280 ± 6.9**	202 ± 5.8**	180 ±4.4**	160 ± 5.8**

Values are presented as mean ± S.E.M.; n = 6 in each group. One way ANOVA followed by *Dunnett's* test **p < 0.01 vs. diabetic control; BNO: Oil of seed of *Brassica nigra*

Effect of BNO on body weight

An increase in the body weight of normal rats was observed whereas the weight of diabetic control rats decrease from day 1 to day 28. BNO at the dose of 500 mg/kg and 1000mg/kg body weight respectively groups when administered to diabetic rats showed a significant change in body weight and it was increase as compared to the diabetic control group. (p<0.01) (Table 4).

Table 4. Effect of *Brassica nigra* oil on body weight in diabetic rats.

Sr. No.	Treatment	Dose	Initial Body Weight (g)	Final Body Weight (g)	Change in weight
1.	Normal	--	220 ± 1.1	240 ± 1.5	+20
2.	Diabetic Control	--	215 ± 1.8	194 ± 2.0	-21[a]
3.	BNO	500 mg/kg p.o	225 ± 2.2	226 ± 1.0	+1
4.	BNO	1000 mg/kg p.o	230 ± 1.3	240 ± 1.4	+10**

Values are presented as mean ± S.E.M.; n = 6 in each group. One way ANOVA followed by *Dunnett's* test [a] p<0.01 vs. normal; **p<0.01 vs. diabetic control; BNO: Oil of seed of *Brassica nigra*

Effect of BNO on insulin level

Table 5 shows the level of plasma insulin in the control and experimental groups of rats. Diabetic rats showed a significant decrease in plasma insulin compared with normal rats. Following dose of oral administration of BNO, plasma insulin level increased when compared to control rats (Table 5).

Effect of BNO on glycosylated hemoglobin (HbA1c)

The effect of BNO on HbA1c in STZ diabetic rats is shown in the Table 5. The level of glycosylated hemoglobin significantly increased (p<0.01) in diabetic rats as compared to normal control group. The diabetic rats when treated with BNO for 28 days showed a significant ($p<0.01$) decreased level of glycosylated Hb as compared to untreated diabetic group. The fall in glycosylated hemoglobin level was found to be dose dependent (Table 5).

Table 5. Effect of *Brassica nigra* oil on glycosylated hemoglobin (HbA1c), hepatic glycogen and insulin in the study.

Treatment	Dose	HbA1c (% of Hb)	Hepatic glycogen (mg/g wt of tissue)	Insulin (micro U/ml)
Normal	--	6 ± 1.4	74 ± 6.6	14 ± 2.1
Diabetic Control	--	11.3 ± 2.4[a]	27 ± 4.5[a]	7.9 ± 1.1[a]
BNO	500 mg/kg	9.5 ± 2.1	45 ± 2.6*	9.8 ± 2.0
BNO	1000 mg/kg	7.8 ± 2.5**	62 ± 4.6**	11.7 ± 2.5*

Values are presented as mean ± S.E.M; n = 6 in each group. One way ANOVA followed by Dunnett's test [a]$p<0.01$ vs. normal; *$p<0.05$; **$p<0.01$ vs. diabetic control; BNO: Oil of seed of *Brassica nigra*

Effect of BNO on hepatic glycogen

The hepatic glycogen content in diabetic rats decreased sharply as compared to control animal (Table 5). After chronic administration of BNO to diabetic rats, a significant increased ($p<0.01$) liver glycogen content as compared to diabetic control group was observed.

Effect of BNO on Lipid profile

Table 6 shows the level of lipids in normal and tested animals. There was a significant decrease in the level of HDL-cholesterol and a significant increase in the levels of total cholesterol and triglycerides in diabetic rats when compared to normal rats. The administration of BNO reverse the level of lipids significantly ($p<0.05$ and $p<0.01$).

Table 6. Effect of *Brassica nigra* oil on Lipid profile.

Treatment	Dose	Cholesterol (mg/dl)	Triglyceride (mg/dl)	HDL (mg/dl)
Normal	--	85 ± 1.5	16 ± 2.5	66 ± 1.9
Diabetic Control	--	232 ± 2.4[a]	43 ± 3.1[a]	37.4 ± 1.2[a]
BNO	500 mg/kg	171 ± 3.6**	30 ± 1.6**	44 ± 2.1
BNO	1000 mg/kg	109 ± 2.5**	20 ± 1.3**	49 ± 1.3*

Values are presented as mean ± S.E.M; n = 6 in each group. One way ANOVA followed by Dunnett's test [a] $p<0.01$ vs. normal; *$p<0.05$; **$p<0.01$ vs. diabetic control; BNO: Oil of seed of *Brassica nigra*

Effect of BNO on in vivo antioxidant parameters

The data depicted in Table 7 show the effect of oil on plasma malondialdehyde and reduced glutathione level. Plasma MDA level was found to be significantly higher in STZ diabetic rats compared to normal rats. The oil at dose 1000 mg/kg body weight p.o significantly reduced the level of MDA in diabetic rats. Plasma GSH level was found to be significantly lowered in STZ diabetic rats as compared to normal rats. The chronic administration of BNO at 1000 mg/kg body weight significantly increased the level of glutathione in diabetic rats.

Table 7. Effect of *Brassica nigra* oil on antioxidant parameters (MDA and GSH).

Treatment	Dose	MDA (nmol/dl)	GSH (μmol/g)
Normal	--	2.8 ± 0.2	41.2 ± 2.8
Diabetic Control	--	5.4 ± 0.4[a]	14 ± 1.15[a]
BNO	500 mg/kg	3.7 ± 0.7	20.6 ± 2.6
BNO	1000 mg/kg	3.2 ± 0.2**	32 ± 2.2**

Values are presented as mean ± S.E.M; n = 6 in each group. One way ANOVA followed by Dunnett's test [a]$p<0.01$ vs. normal; **$p<0.01$ vs. diabetic control; BNO: Oil of seed of *Brassica nigra*

Discussion

The aim of the study was to evaluate the antidiabetic and antioxidant potential of the BNO in STZ induced diabetic rats. Diabetes mellitus causes a disturbance in the uptake of glucose as well as glucose metabolism. A dose of STZ as low as 50 mg/kg produces an incomplete destruction of pancreatic beta cells even though the rats become permanently diabetic.[10] After treatment with a low dose of STZ many beta cells survive and regeneration is also possible.[11] Hyperglycemia generates abnormally high levels of free radicals by autoxidation of glucose and protein glycation, and oxidative stress has been reported to be a positive factor of cardiovascular complications in STZ-induced diabetes mellitus.[12] Hyperglycemia is associated with the generation of reactive oxygen species (ROS) causing oxidative damage particularly to heart, kidney, eyes, nerves, liver, small and large vessels and gastrointestinal system.[13] The increased levels of plasma glucose in STZ-induced diabetic rats were lowered by BNO administration. The plasma glucose lowering activity was compared with glibenclamide, a standard hypoglycemic drug that stimulates insulin secretion from pancreatic beta cells.[14] From the results of the present study, it appears that still insulin producing cells are functioning and the stimulation of insulin release could be responsible for most of the metabolic effects. It may be suggested that the mechanism of action of BNO is similar to glibenclamide. The glucose lowering activity of BNO may be related to both pancreatic (enhancement of insulin secretion) and extra pancreatic (peripheral utilization of glucose) mechanism.

An increase in the level of glycosylated hemoglobin (HbA1c) in the diabetic control group of rats is due to the presence of large amount of blood glucose which reacts with hemoglobin to form glycosylated hemoglobin.[15] Oxidative stress increases due to the activation of transcription factors, advanced glycated end products (AGEs), and protein kinase C. If diabetes is persistent for long time, the glycosylated hemoglobin is found to increase.[16] The level of HbA_1C was decreased after the administration of BNO 1000 mg/kg as compared to diabetic control group.

In STZ induced diabetes mellitus, the loss of body weight is caused by increase in muscle wasting and catabolism of fat and proteins.[17] Due to insulin deficiency protein content is decreased in muscular tissue by proteolysis.[18] A decrease in body weight was registered in case of STZ diabetic control group rats while in tested groups the weight loss was reversed. Fatty acid mobilisation from adipose tissue is sensitive to insulin. Insulin's most potent action is the suppression of adipose tissue lipolysis.[19]A rise in plasma insulin concentration of only 5 IU/mL inhibits lipolysis by 50%, whereas a reduction in basal insulin levels result in a marked acceleration of lipolysis.[20] We demonstrated that BNO increased plasma insulin concentrations in diabetic rats. Insulin levels higher than those of the control group may result in inhibition of lipolysis and decreased plasma triglyceride and cholesterol levels. Some studies suggest that the antihyperglycemic action of traditional antidiabetic plant extracts may be due in part to decreased glucose absorption in vivo.[21] This mechanistic explanation may also apply to the actions of BNO in lowering the triglyceride and cholesterol level.

The conversion of glucose to glycogen in the liver cells is dependent on the extracellular glucose concentration and on the availability of insulin which stimulates glycogen synthesis over a wide range of glucose concentration.[16] Diabetes reduces activity of glycogen synthase thereby affecting the glycogen storage and synthesis in rat liver and skeletal muscle.[22] Oral administration of BNO 1000 mg/kg body weight significantly increased hepatic glycogen levels in STZ diabetic rats possibly because of the reactivation of the glycogen synthase system as a result of increased insulin secretion

In conclusion, the present study showed that oral administration of BNO has potential antidiabetic and antioxidant effect in STZ induced diabetic rats. The potent antioxidant activity may be responsible for the antihyperglycemic effects. This investigation reveals the potential of BNO for use as a natural oral agent with antihyperglycemic and antioxidant effects.

Acknowledgements

The authors are highly grateful to the University grant commission, Delhi (India) for providing research fellowship during research work. The authors have no conflict of interest.

Conflict of Interest

The authors report no conflicts of interest.

References

1. Velisek J, Mikulcova R, Mikova K, Woldie KS, Link J, Davídek J. Chemometric investigation of mustard seed. *Lebenson Wiss Technol* 1995;28(6):620-4.
2. Felter HW, Lloyd JU. King's Dispensatory. USA: Eclectic Medical Publications; 1983.
3. Leung AY. Encyclopedia of Common Natural Ingredients Used in Food, Drugs, and Cosmetics. NewYork: John Wiley & Sons; 1980.
4. Mohan V, Sandeep S, Deepa R, Shah B, Varghese C. Epidemiology of type 2 diabetes: Indian scenario. *Indian J Med Res* 2007;125(3):217-30.
5. Sicree R, Shaw J, Zimmet P. Diabetes and impaired glucose tolerance. In: Gan D, editor. Diabetes Atlas. International Diabetes Federation. 3rd ed. Belgium: International Diabetes Federation; 2006.
6. Pandey A, Tripathi P, Pandey R, Srivatava R, Goswami S. Alternative therapies useful in the management of diabetes: A systematic review. *J Pharm Bioallied Sci* 2011;3(4):504-12.
7. Marudamuthu AS, Leelavinothan P. Effect of pterostilbene on lipids and lipid profiles in Streptozotocin – Nicotinamide induced type 2 diabetes mellitus. *J Appl Biomed* 2008;6:31-7.
8. Seifter S, Dayton S, et al. The estimation of glycogen with the anthrone reagent. *Arch Biochem* 1950;25(1):191-200.
9. Ohkawa H, Ohishi N, Yagi K. Assay for lipid peroxides in animal tissues by thiobarbituric acid reaction. *Anal Biochem* 1979;95(2):351-8.
10. Aybar MJ, Sanchez Riera AN, Grau A, Sanchez SS. Hypoglycemic effect of the water extract of Smallantus sonchifolius (yacon) leaves in normal and diabetic rats. *J Ethnopharmacol* 2001;74(2):125-32.
11. Gomes A, Vedasiromoni JR, Das M, Sharma RM, Ganguly DK. Anti-hyperglycaemic effect of black tea (Camellia sinensis) in rat. *J Ethnopharmacol* 2001;27:243-75.
12. Okutan H, Ozcelik N, Yilmaz HR, Uz E. Effects of caffeic acid phenethyl ester on lipid peroxidation and antioxidant enzymes in diabetic rat heart. *Clin Biochem* 2005;38(2):191-6.
13. Tunali S, Yanardag R. Effect of vanadyl sulfate on the status of lipid parameters and on stomach and

spleen tissues of streptozotocin-induced diabetic rats. *Pharmacol Res* 2006;53(3):271-7.

14. Tian YA, Johnson G, Ashcroft SJ. Sulfonylureas enhance exocytosis from pancreatic beta-cells by a mechanism that does not involve direct activation of protein kinase C. *Diabetes* 1998;47(11):1722-6.
15. Chattopadhyay RR. Possible mechanism of antihyperglycemic effect of Azadirachta indica leaf extract: part V. *J Ethnopharmacol* 1999;67(3):373-6.
16. Sheela CG, Augusti KT. Antidiabetic effects of S-allyl cysteine sulphoxide isolated from garlic Allium sativum Linn. *Indian J Exp Biol* 1992;30(6):523-6.
17. Chakravarti BK, Gupta S, Gambir SS, Gode KD. Pancreatic Beta-cell regeneration in rats by (-)-epicatechin. *The Lancet* 1981;318(8249):759-60.
18. Swanston-Flatt SK, Day C, Bailey CJ, Flatt PR. Traditional plant treatments for diabetes. Studies in normal and streptozotocin diabetic mice. *Diabetologia* 1990;33(8):462-4.
19. Campbell PJ, Carlson MG, Hill JO, Nurjhan N. Regulation of free fatty acid metabolism by insulin in humans: role of lipolysis and reesterification. *Am J Physiol* 1992;263(6 Pt 1):E1063-9.
20. Bonadonna RC, Groop LC, Zych K, Shank M, Defronzo RA. Dose-dependent effect of insulin on plasma free fatty acid turnover and oxidation in humans. *Am J Physiol* 1990;259(5 Pt 1):E736-50.
21. Gallagher AM, Flatt PR, Duffy G, Abdel-Wahab YHA. The effects of traditional antidiabetic plants on in vitro glucose diffusion. *Nutr Res* 2003;23(3):413-24.
22. Kamboj J, Sharma S, Kumar S. In vivo Anti-diabetic and Anti-oxidant potential of *Psoralea corylifolia* seeds in Streptozotocin induced type- 2 diabetic rats. *J Health Sci* 2011;57(3):225-35.

Hypoglycemic Activity of *Fumaria parviflora* in Streptozotocin-Induced Diabetic Rats

Fatemeh Fathiazad[1]*, Sanaz Hamedeyazdan[2], Mohamad Karim Khosropanah[3], Arash Khaki[4]

[1] *Department of Pharmacognosy, Faculty of Pharmacy, Tabriz University of Medical Sciences, Iran.*

[2] *Student's Research Committee, Faculty of pharmacy, Tabriz University of Medical Sciences, Iran.*

[3] *Department of Biology, Faculty of Science, Islamic Azad University of Sanandaj, Sanandaj, Iran.*

[4] *Department of Veterinary Pathology, Tabriz Branch, Islamic Azad University, Tabriz, Iran.*

ARTICLEINFO

Keywords:
Fumaria parviflora
Fumariaceae
Hypoglycemic
Streptozotocin
Anti diabetic

ABSTRACT

Purpose: *Fumaria parviflora* Lam (Fumariaceae) has been used in traditional medicine in the treatment of several diseases such as diabetes. The present work was designed to evaluate the hypoglycaemic effects of methanolic extract (ME) of *F. parviflora* in normal and streptozotocin-induced diabetic rats. ***Methods:*** The rats used were allocated in six (I, II, III, IV, V and VI) experimental groups (n=5). Group I rats served as 'normal control' animals received distilled water and group II rats served as 'diabetic control' animals. Diabetes mellitus was induced in groups II, V and VI rats by intraperitoneal single injection of streptozotocin (STZ, 55 mg kg-1). Group V and VI rats were additionally treated with ME (150 mg kg-1 day-1 and 250 mg kg-1 day-1, i.p. respectively) 24 hour post STZ injection, for seven consecutive days. Groups III and IV rats received only ME 150 mg kg-1 day-1 and 250 mg kg-1 day-1, i.p. respectively for seven days. The levels of blood glucose were determined using a Glucometer. ***Results:*** Administration of *F. parviflora* extract showed a potent glucose lowering effect only on streptozotocin (STZ) induced diabetic rats below 100 mg/dl ($P<0.001$). However, no significant differences in the blood glucose levels were recorded between diabetic rats received 125 or 250 mg/kg of plant extracts. ***Conclusion:*** The findings of the study indicated that *F. parviflora* has significant hypoglycemic effect on STZ-induced diabetic rats with no effects on blood glucose levels of normal rats.

Introduction

Diabetes mellitusa metabolic disorder characterized by an inappropriate hyperglycemia caused by a relative or absolute deficiency of insulin or by a resistance to the action of insulin at the cellular level is found in all parts of the world.[1] If diabetes is not being controlled effectively, the patient would have advanced risks of developing complications, like hypoglycemia, ketoacidosis, and nonketotic hyper-osmolar coma. The longer term complications might be cardiovascular disease, nerve damage, chronic kidney failure, retinal damage, and scanty healing of wounds, followed by gangrene on the feet leading to amputation.[2-5] It has been well recognized that these complications bring about significant morbidity and mortality statistics worldwide, which is affecting negatively the quality of life in patients with diabetes.

From the patient's perspective, the major objective is to design a regimen that will improve the progression of the disease complications. It has been considered very acceptable to include herbal or botanical extracts as a part of medical treatment. Although, herbs for diabetes treatment are not new and the plants and plant extracts since ancient times were used to combat diabetes, administration of herbal remedies in the case of diabetes diseases should certainly not be discounted.[1,6-9] Accordingly, the present study was conducted to analyze one of the herbs, *Fumaria parviflora,* being employed traditionally by native people in the treatment of diabetes with an inadequate knowledge base.

Fumaria parviflora Lam. (Fumariaceae) an annual herbaceous plant that grows in wide variety parts of Iran, Pakistan and Turkey that has been reported to be used traditionally in dermatological diseases, in stimulation of liver function and gall bladder and also as antiscabies, antiscorbite, antibronchite, diuretic, expectorant, antipyretic, diaphoretic, appetizer and laxative.[10] Studies dealing with the bioactivity and potential health benefits of *F. parviflora* in different aspects have been previously reported. The antinoiciceptive and histopathological effects of the percolated and soxhlet methanol extract of *F. parviflora* in formalin test was determined, especially at the late

***Corresponding author:** Fatemeh Fathiazad, Department of Pharmacognosy, Faculty of Pharmacy, Tabriz University of Medical Sciences, Iran. E-mail: fathiazad@tbzmed.ac.ir

phase and hot-plate test in mice and rats.[11] Various species of *Fumaria* have been studied by Orhan et al. which showed anticholinesterase activity for extracts of the aerial parts of *F. parviflora.*[12] Moreover, phytochemical analyses of some plants of genus *Fumaria*, including *F. parviflora* has indicated presence of isoquinoline alkaloids.[13-17] Elsewhere, the antipyretic activity of the hexane, chloroform and water-soluble extracts of *F. parviflora*in rabbits was verified.[18] Akhtar et al. in 1984 published a paper in which they examined the blood glucose levels of the normal and alloxan-diabetic male albino rabbits after oral administration of various doses of the powdered *F. parviflora* and concluded that the plant contained some hypoglycaemic properties.[19] However, firm recommendations for general use of any herbal remedies needs detailed documentations of the glucose or insulin lowering effects of the plants in diabetes. Herein, we have evaluated the effect of the methanol extract of *F. parviflora*on blood glucose level in normal and streptozotocin STZ-induced diabetic rats.

Materials and Methods

Plant Material

The aerial parts of *Fumaria parviflora* Lam were collected during June–July from Aharin East Azerbayjan province in Iran. A voucher specimen of the plant representing this collection has been retained in the herbarium of the Faculty of Pharmacy, Tabriz University of Medical Science, Tabriz, Iran.

Preparation of Plant Extract

Aerial parts of plants (200 g) were air dried, powdered and extracted with maceration in chloroform and methanol (4×1L) consecutively and then evaporated *in vacuo* to afford chloroform and methanol extracts (ME). Since, in our preliminary study chloroform extract showed no effect on blood glucose level in normal and diabetic rats, the assessment of hypoglycemic activity of the plant set out on ME. Without any further purification, the crude methanol extract was refrigerated and subsequently used in this study. Aliquot portions of the crude ME residue was weighed and dissolved in distilled water for use on each day of our experiments.

Animals

Thirty male Wistar albino rats weighing 200-220 g were obtained from animal facility of pasture institute of Iran and were used in this survey. The animals were housed in stainless steel cages under controlled environmental conditions (temperature 25±5 °C, with a light/dark cycle of 12 hours). The cage contained 5 rats and each rat had a tag number. Rats were allowed free access to concentrated animal food and water every day. Housing and caring conditions for the animals and the study protocols for the animal experiments were carried out in accordance with the internationally accepted principles and the national laws concerning the care and the use of laboratory animals.

Induction of Experimental Diabetes

Diabetes type 2 was induced with a single intraperitoneal injection of a freshly prepared solution of streptozotocin (STZ) (55mg/kg), dissolved in cold citrate buffer (0.1M, pH 4.5), immediately before use due to the instability of STZ in aqueous media.

Measurement of Blood Glucose Levels

The blood was drawn from the tail and basal blood glucose levels were determined using an automated blood glucose analyzer (Glucometer One touch, Germany) prior to STZ injection and every 24h after STZ injection in groups II, V and VI and 1h after ME i.p. injection. Rats with blood glucose concentrations above 250 mg/dl were declared diabetic.

Experimental Designand Animal Grouping

The experimental animals were allowed 2-week acclimatization to laboratory environment and they were subsequently divided into 6 groups comprising of 5 animals in each group as follows: Group I, was considered as normal rats (distilled water-treated, Control), group II, diabetic control (STZ-treated), group III, extract-treated (normal + 125 mg/kg body weight/day of ME) rats, group IV extract-treated (normal + 250 mg/kg/day of ME) rats, group V, diabetic + 125 mg/kg/day of ME rats and group VI, diabetic + 250 mg/kg/day of ME rats. In groups V and VI administration of ME commenced 24h after injection of STZ and continued for the next 7 days.

Statistical Analysis

All the data are expressed as Mean ± S.E.M (standard error of means) and a probability level of $P < 0.05$ was taken to be statistically significant in the analyses.

Results

Blood glucose levels in different groups of control and experimental pre and after intra-peritoneal administration of STZ and plant extract were represented in Figure 1. In the control diabetic rats, blood glucose was reached maximum to its peak of about 346.88 mg/dl and remained high up to 192h during the experiment. Whereas, control group of normal rats, group I, did show no changes in mean±SEM blood glucose levels. Additionally, administration of ME in groups III and IV showed no effect on blood glucose levels when compared with normal rats. The findings of the study verified in diabetic treated rats with different concentrations of plant methanol extract (125 mg/kg and 250 mg/kg) levels of blood glucose were markedly controlled below 100 mg/dl at the end of the experiments. However, no significant differences in the blood glucose levels were recorded between diabetic rats received 125 or 250 mg/kg/day of plant extract and they both decreased the blood glucose levels, evidently.

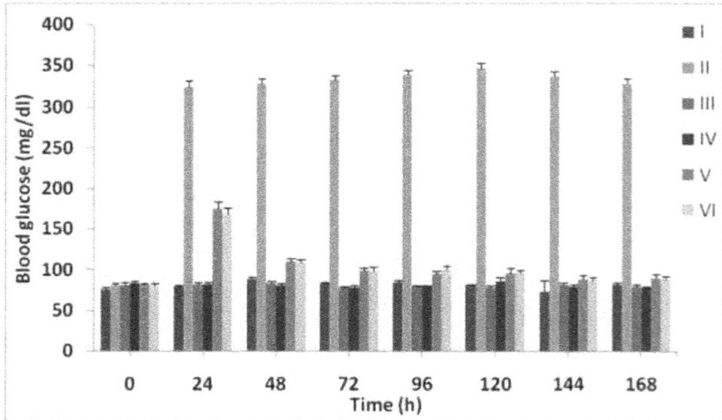

Figure 1. Effect of Methanol extract of *F. parviflora* on blood glucose levels in normal and diabetic rats. Data were given as mean ± SEM for five animals in each group.

* Groups [**I:** Normal controls, **II:** Diabetic controls, **III:** Normal + 125 mg/kg/day of extract, **IV:** Normal + 250 mg/kg/day of extract, **V:** Diabetic + 125 mg/kg/day of extract, **VI:** Diabetic + 250 mg/kg/day of extract].

Discussion

The use of medicinal plants in treatment of diseases have been an important part of medicinal therapy as observed for thousands of years contributing to scientific search of safer phytotherapeutic products, in this regard. Ever-increasing diabetes mellitus draw scores of researchers' attention to this phenomenon as a serious threat to mankind health in all parts of the world. In spite of the traditional use of botanicals in treatment of diabetes, paucity of definitive data on efficacy of these herbal remedies still deals a challenge in this field. In view of the fact that the diabetogenic effect of STZ is the direct consequence of irreversible damage to the pancreatic beta cells, resulting in degradation and loss of insulin secretion, STZ induced hyperglycemia has been recognized as a convenient experimental model to evaluate the activity of hypoglycemic agents.[20,21] Intra-peritoneal administration of STZ (55 mg/kg) effectively induced diabetes in normal rats as reflected by hyperglycaemia when compared with normal rats.[22-24] In our present study we have assessed the hypoglycemic activity of *F. parviflora* on normal and STZ induced diabetic rats.

The results revealed that *F. parviflora*had no effect on the blood glucose level in normal rats (group III and IV). Therefore, it is possible to propose that in addition to insulin-like activity of the ME other mechanism such as alteration in the insulin-resistance pathway may be involved by ME. Hence, this pathway has no role in the normal animals, the extract was not able to change the blood glucose level in groups III and IV. Additionally, it can be suggested that insulin–resistance pathway in the peripheral tissues, possibly is superior to its insulin-like activity. However, this theory should be confirmed with further in vivo and in vitro studies.

Considering the results, administration of the plant extract exhibited a superb blood glucose lowering activity in diabetic rats providing an evidence for the merit of the traditional use of *F. parviflora* among the nations. In all probability, *F. parviflora* do appear to be helpful in diabetic patients as claimed and do have potential anti-diabetic effects in a rat model system of diabetes mellitus since the results are as striking in this study.

Conclusion

The present investigation is an evidence for the anti-diabetic activity of *F. parviflora* in STZ induced diabetic rats. The authors believe that *F. parviflora* could be considered as an excellent candidate for further studies on verifying the mechanisms of hypoglycemic activity, as well as for the isolation and identification of the foremost hypoglycemic phyto-chemical responsible for anti-diabetic activity of the plant. Besides, further comprehensive pharmacological surveys, involving experimental chronic studies, will be of value to assess the possible toxicological effects of this anti-diabetic plant.

Acknowledgments

Financial support of this study by the Research Vice-Chancellor of Tabriz University of Medical Sciences is faithfully appreciated.

Conflict of Interest

The authors report no conflicts of interest in this work.

References

1. Samad A, Shams MS, Ullah Z, Wais M, Nazish I, Sultana Y, et al. Status of herbal medicines in the treatment of diabetes: A review. *Curr Diabetes Rev* 2009;5(2):102-11.
2. Santiago JV. Overview of the complications of diabetes. *Clin Chem* 1986;32(10 Suppl):B48-53.
3. Lundman B, Engstrom L. Diabetes and it's complications in a swedish county. *Diabetes Res Clin Pract* 1998;39(2):157-64.
4. Detournay B, Simon D, Guillausseau PJ, Joly D, Verges B, Attali C, et al. Chronic kidney disease in type 2 diabetes patients in france: Prevalence, influence of glycaemic control and implications for the pharmacological management of diabetes. *Diabetes Metab* 2012;38(2):102-12.
5. Losito A, Pittavini L, Ferri C, De Angelis L. Reduced kidney function and outcome in acute ischaemic stroke: Relationship to arterial hypertension and diabetes. *Nephrol Dial Transplant* 2012;27(3):1054-8.
6. Ceylan-Isik AF, Fliethman RM, Wold LE, Ren J. Herbal and traditional chinese medicine for the treatment of cardiovascular complications in diabetes mellitus. *Curr Diabetes Rev* 2008;4(4):320-8.
7. Wang E, Wylie-Rosett J. Review of selected chinese herbal medicines in the treatment of type 2 diabetes. *Diabetes Educ* 2008;34(4):645-54.
8. Suksomboon N, Poolsup N, Boonkaew S, Suthisisang CC. Meta-analysis of the effect of herbal supplement on glycemic control in type 2 diabetes. *J Ethnopharmacol* 2011;137(3):1328-33.

9. Liu JP, Zhang M, Wang WY, Grimsgaard S. Chinese herbal medicines for type 2 diabetes mellitus. *Cochrane Database Syst Rev* 2004;3:CD003642.
10. Gilani AH, Bashir S, Janbaz KH, Khan A. Pharmacological basis for the use of fumaria indica in constipation and diarrhea. *J Ethnopharmacol* 2005;96(3):585-9.
11. Heidari M, Mandgary A, Enayati M. Antinociceptive effects and toxicity of fumaria parviflora lam. In mice and rats. *Daru* 2004;12(4):136-40.
12. Orhan I, Sener B, Choudhary MI, Khalid A. Acetylcholinesterase and butyrylcholinesterase inhibitory activity of some turkish medicinal plants. *J Ethnopharmacol* 2004;91(1):57-60.
13. Suau R, Cabezudo B, Rico R, Najera F, Lopez-Romero JM. Direct determination of alkaloid contents in fumaria species by gc-ms. *Phytochem Anal* 2002;13(6):363-7.
14. Popova ME, Simanek V, Dolejs L, Smysl B, Preininger V. Alkaloids from fumaria parviflora and f. Kralikii. *Planta Med* 1982;45(2):120-2.
15. Valka I, Walterova D, Popova ME, Preininger V, Simanek V. Separation and quantification of some alkaloids from fumaria parviflora by capillary isotachophoresis1. *Planta Med* 1985;51(4):319-22.
16. Kirjakov H, Panov P. On the alkaloids of fumaria parviflora lam. *Folia Med (Plovdiv)* 1974;16(2):101-3.
17. Valka I, Simanek V. Determination of alkaloids of fumaria parviflora and fumaria capreolata by high-performance liquid chromatography and capillary isotachophoresis. *J Chromatogr* 1988;445(1):258-63.
18. Khattak SG, Gilani SN, Ikram M. Antipyretic studies on some indigenous pakistani medicinal plants. *J Ethnopharmacol* 1985;14(1):45-51.
19. Akhtar MS, Khan QM, Khaliq T. Effects of euphorbia prostrata and fumaria parviflora in normoglycaemic and alloxan-treated hyperglycaemic rabbits. *Planta Med* 1984;50(2):138-42.
20. Szkudelski T. The mechanism of alloxan and streptozotocin action in b cells of the rat pancreas. *Physiol Res* 2001;50(6):537-46.
21. Soon YY, Tan BK. Evaluation of the hypoglycemic and anti-oxidant activities of morinda officinalis in streptozotocin-induced diabetic rats. *Singapore Med J* 2002;43(2):077-85.
22. Perez Gutierrez RM. Evaluation of hypoglycemic activity of the leaves of malva parviflora in streptozotocin-induced diabetic rats. *Food Funct* 2012;3(4):420-7.
23. Venkatesan T, Sorimuthu Pillai S. Antidiabetic activity of gossypin, a pentahydroxyflavone glucoside, in streptozotocin-induced experimental diabetes in rats. *J Diabetes* 2012;4(1):41-6.
24. Jana K, Chatterjee K, Ali KM, De D, Bera TK, Ghosh D. Antihyperglycemic and antioxidative effects of the hydro-methanolic extract of the seeds of caesalpinia bonduc on streptozotocin-induced diabetes in male albino rats. *Pharmacognosy Res* 2012;4(1):57-62.

11

Indomethacin Electrospun Nanofibers for Colonic Drug Delivery: Preparation and Characterization

Abbas Akhgari*, Zohreh Heshmati, Behzad Sharif Makhmalzadeh

Nanotechnology Research Center and School of Pharmacy, Ahvaz Jundishapur University of Medical Sciences, Ahvaz, Iran.

ARTICLE INFO

Keywords:
Electrospun
Nanofiber
Indomethacin
Eudragit

ABSTRACT

Purpose: The objective of this study was to prepare a suitable form of nanofiber for indomethacin using polymers Eudragit RS100 (ERS) and Eudragit S100 (ES) and to evaluate the effect of some variables on the characteristics of resulted electrospunnanofibers. ***Methods:*** Electrospinning process was used for preparation of nanofibers. Different solutions of combinations of ERS, ES and indomethacin in various solvents and different ratios were prepared. The spinning solutions were loaded in 10 mL syringes. The feeding rate was fixed by a syringe pump at 2.0 mL/h and a high voltage supply at range 10-18 kV was applied for electrospinning. Electrospunnanofibers were collected and evaluated by scanning electron microscopy, differential scanning calorimetry and FTIR for possible interaction between materials used in nanofibers. The effect of solvent and viscosity on the characteristics of nanofibers also was investigated. ***Results:*** Fiber formation was successful using a solvent ethanol and mixture of ERS and ES. Increase in viscosity of ethanolic solutions of ERS followed by addition of ES in the solution led to preparation of smooth fibers with larger diameters and less amounts of beads. DSC analysis of fibers certified that indomethacin is evenly distributed in the nanofibers in an amorphous state. FTIR analysis did not indicate significant interaction between drug and polymer. ***Conclusion:*** It was shown that drug-loaded ERS and ES nanofibers could be prepared by exact selection of range of variables such as type of solvent, drug: polymer ratio and solution viscosity and the optimized formulations could be useful for colonic drug delivery.

Introduction

In recent years, drug delivery to colon has gathered a lot of attentions both from pharmaceutical industry and academia. Colonic drug delivery is significantly important not just for the delivery of protein and peptide drugs but also for treatment of diseases associated with colon such as colon cancer, ulcerative Colitis and diarrhea. Colon is believed to be suitable adsorption site especially for poorly absorbed drugs mostly because of its long retention.[1]

Different colon targeted drug delivery systems have been tried where pH, time, pressure dependent and microbially triggered systems are the primary approaches for colon drug delivery.[2,3] Recent researches are mainly based on the combination of two or even more colon-target drug delivery methods. This methodology decreases the effect of physiological changes of gastrointestinal tract and thus facilitates the prediction of drug releasing process in different conditions.

Apart from large diversity in colonic drug delivery systems, nanofibers containing drugs have been less considered in colon-target delivery systems. Various approaches can be used for preparation of nanofibers. Electrospinning is one of the most reliable techniques for nanofiber formation. In this method an electrical charge is applied to draw very fine fiber in nanoscale from a liquid. These electrospun fibers have a high surface to volume ratio which makes them promising candidate in adsorption of less-soluble drugs.[4-6] Electrospinning is mostly applied in tissue engineering,[7] implement materials, wound dressing, prosthesis[8] and drug delivery.[9]

Different parameters significantly affect the process namely: molecular weight, solution characteristics (viscosity, surface tension and conductivity), electric potential, concentration, distance between the capillary and collector screen, temperature, humidity and air velocity in the chamber.[10]

A lot of researches have revealed that indomethacin can be effective in colon cancer treatment. However, indomethacin as a non-steroidal anti-inflammatory drug (NSAIDS) has a lot of adverse effects on gastrointestinal tract. Therefore this drug was chosen in colon-targeted drug delivery process. On the other hand, indomethacin is a less soluble drug which makes that a promising candidate for electrospunnanofibers.

***Corresponding author:** Abbas Akhgari, Nanotechnology Research Center and School of Pharmacy, Ahvaz Jundishapur University of Medical Sciences, Ahvaz, Iran. E-mail: akhgari_a@yahoo.com

The objective of this study was to evaluate the effect of two factors (ratio of Eudragit S100: Eudragit RS100 and ratio of drug: polymer) on morphological characteristics of indomethacin nanofibers and optimize formulation variables such as viscosity of electropinning solutions and type of solvents in order to obtain the best colonic drug delivery system for indomethacin.

Materials and Methods

Materials

Indomethacin (Darupakhsh Pharmaceutical manufacturing *company, Tehran, Iran),* Eudragit S100 (ES) and Eudragit RS100 (ERS) (Rohm Pharma, GmbH, Germany), sodium chloride and potassium di-hydrogen phosphate (Merck, Germany) were obtained from the indicated sources.

Preparation of Electrospinning Solutions

25% (w/v) solution of Eudragit RS and 15% (w/v) dispersion of drug were prepared in water. Then electrospining solution with proportion of 1:1(v/v) for drug and polymer was made. The same work was carried out by ethanol as the solvent. On the other hand, 25% (w/v) solutions of polymethacrylates (ERS and ES) and 15% (w/v) solution of drug were prepared in ethanol as a good solvent. The ratios of ES: ERS were 30:70, 50:50 and 70:30. Then electrospining solution with ratio of 1:1(v/v) for drug and polymers was made. Further formulations with The ratios of 20:80, 80:20 and 100:0 for ES: ERS and the electrospining solution with ratios of drug: polymer at range 1:1,1.5:1, 2:1, and 2.5:1(v/v) were also prepared. Finally, regarding the characteristics and reproducibility of preliminary formulations the least and most levels were considered to design a series of runs according to a 3^2 full factorial design. The ratio of drug to polymer and ES: ERS was considered as the independent variables. Table 1 summarizes the independent variables. The resulted formulations of factorial design are listed in Table 2.

Table 1. Experimental design: factors and responses

Independent variables	-1	0	+1
X_1: Ratio of Eudragit S100: RS100	20:80	60:40	100:0
X_2: Drug:polymer ratio	1:1	1.5:1	2:1

Electrospinning Process

The spinning solutions were loaded in 10 mL syringes. The feeding rate was controlled by a syringe pump (Cole-Pham®, USA) and was fixed at 2.0 mL/h. A high voltage supply fixed at 10-18 kV was applied, and a piece of aluminum foil was used to collect the ultrafine fibers with a horizontal distance of 15 cm from the needle tip. Electrospunnanofibers were collected and stored in desiccator for more studies.

Table 2. Composition of experimental formulations (runs)

Formulation	X_1	X_2
F1	-1	-1
F2	-1	0
F3	-1	+1
F4	0	-1
F5	0	0
F6	0	+1
F7	+1	-1
F8	+1	0
F9	+1	+1

Scanning Electron Microscopy

The surface morphologies of electrospun fibers were assessed using a LEO - rp-1455 scanning electron microscope (SEM). Prior to the examination, the samples were silver sputter-coated under argon to render them electrically conductive. The pictures were then taken at an excitation voltage of 15 kV.

Differential Scanning Calorimetry

DSC analyses were carried out using a Mettler-Ms603s differential scanning calorimeter. Sealed samples were heated at 30 °C/min from 20 to 280 °C.

Fourier Transformed Infrared Spectroscopy

FTIR was conducted using a Nicolet-Nexus 670 FTIR spectrometer. The samples were prepared using the KBr disk method (2 mg sample in 200 mg KBr) and the scanning range was 500–4000 cm^{-1} with a resolution of 2 cm^{-1}.

Results and Discussion

Preparations of Drug-Loaded Nanofibers

Suitable selection of solvent is one of the most important factors for successful preparation of electrospun polymer nanofibers.[11-13] The solvent should be able to dissolve the drug easily as well as maintaining electrospinnability of polymer solutions. Eudragit RS100 could be electrospun into fibers when methanol or ethanol was used as the solvent.[14] In our study, ERS aqueous solutions were unspinnable. Only discrete droplets were observed when they were subjected to the electrospinning process.

Nanofibers from ERS in ethanol showed discrete beads and/or beaded fibers when the viscosity of the solution was low. The formation of half-hollowed beads was thought to be a result of the evaporation of the solvent from the beads. Further increase in solution viscosity by addition of ES resulted in the formation of smooth fibers with larger diameters (Figure 1).

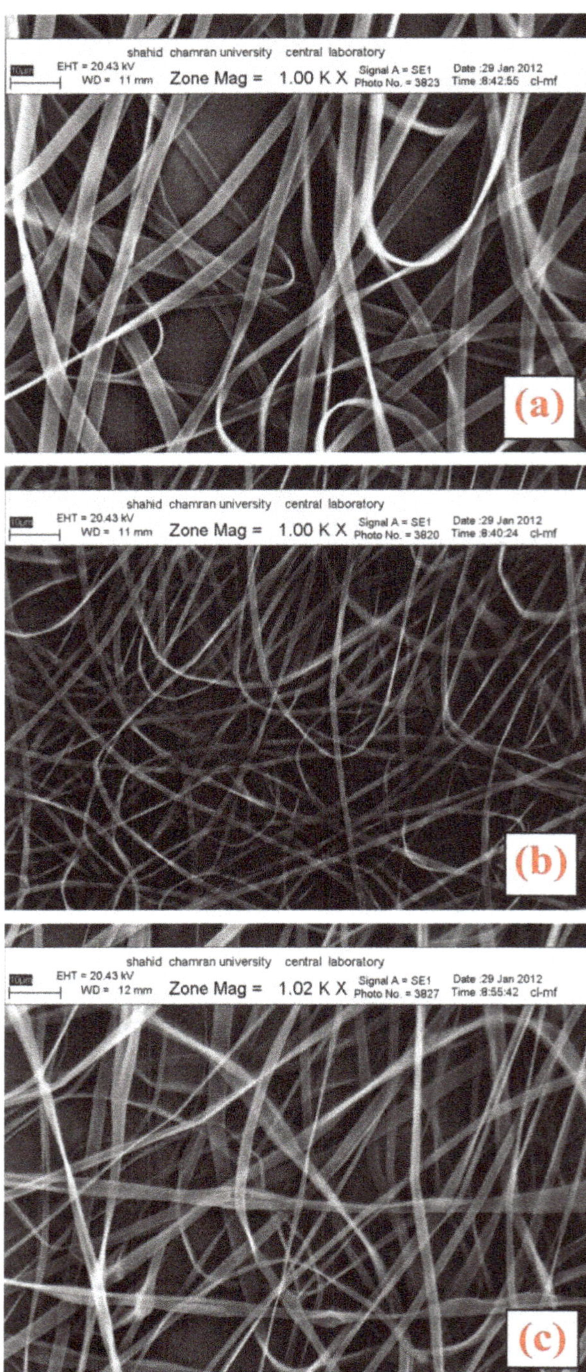

Figure 1. SEM images of formulations with ES: ERS in the ratios of ; (a) 30:70, (b) 50:50 and (c) 70:30 (magnification ×1000).

SEM images of drug loaded nanofibers with different amounts of indomethacin and various ratios of ES: ERS asserted that nanofiber formation is just possible with ratios of drug: polymer in ranges 1:1, 1.5:1 and 2:1 and ratio of 2.5:1 did not form suitable nanofiber in all ratios of polymers. Also, nanofiber formation in formulations with drug: polymer ratios of 2:1 and 1.5:1 was only occurred when the ratio of ES: ERS was in range 20:80 and 100:0. This result could be to the decrease in viscosity of electrospinning solutions affected by increase in amount of drug which in consequence disrupted nanofiber formation process. SEM images of drug loaded nanonfibers are presented in Figure 2. Solution viscosity plays an important role in determining the fiber size and morphology during spinning of polymeric fibers. When the solution viscosity decreases surface tension has the overcoming influence on fiber morphology with the final results of decrease in fiber diameters and bead formation. Correlation between the polymer viscosity and/or concentration and fibers formed from electrospinning has been surveyed in a number of studies.[15-19] Chowdhury et al. investigated the effect of experimental parameters such as polymer concentration, viscosity and surface tension on the morphology of electrospun Nylon 6 fibers. They found that increase in the concentration and viscosity and lowering surface tension manages to formation of the uniform nanofibers.[20]

Finally, according to preformulation studies ratios of 1:1, 1.5:1 and 2:1 for drug: polymer and 20:80, 60:40 and 100:0 for ES: ERS were selected to design 9 formulations based on full factorial design. Figure 3 shows SEM images of formulations containing ES: ERS at the ratio 60:40 ES: ERS and drug: polymer at ranges 1:1, 1.5:1 and 2:1.Comparing SEM Figures 2 and 3 it can be seen that addition of ES could lead to the formation of smooth fibers with larger diameters and low beads which could be illustrated by increase in viscosity of electrospinning solutions.

Physical State of Components in the Nanofibers

DSC thermograms of drug and Eudragits are shown in Figure 4. The DSC curve of pure indomethacin indicated a single endothermic response corresponding to a melting point of 179 °C (Figure 4a). The composed of pure ERS exhibited a single endothermic response in 115 °C, suggesting that Eudragit RS is in amorphous state (Figure 4b). On the other hand, ES showed a single endothermic response in 142 °C (Figure 4c). Figure 5 illustrates thermograms of formulations resulted from factorial design. According to Figure 5, all formulations exhibited a broadband wide endotherm ranging from 190 to 240 ◦C which could be due to polymer melting. In addition, melting point peak of indomethacin was removed in all formulation and it may be caused by the presence of Eudragits that resulted in a loss of crystalline content of indomethacin. The presence of an endothermic peak at 60°C in some formulations (F1, F3, F4 and F5) could be due to lowering of T_g of Eudragits by addition of drug to the formulation composition. This phenomenon was more obvious in formulations containing Eudragit RS. Plasticizing effect of NSAIDs and increase in macromolecular mobilities of polymeric chains due to presence of these drugs has been previously demonstrated.[21,22] DSC studies demonstrated that distribution of drug molecules in the nanonfiber structure was occurred with change in state of drug from crystallinity to amorph status.

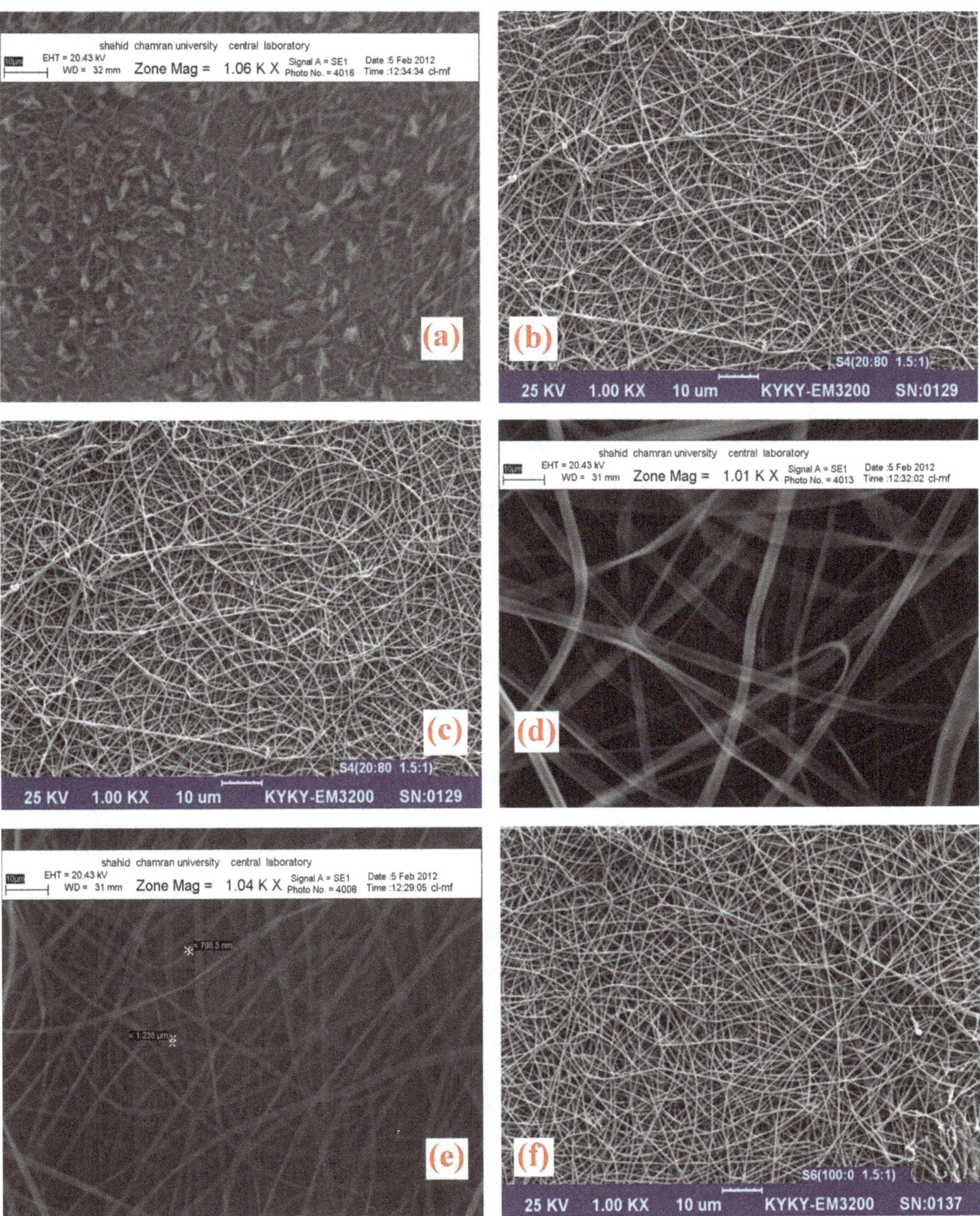

Figure 2. SEM images of formulations; range of ES:ERS and drug:polymer was (a) 20:80 and 1:1, (b) 20:80 and 1.5:1, (c) 20:80 and 2:1, (d) 80:20 and 1:1, (e) 100:0 and 1:1, (f) 100:0 and 1.5:1.

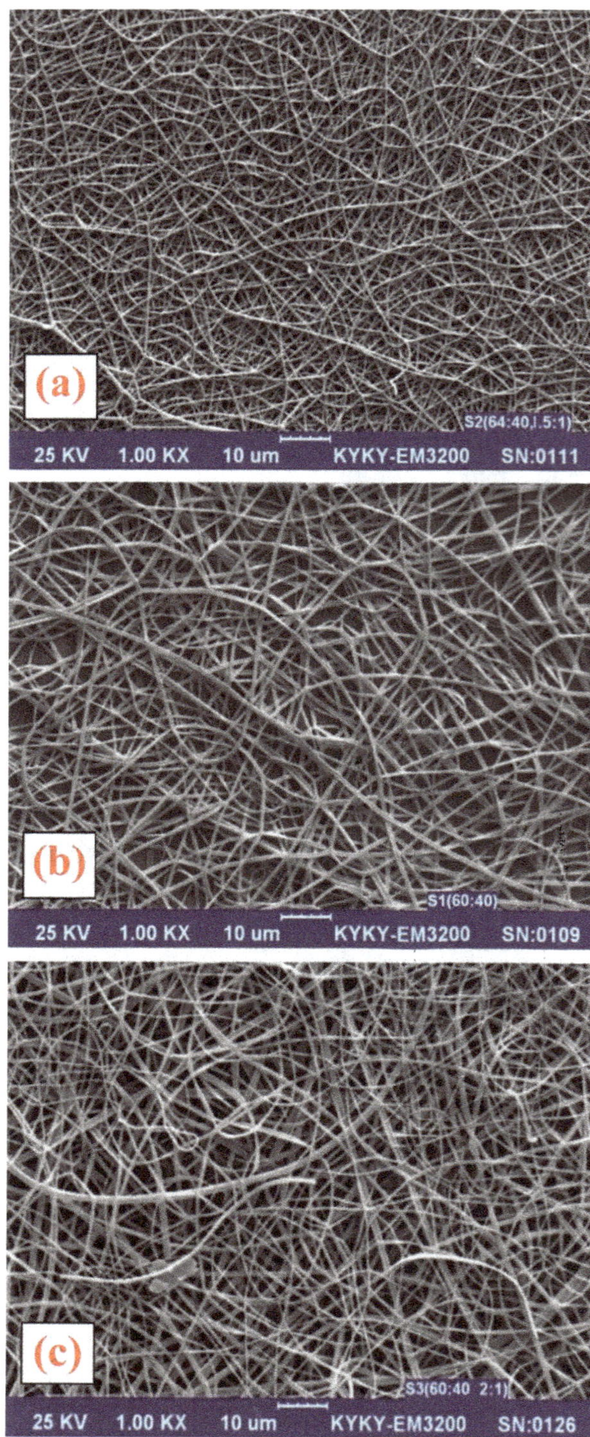

Figure 3. SEM images of formulations with ES:ERS in the ratio of 60:40 and different ratios of drug: polymer; (a) 1:1 ratio, (b) 1.5:1 ratio, and (c) 2:1 ratio.

Compatibility of Nanofiber Components

FTIR spectra of drug, polymers and formulation F1 was shown in Figure 6. Accordingly, the spectrum of indomethacin showed bands characteristic of secondary carbonyl groups (C=O) at 1714 cm^{-1}, (C=O amid) in 1690 cm^{-1}, phenyl groups (C=C stretch vibration) at 1523 cm^{-1} and (O-H stretch vibration) at 3022 cm^{-1}. The spectrum of ERS had a broad band characteristic of groups carbonyl (C=O) at 1723 cm^{-1}, and ester linkages (C-O stretch vibration) at 1149 cm^{-1}. The spectrum of ES showed a broad band characteristic of carbonyl groups (C=O) at 1727 cm^{-1}, characteristic bands of hydroxyl groups (C-H stretch vibration) at 2957 cm^{-1}. Two other spectra at 1152 and 3087 cm^{-1} were also indicative of C-O and O-H stretch vibration, respectively. FTIR of formulation F1 exhibited the same spectra which in result there would be no significant shift in spectra and interactions between drug and polymer was not seen. Interaction between ionizable drugs and eudragits was investigated in some researches. For example Heun et al. foundinteractions between drugs and Eudragits RL/RS resins in aqueous environment.[23] Also in the other study ionic interaction between propranolol hydrochloride and three different anionic polymers Eudragit S 100, Eudragit L 100-55 and sodium carboxymethylcellulose was demonstrated.[24] However, in our study there was no any significant ionic or hydrogenic interaction between drug and polymers.

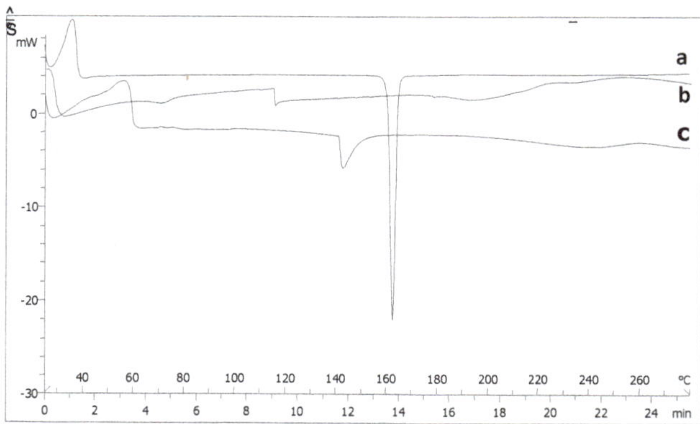

Figure 4. DSC thermograms of (a) drug, (b) Eudragit RS100 and (c) Eudragit S100.

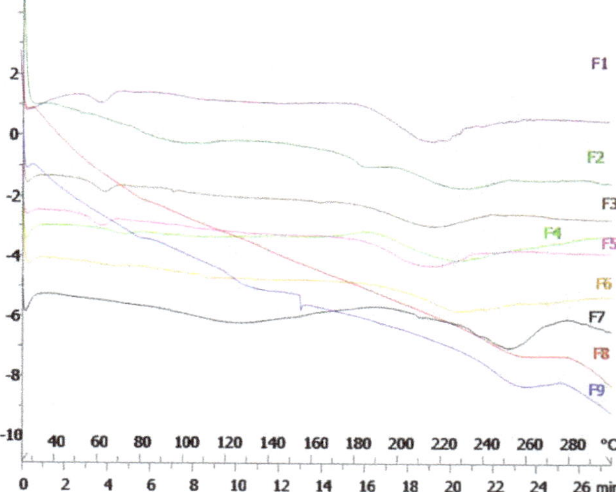

Figure 5. DSC thermograms of formulations resulted from factorial design

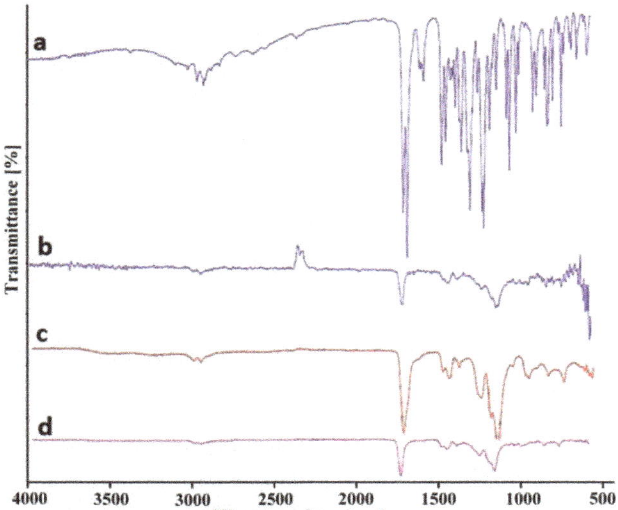

Figure 6. FTIR spectra of (a) indomethacin, (b) Eudragit RS, (c) Eudragit S, and (d) formulation F_1

Conclusion

Combination of Eudragit RS and Eudragit S for prepration of nanofibers containing indomethacin using electrospinning method was successfully tried. Accurate selection of solvent, viscosity, and ratios of ERS: ES and drug: polymer was important for successful preparation of electrospunnanofibers. In the entire composite nanofibers drug was present in an amorphous state. The optimized formulations were capable of drug loading up to 66% and could be useful for further studies on possible colonic delivery of indomethacin.

Acknowledgments

This work is the Pharm. D thesis of Mrs Z. Heshmati which is supported by a grant from research chancellor of Ahvaz Jundishapur University of Medical Sciences. The authors would like to thank Darupakhsh pharmaceutical co. for their collaboration and providing samples used in this paper.

Conflict of Interest

There is no conflict of interest in this study.

References

1. Watts PJ, Illum L. Colonic drug delivery. *Drug Dev Ind Pharm* 1997;23:893-913.
2. Goskonda SR, Upadrashta SM. Avicel RC-591/Chitosan beads by extrusion-spheronization technology. *Drug Dev Ind Pharm* 1994;19:915-27.
3. Rodriguez M, Vila-Jato JL, Torres D. Design of a new multiparticulate system for potential site-specific and controlled drug delivery to the colonic region. *J Control Release* 1998;55:67-77.
4. Ahn YC, Park SK, Kim GT, Hwang YJ, Lee CG, Shin HS, et al. Development of high efficiency nanofilters made of nanofibers. *Curr Appl Phys* 2006;6:1030-5.
5. Lannutti J, Reneker D, Ma T, Tomasko D, Farson D. Electrospinning for tissue engineering scaffolds. *Mater Sci Eng* C 2007;27(3):504-9.
6. Hunley MT, Long TE. Electrospinning functional nanoscale fibers: a perspective for the future. *Polym Int* 2008;57:385-9.
7. Chong EJ, Phan TT, Lim IJ, Zhang YZ, Bay BH, Ramakrishna S, et al. Evaluation of electrospun PCL/gelatin nano fibrous scaffold for wound healing and layered dermal reconstitution. *Acta Biomater* 2007;3:321-30.
8. Thomas S. Wound Management and Dressings. London: Pharmaceutical Press;1990.
9. Kenawy el R, Bowlin GL, Mansfield K, Layman J, Simpson DG, Sanders EH, et al. Release of tetracycline hydrochloride from electrospun poly(ethylene-co-vinylacetate), poly(lactic acid), and a blend. *J Control Release* 2002;81(1-2):57-64.
10. Chen Z, Mo X, Qing F. Electrospinning of collagen-chitosan complex. *Mater Lett* 2007;61:3490-4.
11. Moghe AK, Gupta BS. Co-axial electrospinning for nanofiber structures: preparation and applications. *Polym Rev* 2008; 48:353-77.
12. Qi H, Sui X, Yuan J, Wei Y, Zhang L. Electrospinning of cellulose-based fibers from NaOH/urea aqueous system. *Macromol Mater Eng* 2010;295:695-700.
13. Liu Y, Ma G, Fang D, Xu J, Zhang H, Nie J. Effects of solution properties and electric field on the electrospinning of hyaluronic acid. *Carbohyd Polym* 2011;83(2):1011-5.
14. Shen X, Yu D, Zhu L. Electrospundiclofenac sodium loaded Eudragit® L 100-55 nanofibers for colon-targeted drug delivery. *Int J Pharm* 2011;408:200-7.
15. Kim KH, Jeong L, Park HN, Shin SY, Park WH, Lee SC, et al. Biological efficacy of silk fibroin nanofiber membranes for guided bone regeneration. *J Biotechnol* 2005;120: 327-39.
16. Huang L, Nagapudi K, Apkarian RP, Chaikof EL. Engineered collagen-PEO nanofibers and fabrics. *J Biomat Sci Polym E* 2001;12:979-93.
17. Son WK, Youk JH, Lee TS, Park WH. The effects of solution properties and polyelectrolyte on electrospinning of ultrafine poly (ethylene oxide) fibers. *Polymer* 2004;45:2959-66.
18. Ding B, Kim HY, Lee SC, Shao CL, Lee DR, Park SJ, et al. Preparation and characterization of a nanoscale poly (vinyl alcohol) fiber aggregate produced by an electrospinning method. *J Polym Sci Part B: Polym Phys* 2002;40:1261-8.
19. Koski A, Yim K, Shivkumar S. Effect of molecular weight on fibrous PVA produced by electrospinning. *Mater Lett* 2004;58:493-7.
20. Chowdhury M, Stylios G. The effect of experimental parameters on the morphology of electrospun Nylon 6 fibres. *Int J Bas Appl Sci* 2010;10 (6):116-31.
21. Siepmann F, Le Brun V, Siepmann J. Drug acting as plasticizers in polymeric systems: a quantitative treatment. *J Control Release* 2006;115:298-306.
22. Yu DG, Shen XX, Branford-White C, White K, Zhu LM, Bligh SW. Oral fast-dissolving drug delivery membranes prepared from electrospun polyvinylpyrrolidone ultrafine fibers. *Nanotechnology* 2009;20(5):055104.
23. Heun G, Lambov N, Groning R. Experimental and molecular modeling studies on interactions between drugs and Eudragit RL/RS resins in aqueous environment. *Pharm Act Helv* 1998;73:57-62.
24. Takka S. Propranolol hydrochloride-anionic polymer binding interaction. *Il Farmaco* 2003;58(10):1051-6.

12

Study on Phytochemical Composition, Antibacterial and Antioxidant Properties of Different Parts of *Alstonia scholaris* Linn.

Deepak Ganjewala*, Ashish Kumar Gupta

Amity Institute of Biotechnology, Amity University Uttar Pradesh, Sector-125, Noida-201303 (UP), India.

ARTICLEINFO

Keywords:
Alstonia scholaris
Antibacterial
Antioxidant
Follicles
Latex
Phenolics

ABSTRACT

Purpose: To evaluate phytochemical composition, antibacterial and antioxidant properties of methanolic extracts of different parts *viz.*, leaves, follicles and latex of Indian devil tree (*Alstonia scholaris* Linn.) R. Br. ***Methods:*** Antibacterial activities of the methanol extracts against Gram +ve (*Bacillus subtilis* and *Staphylococcus aureus*) and Gram -ve (*Escherichia coli, Pseudomonas aeruginosa*) bacteria were determined by well diffusion techniques. Aantioxidant profiles of methanol extracts were determined by 1,1-diphenyl-2-picryl-hydrazil (DPPH) free radical scavenging, superoxide anion radial scavenging and ferric thiocyanate reducing assays. ***Results:*** Phytochemical composition revealed abundance of flavonoids (97.3 mg QE/g DW), proanthocynidins (99.3 mg CE/g DW) and phenolics (49.7 mgGAE/g DW) in the leaf extract. Extracts of follicles and latex had comparatively very content of phenolics, flavonoids and proanthocyanidins. However, in follicle extract level of proanthocyanidins was significantly higher (46.8 mg CE/gDW). Latex extract among others exhibited most potent antibacterial activity. All the extracts displayed strong DPPH free radical and superoxide anion scavenging activities, only leaf extract displayed powerful reducing and ferrous ion chelating activities. ***Conclusion:*** Study revealed significant antioxidant activities of *A. scholaris* leaf, follicles and latex extracts and potential antibacterial activity of latex extract.

Introduction

Medicinal plants play important roles in our daily life to treat many diseases and ailments. Research in medicinal plants reflects the recognition of the validity of many herbal products.[1] Plants has been a major source of natural products and medicines since Ayurveda one of the world's oldest systems of medicine practiced in India.[2,3] In developing countries like India several plants based medicine, also known as herbal medicine are used. *Alstonia scholaris* (L.) R. Br. belong to family Apocynaceae commonly called as Indian devil tree has been used as folklore medicines,[1] possesses different pharmacological activities[4,5] and potentially used as antimalaria drug Ayush-64, NRDC, India.[6] Different parts of *A. scholaris viz;* leaves, follicles and latex a milky white secretion from folicles[3] are used in the treatment of various types of disorders in different medicinal system.[8] In alternative medicinal systems it is effective against different ailments such as asthma, malaria, fever, dysentery, diarrhoea, epilepsy, skin diseases and snakebite.[5] Latex is useful in application in ulcers, sores, tumors and rheumatoid pain.[2] Fruits are useful in syphilis and epilepsy and also used a tonic, antiperiodic and anthelmintic.[8]

Previous studies on *A. scholaris* have revealed the presence of different phytoconstituents[1,3] as well as the antibacterial and antioxidant properties.[2,6,8,9] While the antimicrobial properties of *A. scholaris* are well known[2,8,10-12] only little is known about the phytochemical compositions of the leaf, fruit and latex and their antibacterial and antioxidant properties. Therefore the present study was undertaken to investigate the phytochemical compositions, and antioxidant and antibacterial properties of leaves, follicles and latex parts of *A. scholaris*.

Materials and Methods

Plant material and extraction

Fresh leaves were collected from *A. scholaris* trees (8-12 feet) grown wild in the campus of Amity University and nearby areas in Noida (U.P.) India. Follicles were collected during the month February to March when the tree is laden of follicles. Follicles were cut with sharp blade and compressed to collect milky white latex in a beaker. Latex was stored at 0-4°C in refrigerator until used.

***Corresponding author:** Deepak Ganjewala, Amity Institute of Biotechnology, Amity University Uttar Pradesh, Sector 125, Noida-201303 (UP), India. Email: deepakganjawala73@yahoo.com; dganjwala@amity.edu

A known amount of leaves and follicles (100 g each) were kept in an oven at 40 °C for drying. Dried leaves and follicles were powdered by using mortar and pestle. The powder (10 g) of leaves and follicles were separately extracted with methanol (25-50 ml) for 24 h in separate Erlenmeyer flasks. Extraction process was repeated three times and each time the extract obtained were filtered through 0.45-μm filter paper and collected in a beaker. The extract thus obtained was dried over reflection water bath. Dried extracts were stored at 4 °C.

Antibacterial assay

Antibacterial activities of methanolic extracts of leaves, follicles and latex were assessed against Gram +ve (*Bacillus subtilis* and *Staphylococcus aureus*) and Gram -ve (*Escherichia coli, Pseudomonas aeruginosa*) bacteria by agar well diffusion method.[11] The culture plates were prepared by first sterilizing the nutrient agar (36 gm in 1000 ml) in an autoclave at 121 °C at 15 lb for 15 minutes and then by pouring 20 ml of media into sterilized Petri dishes. 1 ml inoculums suspension was spread uniformly over the agar in Petri dishes using sterile glass rod. Wells were made by sterile cork borer (6 mm) in each plate. Extracts 100 µl (at concentration of 50, 100 mg/ml) dissolved in dimethyl sulfoxide (DMSO) was added aseptically into the well. Simultaneously, a control with DMSO was also run. Plates were incubated at 37 °C for 24 hrs. After incubation, microbial growth was observed in the Petri dishes. The antibacterial activity was expressed as the mean of diameter of the inhibition.

Determination of phenolics content

Total content of phenolics, flavonoids and proanthocynidins were determined according to previously published report.[13] 0.5 ml of methanol extract of each sample (concentration 1 mg/ml) were taken in separate test tubes and 0.5 ml of the Folin-Ciocalteu reagent was added. Contents were mixed gently. After 2 min, 0.5 ml of sodium carbonate (100 mg/ml) was added gently to the content and allowed to stand for 2 h. The optical density of the solution turned blue was measured at 765 nm. Total phenolic contents were expressed as mg gallic acid equivalent (GAE)/g dry weight of the sample.

Flavonoids content was measured by the method of Jia et al.[14] 250 μl of extract from stock (1 mg/ml) was taken in a test tube containing 1.25 ml of distilled water. To this, added 75 μl of 5% sodium nitrate solution and left for 5 min. Then added 150 μl of 10% ammonium chloride followed and after 6 min 500 μl of 1 M sodium hydroxide was added. The content was diluted with 275 μl of distilled water. Absorbance of the solution was measured at 510 nm. Total flavonoids content was expressed as milligrams of quercetin equivalent (QE)/g dry weight of sample.

Proanthocyanidin content was measured according to the previously published method.[15] 0.5 ml of extract was mixed with 3 ml of 4% vanillin methanol and 1.5 ml of hydrochloric acid in a test tube. The content was mixed well and left at room temperature for 15 min. The absorbance of the solution was measured at 500 nm. Total proanthocyanidins content was expressed as milligrams of catechin equivalent (QE)/g dry weight of sample.

DPPH assay

The antioxidant activity of the each sample extract was assessed by the ability of the extract to scavenge 2, 2-diphenyl-1-picrylhydrazyl (DPPH) free radicals.[13] The extracts were taken in separate test tubes and allowed to react with DPPH. DPPH free radical scavenging activity was monitored by measurement of decline in absorbance at 517 nm. Butylated hydroxyanisole (BHA) was used as the standard compound.

Superoxide anion scavenging assay

Superoxide anion scavenging activity was determined using riboflavin–light NBT system.[16] The assay system consists of 0.5 ml phosphate buffer (50 mM pH 7.6), 0.3 ml riboflavin (50 μM), 0.25 ml PMS (20 mM), 0.1 ml NBT (0.5 mM) and 1 ml methanol extract of each sample. The reaction was initiated by illuminating fluorescence lamp. After 20 min of incubation, the absorbance was recorded at 560 nm. Superoxide anion scavenging activity was calculated using the formula of scavenging activity (%) = $[(A_{560}$ of control $- A_{560}$ of sample$)/A_{560}$ of control$] \times 100$. Quercetin and BHA were used as standards.

Determination of reducing power

Reducing power of each sample extract was determined in accordance with previous report.[17] In a test tube, 2 ml of methanol extract was mixed with 2 ml of 0.2M (pH 6.6) phosphate buffer and 2 ml of potassium ferricyanide (10 mg/ml). The mixture was incubated at 50°C for 20 min followed by addition of 2 ml of trichloroacetic acid (100 mg/ml). 2 ml aliquot from this mixture was transferred to fresh test tube and diluted with 2 ml of distilled water. To the diluted solution, added 0.4 ml of 0.1% ferric chloride and kept for 10 min The absorbance was measured at 700 nm.

Determination of ferrous ions chelating activity

Ferrous ion Fe^{2+} chelating ability of the methanol extract of each sample was measured determined by the ferrous iron-ferrozine complex method.[18] Various dilution (10, 8, 6, 4, and 2 mg/ml) of the of the extracts were prepared in methanol. An aliquot (0.8 ml) of diluted extract was taken in a test tube and mixed with 50 μl (2mM) of $FeCl_2$, 200 μl (5 mM) ferrozine and incubated at 25 ± 2 °C for 10 min. Absorbance was measured at 562 nm against methanol as blank. Ferrous ion chelating activity was calculated by the formula: Chelating ferrous ion (%) = [(A_{562} of control–A_{562} of sample/A_{517} of control] × 100.

Results

Phytochemical constituents

Total phenolics content including flavonoids and proanthocyanidins of leaves, follicles and latex extracts are presented in Table 1. The results revealed marked variation in overall content of phenolics in leaf, follicle and latex extracts. The leaf extract had highest content of overall phenolics followed by follicle and latex extracts. In the leaf extract, flavonoids and proanthocyanidins were present in abundance with values observed 97 mgQE/g DW and 99 mgCE/g DW, respectively, whereas the phenolics were only 50 mgGAE/gDW. In the follicle extract, level of flavonoids and phenolics were comparatively lower than leaf extract, however proanthocynidins (47 mgCE/g DW) was found significant. Latext extract had lowest content of phenolics (17 mgGAE/g DW), flavonoids (11 mgQE/g DW) and proanthocynidins (18mgCE/g DW).

Table 1. Phenolics content of methanolic extracts of leaves, follicles and latex of *A. scholaris*.

Phytoconstituents	Plant parts		
	Leaves	Follicles	Latex
Phenolics (mg GAE/g)	49.66±1.52	18.68±1.53	17.0±2.0
Flavonoids (mg QE/g)	97.33±1.52	15.86±01.64	11±1.0
Proanthocyanidins (mg CE/g)	99.33±1.52	46.86±1.75	18.33±.57

Antibacterial properties

The antibacterial profiles of the three extracts *viz.,* leaves, follicles and latex are presented in Table 2. Results revealed that all the extracts tested showed fairly well bactericidal activity against a set of Gram +ve than Gram –ve bacteria. However, the latex extract exhibited more potent antibacterial activity than the leaf and follicle extracts. Extract of latex (100 mg/ml) did best against *B. subtilis* with zone of inhibition 21 mm. However, extracts tested were found least effective against *P. aeruginosa* with measured zone of inhibition of 8 mm. In comparison to the standard antibiotics used, antibacterial potential of the extracts of the samples were found moderately effective.

Table 2. Antibacterial activity of methanolic extracts of leaves, follicles and latex of *A. scholaris.*

Extracts / Standard	Concentration (mg/ml)	Zone of inhibition (mm)			
		S. aureus	*B. subtilis*	*P. aeruginosa*	*E.coli*
Leaves	50	12	15	8	11
	100	15	18	12	14
Follicles	50	11	15	9	10
	100	13	17	11	13
Latex	50	13	17	10	12
	100	18	21	13	16
Ampicillin	**10**	**23**	**21**	**17**	**16**

DPPH free radical and superoxide anion scavenging activities

Antioxidant profiles of methanol extracts of leaves, follicles and latex in terms of their ability to scavenge DPPH free radicals are depicted in Figure 1. Among the extracts tested, leaf extract displayed most potent antioxidant activity (70-80%) followed by follicle (50-80%) and latex (40-58%). However, leaf and follicle extracts exhibited similar antioxidant (75-80%) activities at concentrations, 20 and 50 mg/ml. The riboflavin–light NBT system revealed almost similar superoxide anion radical scavenging profiles (80-90%) for all the three extracts (Figure 2). Interestingly, lower concentration of the extracts (10-20 mg/ml) displayed higher superoxide anion radical-scavenging

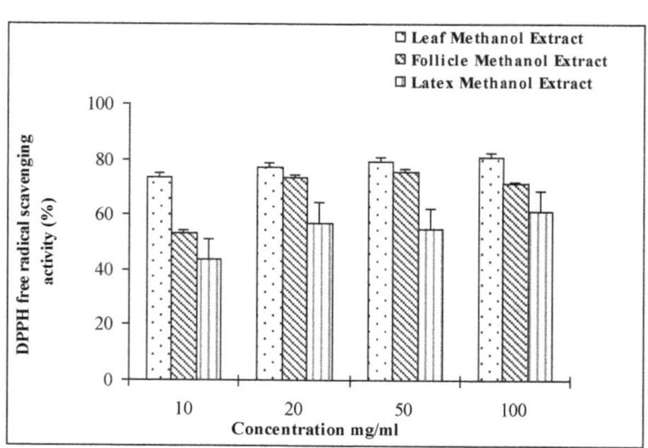

Figure 1. DDPH free radical scavenging activity of methanolic extracts leaves, follicles and latex of *A. scholaris*.

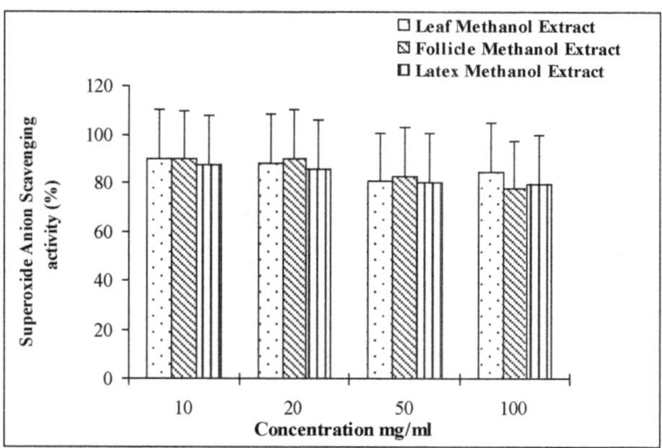

Figure 2. Superoxide anion scavenging activities of methanolic extracts of leaves, follicles and latex of *A. scholaris.*

Ferrous ion chelating and reducing activities

As shown in the Figure 3, ability of the leaf extract to chelate ferrous ion was the highest followed by follicles and latex extracts. Ferrous ion chelating activity increased linearly with increase in the concentration (1-8 mg/ml) of extracts. Higher ferrous ion chelating activities 80, 68 and 57 %, respectively of leaves, follicles and latex were observed at a concentration 8 mg/ml. A similar trend of the reducing activities was observed for the three extracts with leaves extract displaying highest reducing activity (Figure 4).

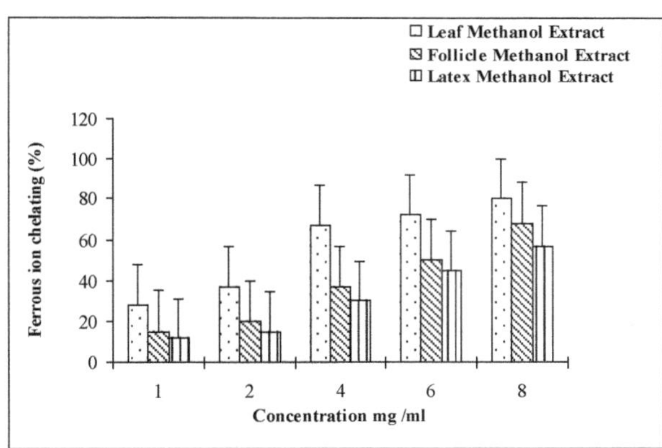

Figure 3. Ferrous ion chelating abilities of methanolic extracts of leaves, follicles and latex of *A. scholaris.*

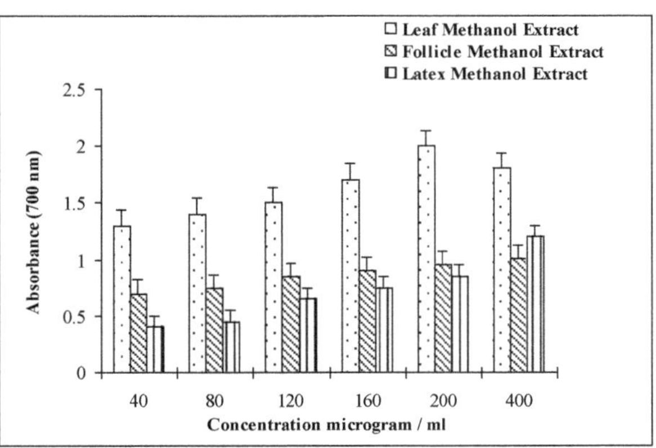

Figure 4. Reducing power of methanolic extracts of leaves, follicles and latex of *A. scholaris.*

Discussion

Previously, several reports have been published on phytochemical composition and antimicrobial properties of different parts *viz.,* leaves, flowers, fruits, roots, latex and bark of *A. scholaris* from different regions. Still reports on antioxidant properties of *A. scholaris* are limited. Since awareness towards natural products in healthcare is rapidly increasing, interest in medicinal plants has been multiply increased.[1] Plants produce many important compounds such as phenolics and flavonoids which possesses antioxidant and antimicrobial properties.[6] Phenolics and flavonoids provide protection against free radicals and regulate various oxidative reactions occurring naturally. Also, they are used to protect food quality mainly by the prevention of oxidative deterioration of constituents of lipids.[9]

Here we have reported phytochemical composition of leaves, follicles and latex of *A. scholaris* along with their antibacterial and antioxidant properties. Study revealed that *A. scholaris* leaves accumulated high content of phenolics including flavonoids and proanthocynidins whereas follicles and latex had comparatively lesser phenolics content. Higher levels of phenolics accumulated in the green tissues (leaves) may be due to higher rates at which photosynthesis proceeds in these parts. Total phenolic contents (49.7mg/ml) of *A. scholaris* leaf extract reported here matches with phenolics content (35-36 mg/ml) of *A. scholaris* from Karnataka region, however, flvonoids and proanthocynidins content were significantly higher.[8,9] Kumar et al.[19] have also reported significantly higher (80mg/ml) phenolics content in leaf methanolic extract of *A. scholaris* than the levels observed in the present study *A. scholaris* bark methanolic extract also contained significantly higher (46 mg/ml) phenolics content.[20] Here we have not investigated the bark extract for phenolics. Variations in the phytochemical compositions of the different plant parts of *A. scholaris* are typical of many other plant species reported previously.[21-24] Phytochemical contents are also reported to be influenced by several other factors such as geographical, genetic, environmental, degree of maturity at the time of harvest. Higher levels of phenolics accumulated in the green tissues (leaves) may be due to higher rates at which photosynthesis proceeds in these parts.

Phenolics content of the plants/parts are often correlated with their strong antioxidant activities.[25,26] In the present study, methanol extracts of *A. scholaris* leaves, follicles and latex extracts prepared with methanol exhibited strong antioxidant activities in terms of scavenging DPPH free radicals and superoxide anions. Leaf extract also had significant ferrous ion chelating and reducing abilities than follicle and latex extracts. The hydrogen donating potential is known to be one of the various mechanisms for measuring antioxidant activity. In DPPH assay, the radical scavenging ability of the extract was determined by the

DPPH which itself is a stable nitrogen-centered free radical. The color of ethanolic DPPH solution changes from purple to yellow due to the formation of diphenyl picryl hydrazine, a stable diamagnetic molecule upon reduction by either the process of hydrogen radical or electron-donation.[27,28] Superoxide anions are weak oxidants that produce very strong and harmful hydroxyl radicals and singlet oxygen causative agents of the oxidative stress.[29] Polyphenols are well-known to chelate pro-oxidant metal ions (ferrous ions) and prevent free radical formation from this pro-oxidants.[30]. Here, the leaf extract showed 78 % DPPH free radical scavenging activity, much higher than that reported previously.[31] Whereas, superoxide anion scavenging activity (89%) was only slightly higher than (73%) that reported in leaf methanol extract of *A. scholaris*.[9] The methanolic extract of bark also displayed strong antioxidant (90%) activity.[20]Also, higher antioxidant activities of *A. scholaris* plant parts reported here also coincide with the previous study reported significant amount of phyto constituents as well as antioxidant activities of *A. scholaris*.[8] However, no report is available on antioxidant activity of *A. scholaris* follicles and latex methanolic extracts except that by James et al.[32]

Similarly, the antibacterial activities of the methanol extracts of latex and follicles are studied for the first time. Latex extract among others showed stronger antibacterial activity against bacteria, particularly *B. subtilis*. Several other studies have also reported more or less similar antibacterial potential of the leaf meathonic extracts.[2,11] Stronger antibacterial effects of the extracts against Gram +ve bacteria might be due to absence of phospholipid membrane in Gram +ve bacteria.[12] Antibacterial activity of *A. scholaris* plant parts reported here are comparatively lesser than the standard antibiotic used. In conclusion, methanolic extracts of *A. scholaris* plant parts leaf, follicles and latex exhibited significant antioxidant and antibacterial activity.

Acknowledgments
Corresponding author of this article is grateful to Dr. Ashok Kumar Chauhan, Founder President and Atul Chauhan, Chancellor, Amity University, Uttar Pradesh, Noida, India for providing necessary facilities and support. Also, I duly acknowledge research grant from Council of Scientific and Industrial Research (CSIR), New Delhi.

Conflict of Interest
No conflicts of interest among the authors

References

1. Saxena N, Shrivastava PN, Saxena RC. Preliminary physcio-phytochemical study of stem bark of *Alstonia scholaris* (L.) R. BR.-A medicinal plant. *Int J Pharma Sci Res* 2012;3(4):1071-5.
2. Misra CS, Pratyush K, Dev LMS, James J, Vettil AKT, Thankamani V. A comparative study on phytochemical screening and antibacterial activity of roots of *Alstonia scholaris* with roots, leaves and stem bark. *Int J Res Phytochem Pharmacol* 2011;1(2):77-82.
3. Kaushik P, Kaushik D, Sharma N, Rana AC. *Alstonia scholaris*: It's phytochemistry and pharmacology. *Chron Young Sci* 2011;2(2):71-8.
4. Pratyush K, Misra CS, James J, Dev LMS, Veettil AKT, Thankamani V. Ethnobotanical and pharmacological study of *Alstonia* (Apocynaceae) - A Review. *J Pharm Sci Res* 2011;3(8):1394-403.
5. Dey A. *Alstonia scholaris* R.Br. (Apocynaceae): Phytochemistry and pharmacology: A concise review. *J Appl Pharm Sci* 2011;1(6):51-7.
6. Arulmozhi S, Mazumder PM, Narayanan LS, Thakurdesai PA. In vitro antioxidant and free radical scavenging activity of fractions from *Alstonia scholaris* Linn.R.Br. *Int J Pharm Tech Res* 2010;2(1):18-25.
7. Meena AK, Nitika G,Jaspreet N, Meena RP, Rao MM. Review on ethanobotany, phytochemical and pharmacological profile of *Alstonia scholaris*. *Int Res J Pharm* 2011;2(1):49-54.
8. Pankti K, Payal G, Manodeep C, Jagadish K. A phytopharmocological review of *Alstonia scholaris*: A panoramic herbal medicine. *Int J Res Ayu Pharm* 2012;3(3):367-71.
9. Ramachandra YL, Ashajyothi C, Padmalatha RS. Antioxidant activity of *Alstonia scholaris* extracts containing flavonoids and phenolic compounds. *Int J Pharm Pharma Sci* 2012;4(3):424-6.
10. Khan MR, Omoloso AD, Kihara M. Antibacterial activity of *Alstonia scholaris* and *Leea tetramera*. *Fitoterapia* 2013;74(8):736-40.
11. Khyade MS, Vaikos NP. Phytochemical and antibacterial properties of leaves of *Alstonia scholaris* R. Br. *Afr J Biotechnol* 2009;8(22):6434-6.
12. Patel JP, Gami B, Patel K, Solanki R. Antibacterial activity of methanolic and acetone extract of some medicinal plants used in indian folklore. *Int J Phytoremediation* 2011;3(2):261-9.
13. Liu X, Zhao M, Wang J, Yang B, Jiang Y. Antioxidant activity of methanolic extract of emblica fruit (*Phyllanthus emblica* L.) from six regions in China. *J Food Compos Anal* 2008;21(3):219-28.
14. Jia Z, Tang M, Wu J. The determination of flavonoid contents in mulberry and their scavenging effects on superoxide radicals. *Food Chem* 1999;64(4):555-9.
15. Manikandan S, Devi RS. Antioxidant property of alpha-asarone against noise-stress-induced changes in different regions of rat brain. *Pharmacol Res* 2005;52(6):467-74.
16. Mehrotra S, Mishra KP, Maurya R, Srimal RC, Yadav VS, Pandey R, et al. Anticellular and

immunosuppressive properties of ethanolic extract of Acorus calamus rhizome. *Int Immunopharmacol* 2003;3(1):53-61.

17. Oyaizu M. Antioxidative activities of browning products of glucosamine fractionated by organic solvent and thin-layer chromatography. *J Jpn Soc Food Sci Technol* 1998;35(11):771-5.
18. Meyer AS, Isaksen A. Application of enzymes as food antioxidants. *Trends Food Sci Technol* 1995;6(9):300-4.
19. Kumar A, Kaur R, Arora S. Free radical scavenging potential of some Indian medicinal plants. *J Med Plant Res* 2010;4(19):2034-42.
20. Kulkarni PM, Juvekar AP. Effect of *Alstonia scholaris* R. Br. on stress and cognition in mice. *Indian J Exp Biol* 2008;47(1):47-52.
21. Kannan P, Ganjewala D. Antibacterial Activity of *Nyctanthes Arbor-tristis* (Lour.) flowers, leaves, fruits and seeds. *Res J Phytol* 2007;1(2):61-7.
22. Song W, Wang HJ, Bucheli P, Zhang PF, Wei DZ, Lu YH. Phytochemical profiles of different mulberry (Morus sp.) species from China. *J Agric Food Chem* 2009;57(19):9133-40.
23. Asha D, Ganjewala D. Antioxidant activities of methanolic extracts of *Acorus calamus* (L.) rhizome and leaves. *J Herb Spic Med Plant* 2011;17(1):1-11.
24. Bhakta D, Ganjewala D. Effects of leaf position on total phenolics, flavonoids and proanthocynidines and their antioxidant activities in *Lantana camara* (L.). *J Sci Res* 2009;1(2):363-9.
25. Rice-Evans CA, Miller NJ, Paganga G. Structure-antioxidant activity relationships of flavonoids and phenolic acids. *Free Radic Biol Med* 1996;20(7):933-56.
26. Sim KS, Nurestri AM, Norhanom AW. Phenolic content and antioxidant activity of Pereskia grandifolia Haw. (Cactaceae) extracts. *Pharmacogn Mag* 2010;6(23):248-54.
27. Kris-Etherton PM, Hecker KD, Bonanome A, Coval SM, Binkoski AE, Hilpert KF, et al. Bioactive compounds in foods: their role in the prevention of cardiovascular disease and cancer. *Am J Med* 2002;113 Suppl 9B:71S-88S.
28. Oktay M, Gulcin I, Kufrevioglu OI. Determination of in vitro antioxidant activity of fennel (*Foeniculum vulgare*) seed extract. *LWT-Food Sci Technol* 2003;36(2):263-71.
29. Tepe B, Sokmen A. Screening of the antioxidative properties and total phenolic contents of three endemic Tanacetum subspecies from Turkish flora. *Bioresour Technol* 2007;98(16):3076-9.
30. Wang HZ, Cheng YG, Fan CS. Review of studies on chemical constituents and pharmacology of genus *Acorus* in China. *Acta Bot Yunnanica* 1998;20:96-100.
31. Kumar V, Gogoi BJ, Meghvansi MK, Singh L, Srivastava RB, Deka DC. Determining the antioxidant activity of certain medicinal plants of Sonitpur, (Assam), India using DPPH assay. *J Phytol* 2009;1(1):49-56.
32. James J, Veettil AKT, Pratyush K, Misra CS, Sahadevan LDM, Thankamani V. In vitro antioxidant activity of flowers and fruits of *Alstonia scholaris*. *Int J Phytomed* 2011;3(4):475-9.

Formulation, Characterization and Physicochemical Evaluation of Potassium Citrate Effervescent Tablets

Abolfazl Aslani*, Fatemeh Fattahi

Department of Pharmaceutics, School of Pharmacy and Novel Drug Delivery Systems Research Center, Isfahan University of Medical Sciences, Isfahan, Iran.

ARTICLEINFO

Keywords:
Effervescent tablets
Potassium citrate
Direct compression method
Fusion method
Wet granulation method

ABSTRACT

Purpose: The aim of this study was to design and formulation of potassium citrate effervescent tablet for reduction of calcium oxalate and urate kidney stones in patients suffering from kidney stones. ***Methods:*** In this study, 13 formulations were prepared from potassium citrate and effervescent base in different concentration. The flowability of powders and granules was studied. Then effervescent tablets were prepared by direct compression, fusion and wet granulation methods. The prepared tablets were evaluated for hardness, friability, effervescent time, pH, content uniformity. To amend taste of formulations, different flavoring agents were used and then panel test was done by using Latin Square method by 30 volunteers. ***Results:*** Formulations obtained from direct compression and fusion methods had good flow but low hardness. Wet granulation improves flowability and other physicochemical properties such as acceptable hardness, effervescence time ≤3 minutes, pH<6, friability < 1%, water percentage < 0.5% and accurate content uniformity. In panel test, both of combination flavors; (orange - lemon) and (strawberry - raspberry) had good acceptability. ***Conclusion:*** The prepared tablets by wet granulation method using PVP solution had more tablet hardness. It is a reproducible process and suitable to produce granules that are compressed into effervescent tablets due to larger agglomerates.

Introduction

Effervescent tablets were designed to produce solutions that release carbon dioxide simultaneously. Usually, these tablets are prepared by compressing the active ingredients with mixture of sodium bicarbonate and organic acids such as citric and tartaric acid.[1]

Generally, these tablets are included drugs that are solved rapidly when entered to water and they are recommended as a clear and palatable solution.[2] So, they can be prescribed to patients who suffered from swallow capsules or tablets.[3]The main advantages of effervescent tablets are quick production of solution. Thus, it is faster and better to absorb.[4]

As a source of acid, citric acid is the most used acid. Also other acids such as tartaric, fumaric, adipic, malic acid and anhydrides and salts of acid can be used. Potassium and sodium carbonate, sodium and potassium bicarbonate, arginine carbonate are used as a sources of alkali. Sodium bicarbonate is one of the most used carbonate because of high solubility, severe reaction and low cost.[5] So, excepients such as water soluble lubricants (e.g. PEG 4000, 6000 and sodium benzoate), sweeteners, flavorings and water-soluble colors are applied.[5]

Polyvinylpyrolidone (PVP) is an effective binder of effervescent tablets. It can be added as dry powder or in a wet form as an aqueous or hydroalcoholic solution. Mannitol, PEG 6000 and water in small amounts can be used as effective binder.[5,6]

Low relative humidity (maximum of 25% or less) and moderate to cool temperatures (about 25 °C or 77 °F) in the environment are essential to prevent sticking granule or tablets to tablet press machine.[5]

In producing direct compression method, the mixtures of powder with excellent flowability, and without particles segregation are needed and particle size of all raw materials should be equal. It is necessary to prepare granules, if particle size is small.[3,7]

In fusion method, mostly monohydrate citric acid, released its water at 54 °C in order to obtain the granules by agglomeration of the particles. Granulation with nonreactive solution contain of ethanol or isopropanol, that the most components of tablets are insoluble in them. So, a very small amount of water (0.1-0.5%) is active solution.[5]

Effervescent tablets are produced and controlled same as conventional tablets. These controls are included physicochemical properties such as hardness, weight variation, friability, solution time, pH and content uniformity.[5]

***Corresponding author:** Abolfazl Aslani, Department of Pharmaceutics, School of Pharmacy and Pharmaceutical Sciences, Isfahan University of Medical Sciences, Isfahan, Iran. Email: aslani@pharm.mui.ac.ir

Potassium citrate is very soluble in water and almost insoluble in alcohol with very salty taste. Each g of potassium citrate (monohydrate) consists of about 9.3 mmol of potassium and 3.08 mmol of citrate.[8]

Potassium citrate is used to replace sodium bicarbonate in the treatment of metabolic acidosis in patients, alkalizing agent of urine and symptomatic relief of mild urinary tract infections. Studies were shown that it is effective in reduction of calcium oxalate and urate kidney stones formation and prevent from bone loss.[9-12] So, studies are shown that oral supplements of potassium prevents hyperkalaemia from it due to the high absorption from the gastrointestinal tract but slowly.[12]

Products of potassium citrate are available in pharmaceutical world market in the forms of: tablet (5, 10, and 15 mEq potassium citrate, Urocit®-K), effervescent powder (1500 mg equivalent to 13 mEq potassium citrate, Effercitrate®) and oral solution.[8] Although the mentioned dosage form are available in the pharmaceutical market, none of them are held accountable for patient requirement, because high doses of drug are needed for patients with calcium and urate kidney stones.

These patients are using the drug into two forms: 1) a pharmaceutical dosage form with a low dose and high frequency consumption or 2) the bulk of the raw materials. Until now in the pharmaceutical market, this potassium citrate effervescent tablet with 25 meq does not exist. It is a new and applications design.

The aim of this study is design, formulation and preparation of the potassium citrate effervescent tablets containing 25 mEq monohydrate potassium citrate. These tablets will help to physicians prescribing and convenience consumption for patients suffering from calcium oxalate and urate kidney stones.

Materials and Methods

Material

Potassium citrate (monohydrate), sodium bicarbonate, citric acid (monohydrate), tartaric acid, PEG 6000, sodium benzoate, manitol, sorbitol and aspartame were procured by Merck (Darmstadt, Germany). Povidon k-30 (PVP) was purchased from Rahavard Tamin (Tehran, Iran). Orange flavoring agent was procured from Kagawa (China) and raspberry, strawberry, cherry and lemon flavoring agents were prepared by Farabi pharmaceutical Company, (Isfahan, Iran).

Preformulation

Firstly, the formulas were made up in the different stoichiometric ratios from tartaric acid, citric acid and sodium bicarbonate based on below reactions. According to Table 1, materials of each formulation were weighed and then 2700 mg of monohydrate potassium citrate was added to each formulation. Finally, after preparation of appropriate mixture, the lubricants including 30 mg of PEG 6000 and 10 mg of sodium benzoate were added the mixture and then the tablets compressed by using a single-punch press machine (KILIAN & CO, Germany). For next stages, the better stoichiometric ratios were selected with regard to three factors: solubility, effervescence time and pH.

$$H_3C_6H_5O_7.H_2O+3NaHCO_3 \longrightarrow Na_3C_6H_5O_7+4H_2O+3\ CO_2$$

$$H_2C_4H_4O_6 + 2NaHCO_3 \longrightarrow Na_2C_4H_4O_6 + 2H_2O + 2CO_2$$

Table 1. Composition of preliminary formulations (ratio) with their effervescence time, pH and solubility (Mean ± SD).

Formulations	Tartaric acid	Citric acid	Na bicarbonate	Effervescent time(s)	pH	*Solubility
S_1	-	0.5	0.5	105 ± 2.08	5.9 ± 0.05	3
S_2	-	0.5	1	40 ± 1.52	6.2 ± 0.1	3
S_3	1	0.5	1	39 ± 1.51	6.1 ± 0.04	1
S_4	0.5	1	1	36 ± 2	6.1 ± 0.05	2
S_5	-	1	1	50 ± 2.13	5.9 ± 0.06	5
S_6	1	1	1	48 ± 2.01	6.1 ± 0.06	2
S_7	1.5	0.5	1	52 ± 1.8	6.1 ± 0.1	2
S_8	2	0	1	55 ± 1.83	6.1 ± 0.08	1
S_9	-	1	1.5	43 ± 1.51	6.1 ± 0.7	4
S_{10}	-	1	0.5	30 ± 3.11	5.6 ± 0.4	4
S_{11}	-	1.5	1.5	25 ± 2.13	5.6 ± 0.05	5
S_{12}	-	1.5	1	49 ± 1	5.6 ± 0.04	4
S_{13}	-	2	2	20 ± 2.07	5.5 ± 0.06	4

*Solubility was defined by Likert Scale from 1= very poor, 2 = poor, 3 = average, 4 = good and 5 = excellent

Methods of Potassium Citrate Effervescent Tablets Production

Direct Compression

According to Table 2, raw materials of each formulation were weighed and were mixed in a tumbling cubic blender for 15 minutes.

After the preparation of the primary powder mixtures, sweeteners including aspartame, sorbitol, mannitol and fruit flavoring agents were passed through the appropriate mesh and were added to the powders and these were mixed altogether for 5 minutes. Finally, the selective lubricants including sodium benzoate (10 mg) and PEG 6000 (30 mg) were added and again mixed for about 2-5 minutes with other material.

Then, the powders were compressed into tablets by using a single-punch press machine (KILIAN & CO, Germany), with 25 mm punch set. Weight of each tablet was considered about 4.5 g. At the end, the tablets were dried in an oven with air circulation at 54°C for 1 hr and after cooling were packed in plastic tubes.

Table 2. Different components of prepared tablets from the direct compression (D) and fusion (f) methods.

Ingredients (mg)	Formulations					
	F_1	F_2	F_3	F_4	F_5	F_6
K citrate	2700	2700	2700	2700	2700	2700
Citric acid	570	850	850	850	850	850
Na bicarbonate	500	750	750	750	750	750
Mannitol	-	-	60	120	-	60
Sorbitol	-	-	-	-	60	-
Aspartame	-	-	-	-	-	1.5

Fusion Method

According to the formulations which are shown in Table 2, amounts of citric acid, sodium bicarbonate, potassium citrate and mannitol (sorbitol) were weighted accurately and were mixed for about 15 minutes in a tumbling cubic blender. Then, the obtained mixture was placed in an oven at 54 °C. The powder was mixed regularly until the crystallization water of citric acid was released as binder factor (approximately 30 minutes). After obtaining an appropriate pasty mass, this wet mass was passed through sieve No. 20 and the obtained granules were dried in an oven at 54 °C for 1 hr. After drying, for second times the granules were passed through sieve No. 20.

In the next stage, sweeteners and flavors were added with the granule mass and mixed for 5 minutes with other material.

At last, the lubricants including sodium benzoate (10 mg) and polyethylene glycol 6000 (30 mg) were added and mixed for 2-5 minutes with other material. The granule mixtures compressed into tablets by a single-punch press machine (KILIAN & CO, Germany), with 25 mm punch set. Finally, they were dried and packed with the previous methods.

Wet granulation Method

Wet granulation was performed on F_5 and F_6 formulations. First, citric acid and sodium bicarbonate and potassium citrate were milled by using miller so that all powders were passed through sieve No. 35 and were blended for 10 minutes. Then 9.5 % w/v PVP solution in absolute ethanol was added with the mixture, so that white pasty mass was formed. This wet mass was passed through sieve No. 20 and the granules were dried in an oven at 54 °C for 75 minutes. So, the dried mass was passed through sieve No. 20 and the other ingredients were added to them like as fusion method. The granule mixtures were compressed into tablets by using a single-punch press machine (KILIAN & CO, Germany), with 25 mm punch set. Prepared tablets were dried in an oven with air circulation at 54 ° C for 90 minutes, then were wrapped in Aluminum foil and were packaged in plastic tubes.

Precompression Tests

Particle Size Analysis

The average particle size of powder mixture was determined by sieve analysis method. 100 grams of powder mixtures and granules poured on the upper sieve. Series of sieve were placed on ERWEKA shaking apparatus for 10 minutes after this period; the amount remaining on each sieve was measured.[13]

The mean diameter of the powders was calculated by equation (1).

$$d = \sum \frac{X_i d_i}{100} \qquad \text{Eq.1}$$

x_i = The average size of both upper and lower sieve

d_i = The percentage of the amount of i in limited area by two sieves.

Flowability

For evaluation of powder flow, the angle of repose, compressibility index and Hausner´s ratio can be used.

Angle of Repose (α): The powder or granule mass was passed from the funnel. Angle of repose was determined by equation 2.

The average of three measurements was interpreted according to USP NF. 2008.[14]

$$\tan(\alpha) = \frac{Height}{0.5\ Base} \qquad \text{Eq. 2}$$

Height: The height of the formed cone

Base: Diameter of the formed cone

Compressibility Index and Hausner´s Ratio: For measurement of bulk density, 100 grams of powders and granules was poured into the graduated cylinder (250 ml) using a glass funnel and its volume is recorded.

$$\rho\ bulk = \frac{m}{V\ bulk} \qquad \text{Eq. 3}$$

Tapping to cylinder containing the powder continued until no further volume changes occur. Tapped density is obtained from the following equation.

$$\rho \text{ tapped} = \frac{m}{V \text{ tapped}} \quad \text{Eq. 4}$$

Compressibility Index and Hausner´s ratio parameters obtained by using the mean of three measurements from ρ_{bulk} and ρ_{tapped} and were compared according to the USP NF.2008.[14]

$$\text{Compressibility Index} = 100 \times \left[\frac{\rho \text{ tapped} - \rho \text{ bulk}}{\rho \text{ tapped}}\right] \quad \text{Eq. 5}$$

$$\text{Hausner's Ratio} = \frac{\rho \text{ tapped}}{\rho \text{ bulk}} \quad \text{Eq. 6}$$

Post compression Tests

Measurement of Tablet Hardness

Hardness of tablets was determined according to the USP for 10 tablets of each formulation by using a hardness tester (Erweka, 24-TB, Germany).

Hardness of effervescent tablets is usually lower than conventional tablets and minimum of acceptable hardness of uncoated tablets is 40 N approximately.[1]

Measurement of Tablet Thickness

The thickness of 10 tablets from each formulation was determined by using calibrated collies. Average fluctuations of thickness, should not exceed more than 5 % of its normal limits.[1]

Friability

20 tablets of each formulation was taken randomly and after weighting altogether, were placed in the friabilator chamber (Erweka, TAP, Germany) for 4 minutes at 25 rpm. If weight loss is greater than 1% is unacceptable.[1]

Evaluation of Weight Variation

20 tablets of each formulation were weighed individually and the mean of weight were determined. According to the USP for tablets with weight more than 324 mg, among 20 tablets; just two tablets can be out of the 5% of the average weight and none deviated by more than twice that percentage.[14]

Measurement of Effervescence Time

A single tablet was placed in a beaker containing 200 ml of purified water at 20 °C ± 1 °C. Whenever a clear solution without particles was obtained effervescence time has finished.[15]

The mean of three measurements of each formulation was reported.

Determination of Effervescent Solution pH

pH solution was determined with one tablet in 200 ml of purified water at 20 ± 1 °C by using pH meter (Metrohm, 632, Switzerland), immediately after completing the dissolution time.[15] This experiment was repeated 3 times for each formulation.

Measurement of CO_2 Content

One effervescent tablet solved in 100 ml of 1N sulfuric acid solution and weight changes were determined after dissolution end. The obtained weight difference was shown the amount (mg) of CO_2 per tablet. The CO_2 content reports are averages of 3 determinations.[15]

Evaluation of the Water Content

10 tablets of each formulation were dried in a desiccator containing of activated silica gel for 4 hours. Water content of 0.5% or less is acceptable.[15]

Assay

The first, 3 effervescent tablets of potassium citrate was triturated and 347 mg of crushed powder (Equivalent to 200 mg of anhydrous potassium citrate) accurately weighed and was dissolved in 25 ml of acetic acid glacial. Added 2 drops of crystal violet TS solution and titrated with 0.1N perchloric acid VS (USP) to a green end point. The same steps was done on a blank solution prepared from effervescent tablets of potassium citrate without active ingredient and was made any necessary correction. In the titration, the prepared blank was consumed perchloric acid and corrected volumes were required. Each ml of 0.1N perchloric acid is equivalent to 10.21 mg of anhydrous potassium citrate.[14] 2700 mg of hydrated potassium citrate is equivalent to 2550.194 anhydrous potassium citrate. Of course, in this assay other alternative methods such as atomic absorption can also be used.

$$N \times V(\text{corrected by blank}) = \frac{mg}{108.14} \quad \text{Eq.7}$$

N: Normality of standardized acid by potassium biphthalate according to USP

mg: milligram of hydrated potassium citrate

108.14: Eq of hydrated potassium citrate

Evaluation of Content Uniformity

10 tablets of each formulation were selected at random to measurement of the active ingredient amount. None of the tablets should not be out of range (90-110 %) of mention amounts in formula, and coefficient of variation (CV) should not be more than 6. If only one tablet was out of previous range and range of 80 – 120 %, 20 tablets must be tested. Among these 20 tablets, anything of them should not be out of range 90-110 percent.[14]

Determination of the Equilibrium Moisture Content

Three desiccators were prepared containing saturated salt solutions of potassium nitrate (for creation 90% RH, at 18 °C), sodium chloride (for creation 71% RH, at 18 °C) and sodium nitrite (for creation 60% RH, at 18 °C). Three tablets of each formulation were placed in desiccators. Then, the equilibrium moisture content was determined by Karl Fischer method and the autotitrator device (Mettler, TOLEDO-DL53, Switzerland) in the first day and after 7 day.[14]

Evaluation of Prepared Tablets Taste

Before beginning the evaluation, the taste ability of volunteers was measured by four base tastes (salt, sweet, sour, bitter) by 20 ml of 0.2% sodium chloride, 2% sucrose, 0.07% citric acid, and 0.07% caffeine in water respectively.[16]

To evaluate the taste, panel tests were performed by Latin Square method. The first, with the help of 5 volunteers, 7 flavors which were added to F_6 formulation (optimum formulation), were examined (Table 3). Thus, the volunteers were asked to score each of the formulation from 1 = very bad, 2 = bad, 3 = no taste, 4 = good and 5 = excellent taste based on Likert Scale.

At next stage, another 30 volunteers were asked to give points to the 2 selected flavors of early stages from 1 = very bad, 2 = bad, 3 = no taste, 4 = good and 5 = excellent taste based on Likert Scale.

Table 3. Different flavors were used for panel test of potassium citrate effervescent tablets.

Code	Flavoring agent	Amount (mg)
A	Raspberry	4.4
B	Strawberry	4.4
C	Cherry	4.4
D	Orange	4.4
E	Lemon	8.8
F	Orange & Lemon	4.4 & 8.8
G	Raspberry & strawberry	4.4 & 4.4

In all time of experiments, the standard conditions of panel test were considered such as temperature equal to 21°C, 20 minutes distance from the previous samples, samples with similar concentrations of drugs and have been done without exchanging the volunteers' idea.[16]

Results

Results of preformulation study is shown that formulations with stoichiometric ratios 1:1 and 1.5:1.5 (S_5, S_{11}) were selected as the appropriate base formulations in tableting process, and with better physicochemical characteristics.

Results from characterization of the powder formulations containing of the particle size distribution, angle of repose, compressibility index and Hausner′s ratio are given in the Tables 4, 5 and Figure 1.

The results of obtained from tablets evaluation are presented for hardness, friability, tablet thickness, effervescence time, pH, weight variation, water and CO_2 content, content uniformity and equilibrium moisture content properties are given in the Tables 5,6,8, too.

The particle size distribution of three manufacturing methods is listed in Tables 4 and 5. The mean diameters of granules were greater than the powders. Figure 1 shows the particle size distribution diagram of F_5 formulation which has normal distribution.

Table 4. The mean diameter, particle size distribution and percentage on each sieve of the obtained formulations from direct compression (D) and fusion (f) methods.

Formulations	Sieve number								Mean diameter(μ)
	<20	20-25	25-30	30-35	35-40	40-70	70-100	>100	
D_1	1.69	1.46	5.64	5.29	1.62	47.9	16.13	20.28	311.42
f_1	2.59	3.08	8.06	5.74	1.25	48.41	12.73	18.15	340.63
D_2	1.9	2.73	6.62	6.66	1.28	45.42	16.1	19.29	326.08
f_2	2.33	2.17	6.57	6.62	1.44	67.74	7.08	6.05	360.47
D_3	1.52	2.01	4.59	5.67	1.17	48.04	13.63	23.38	307.95
f_3	3.05	3.47	7.69	7.91	1.92	55.45	12.41	8.09	367.03
D_4	1.8	2.09	5.25	4.52	1.6	44.47	13.85	26.42	304.59
f_4	7.02	4.31	7.39	6.64	0.62	51.63	8.76	13.62	381.84
D_5	1.84	2.24	3.06	6.56	12.55	50.86	12.51	10.38	347.48
f_5	3.02	2.74	3.9	6.26	12.94	57.55	8.08	5.51	373.05
D_6	1.41	2.06	4.5	4.43	1.77	44.66	16.36	24.82	299.12
f_6	8.53	3.07	6.33	5.04	0.75	44.93	13.36	17.98	363.39

Table 5. Particle size distribution, mean diameter and flowability of obtained granules in wet granulation method together with tablets characteristics for G_5 and G_6 formulations.

Formulations	-	G_5	G_6
Sieve number	<16	0.28	0.04
	16-20	2.26	2.68
	20-25	7.73	21.17
	25-30	11.09	33
	30-35	16.08	6.74
	35-40	22	0.51
	40-70	33.66	30.33
	>70	6.9	5.52
	Mean diameter (µ)	471.2	556.71
Flow Properties	Hausner´s ratio	1.06±0.01	1.08±0.02
	Compressibility index	5.73±0.66	7.6±2.14
	Angle of repose	15.076±0.12	14.713±0.59
Tablets characteristics	Weight variation	4.401 ± 0.113	4.416 ± 0.063
	Hardness	78.85 ± 2.26	65.05 ± 2.72
	Content uniformity, (%CV)	2744 ± 97.5 (3.55)	2742 ± 54.9 (2.0)
	Water content	0.0405 ± 0.01	0.0096 ± 0.005
	Tablet thickness	5.97 ± 0.06	6.048 ± 0.06
	Effervescence time(s)	132 ± 2	112.7 ± 2.52
	pH solution	5.8 ± 0.02	5.8 ± 0.02
	CO_2 content	313 ± 13	423 ± 16
	Assay (mg)	2700 ± 40	2720 ± 20
	Friability (%)	0.973±0.02	0.936±0.05

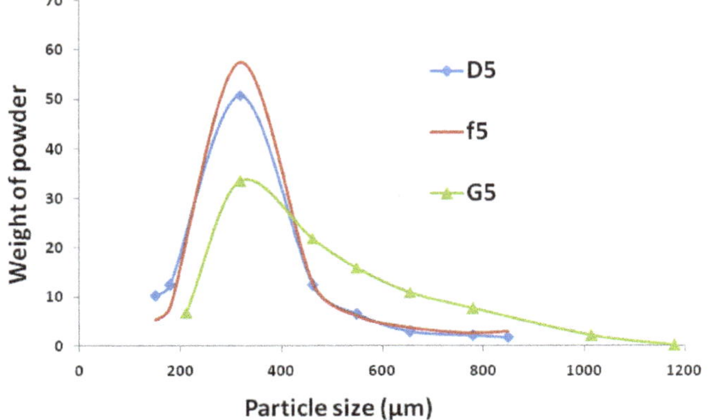

Figure 1. Particle size distribution diagram of F_5 in direct compression (D), fusion (f) and wet granulation (G) methods

According to the results in Table 7, PVP 0.5 % (w/w) and sieve No. 20 were chosen considering hardness and effervescence time.

Range of hardness in obtained formulations of direct compression method (D) was varied from 15 N to 22 N and obtained granules from the fusion method (f) were shown a slight increase from 20 - 25 N (Table 6).

Produced tablets were evaluated by hardness, weight variation, tablet thickness, friability, effervescent time, pH, content uniformity, water and CO_2 content. These values are reported in Table 5. In Table 5, hardness was shown threefold increase in wet granulation method.

In this study, at 60 % RH and 18°C, the variation in percentage of equilibrium moisture content after 7 days was nothing, but, at 90 % RH and 18°C, it was most.

For correcting the potassium citrate effervescent tablet tastes, in the first stage, volunteers selected orange – lemon and strawberry - raspberry flavors. Figure 2 is shown means of obtained results from the 30 volunteers in the panel test by Latin Square method. Both of desirable flavors had good acceptability.

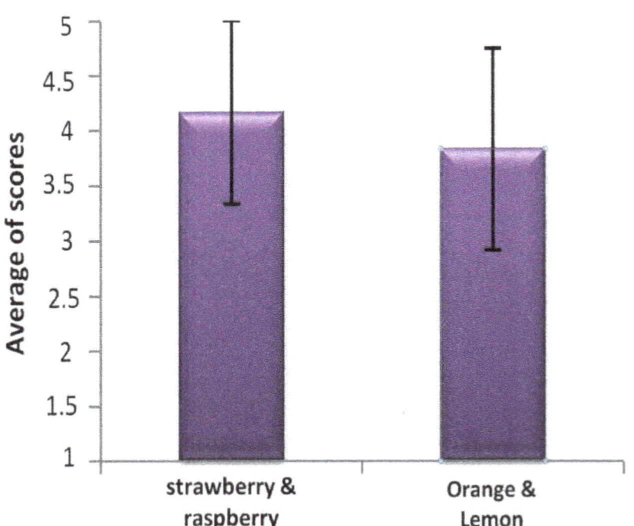

Figure 2. Evaluation of prepared tablets taste by Latin Square method.

Discussion

The pharmaceuticals which are suitable for formulation of the effervescent tablets should have specific particulars such as quick absorption of drug, good dissolution in water and high dose.[17] These particulars were existed in potassium citrate.

Potassium citrate recommended for the people who suffer from urate and calcium kidney stones. One study which was done on 500 patients with recurrent kidney stones showed potassium citrate have been reduced the prevalence of kidney stones from two stone to half stone in a year.[8] Also, these patients need to consume large amount of water daily, thus, solution of effervescent tablet in the water could remove this need. Currently, patients are taking potassium citrate into form of raw material powder. This kind of usage is not desirable for flavor and is not the exact for the consumption dosage. Therefore, the main objective of this study is design and formulation of potassium citrate effervescent tablets which have good taste and also have certain dosage. The main uses of these tablets are reduction of calcium oxalete and urate stones in patients with kidney stones.

Table 6. Flowability properties and hardness of tablets obtained from direct compression (D) and fusion (f) methods (Mean ± SD).

Flowability properties	Formulations					
	F_1	F_2	F_3	F_4	F_5	F_6
Angle of repose (D)	27.42±1.06	29.9±0.75	26.7±0.02	26.06±0.85	27.05±0.0	26.38±1.37
Angle of repose (f)	24.03±1.17	25.17±1.13	24.48±1.33	24.12±1.73	26.06±0.99	24.9±1.76
Hausner´s ratio(D)	1.103±0.06	1.142±0.0	1.099±0.01	1.087±0.01	1.13±0.01	1.12±0.0
Hausner´s ratio (f)	1.083±0.01	1.095±0.01	1.073±0.01	1.066±0.0	1.083±0.01	1.08±0.01
Compressibility index (D)	9.33±1.94	12.48±0.64	9.08±1.33	7.99±0.66	11.50±1.02	11.07±0.65
Compressibility index (f)	8±0.78	8.75±1.26	6.813±0.75	6.2±0.62	7.677±0.7	7.437±0.64
Hardness (Newton) (D)	15±2.34	17±3.54	17±3.96	17.5±5.11	22±4.26	17.5±5.16
Hardness (Newton) (f)	20±4.81	20±5.21	20±2.85	23±3.49	25±6.53	22±4.73

Table 7. Relationships between (%PVP /tablet, Sieve No) and (hardness, effervescence time) in formulation G_6 (Mean ± SD).

Independent properties		Dependent properties	
PVP (% W/W) /tablet	Sieve No.	Hardness (N)	Effervescence time (s)
0.34	20	52.9±6.5	125±1.11
0.36	20	55.5±4.81	138±1.52
0.43	40	68.25±5.49	180±1.83
0.43	20	68.75±3.51	162±1.74
0.45	16&20	53.5±4.16	140±2.21
0.45	20&25	36.66±2.32	130±1
0.5	20	66.75±2.12	170±2.03
0.67	16&20	112.4±3.95	187±0.57
1	20	90.83±4.45	240±1.51

Table 8. Equilibrium Moisture Content (%) in the G_5 and G6 effervescent tablets (Mean ± SD).

Microclimates	G_5			G_6		
	1st Day	7th Day	Variation	1st Day	7th Day	Variation
60% RH, 18°C	11.31±0.96	11.42±0.77	0.10	10.02±0.46	10.13±0.74	0.11
71% RH, 18°C	11.81±0.47	14.86±0.51	3.05	10.64±0.84	13.51±1.43	2.88
90% RH,18°C	12.09±1.1	22.39±0.96	10.30	11.28±0.61	14.44±0.82	3.15

Ratios of effervescent components in the formulations of S_5 and S_{11} were led to better solubility, pH less than 6, and an appropriate effervescent reaction. In the next steps, this stoichiometric ratios were used for the preparation of effervescent tablets (Table 1). In comparison of formulations containing tartaric acid, this result was obtained: tartaric acid should remove from the formulations because of low solubility and much precipitation.

The mean diameter of particles in the wet granulation method is larger than the average diameter of the particles in the two other methods due to the adhesion of smaller particles and formation of larger particles (Tables 4 and 5).

Accordingly to Figure 1, diagram peak of f_5 is drawn upward and is drawn to the right for G_5 which is representative of particle size increase in granulation.

Angle of repose is lessened in the produced granules due to shape changing into sphere and contact level deduction.

As results showed, angle of repose reduced in fusion and wet granulation methods. For example, angles of repose of D_6, f_6, G_6 (the same formulations, but different manufacturing methods) report: 26.38, 24.496 and 14.713, respectively (Tables 5 and 6). Hausner's ratio and compressibility index are reduced in fusion and wet granulation methods. Granulation (fusion or wet) increases flowability and decreases angle of repose due to increasing of particle size and shape changing into sphere, but these changes are higher in the wet granulation. In other study, the results were extracted similar to our results.[18]

Tablets' hardness of D_5, f_5 and G_5 (the same formulations but different manufacturing methods) were 22, 25, and 78.85 respectively. Wet granulation improves hardness of tablet due to internal porosity granules and the plastic deformation.[18] Also, for hardness increasing, the dry forms of binder such as mannitol , sorbitol and PVP were used, but, the desired results were not found. Then wet granulation method using PVP was performed on the best formulations (G_5 and G_6).These formulations were better because of flowability and they had not capping and sticking in the manufacturing process. Increasing PVP percentage was found to enhance the hardness and effervescence time (Table 7). In the other study was shown that wet granulation technique could improve compressibility and flowability properties and hardness that the results were in agreement with this study.[15]

Thickness of the tablets must be between 6.1 ± 0.3 mm, that the results are acceptable regarding to pharmacopoeia standards (USP NF.2008).

According to the USP, in the tablets which their weight are more than 324 mg, among 20 tablets, just 2 tablets can be exceed from ± 5 % of the weight average (for G_5 ± 221.14 and for G_6 ± 221.21) that the result are acceptable.[14]

pH less than 6 is necessary to increase the absorption of effervescent tablets, that pH of two optimum formulations is less than 6. The equal pHs in different samples of one formulation indicate that granule mixtures are uniform. In other study on effervescent granules containing citric acid and sodium bicarbonate has been done, solution pH which is obtained from dissolving granules was measured at 5.64. It is comparable with the results in this study.[15]

Effervescence time of tablet must be less than 3 minutes that the results are indicated this subject.[15]

In the studied formulations, CO_2 contents of G_5 and G_6 were 313 and 423 mg, respectively. One study has been shown that amount of carbon dioxide in 2.5 g effervescent tablets containing of aspirin (prepared by direct compression method) were measured at 242 mg[19] and other study reported that in each grams of formulas containing of citric acid and sodium bicarbonate CO_2 content was 292 mg which is comparable with the results.[15] In the formulation G_5, lower level of CO_2 was obtained. In this formulation, sorbitol exists which is a hygroscopic matter. Absorbed moisture by sorbitol causes beginning of an effervescent reaction in the small scale.

As Table 5 shows, the friability of tablets was satisfactory, attributed by the acceptable hardness.

In the formulation G_5 and G_6, water content was gained 0.0405 and 0.0096, respectively. Reason of higher water content in formulation G_5 is the presence of sorbitol and the absorption of moisture. The prepared tablets by the wet granulation have very low water content due to getting temperate during drying process.

Effervescent materials are hygroscope highly and they are susceptible for degradation by air humidity. Of course potassium citrate is a hygroscopic substance since potassium citrate effervescent tablets are containing large amounts of active ingredient; much ability will have to absorb moisture. Consequently, possibility of effervescent reaction beginning and instability is high in these tablets. So it is necessary to determined that the provided tablets are stable up to what moisture percent. At 60 % RH and 18°C, the variation in percentage of equilibrium moisture content after 7 days was alittle, thus, the granules ready to be compressed into tablets aren't hygroscopic mostly up to 60 % RH at 18°C. Also G_5 formulation equilibrium moisture content after 7 days showed more variation because the presence of sorbitol that is a hygroscopic substance.

Since, the amount of active ingredient (hydrated potassium citrate) can fluctuate in ranges from 2430 to 2970 mg and coefficient of variation percents (CV %) were not upper than 6%, content uniformity of G_5 and G_6 were in the acceptable range and the prepared tablets have USP standard about amount of active ingredient and the content uniformity.

As depicted in Figure 2, volunteer gave more scores to both the combination flavor of orange-lemon and raspberry-strawberry. Strawberry-raspberry flavors took more scores compare to orange–lemon but closed results showed, selection of flavor is depending on individual relish.

Conclusion

In this work, it was tried to produce potassium citrate effervescent tablets by using direct compression, fusion and wet granulation techniques. The results of this study show that wet granulation is a suitable method to produce effervescent tablets of potassium citrate due to the large size of these tablets in the pharmaceutical industry. Wet granulation is one of the most common methods used for granulation in the industry. This method is obtained by adding a solution with (or without) adhesive to the powder to form a wet mass. In this study, the prepared tablets were acceptable under the terms of pharmacopoeia standards only when PVP was added as a binder during the granulation process.

Due to particle adhesion, the prepared tablets through wet granulation technique had better compression and uniformity. They had not processing problems such as sticking, capping, and friction.

Among the studied formulations, only the formulation G_6 was desirable for all physiochemical characteristics, including effervescent time under 3 minutes or less, pH <6, friability under 1 percentage, the water content below 0.5 percentage, low weight variation, and correct content uniformity. Finally, its taste was also amended by adding strawberry - raspberry flavor.

These tablets will help to convenience consumption of potassium citrate and more acceptances of patients who are affected by urate and calcium kidney stones.

Conflict of Interest

The authors report no conflicts of interest in this work.

References

1. Lachman L, Liberman HA, Kanig JL. The theory and practice of industrial pharmacy. 3rd ed. Philadelphia: lea and febiger; 1986.
2. Allen LV, Popovich NG, Ansel HC. Ansel's pharmaceutical dosage forms and drug delivery systems. 8th ed. Philladelphia: Lippincott Williams & Wilkins; 2010.
3. Swarbrick J, Boylan JC. Encyclopedia of pharmaceutical technology. New York: Marcel Dekker; 2002.
4. Altomare E, Vendemiale G, Benvenuti C, Andreatta P. Bioavailability of a new effervescent tablet of ibuprofen in healthy volunteers. *Eur J Clin Pharmacol* 1997;52(6):505-6.
5. Monrle R. Effervescent tablet in: Liberman HA, Lachman I, Schwartz J. Pharmaceutical dosage form: tablets, 2nd ed. New York: Marcel Dekker Inc; 1980.
6. Callhan JC, Cleary GW, Elafant M, Kaplan G, Kensler T, Nash RA. Equilibrium Moisture Content of Pharmaceutical Excipients. *Drug Dev Ind Pharm* 1982 8(2):355-69.
7. Saleh SI, Boymond C, Stamm A. Preparation of direct compressible effervescent components: spray- dried sodium bicarbonate. *Int J pharmaceut 1988*; 45(1-2):19-26.
8. Sweetman SC. Martindle: The complete drug refrence, 35th ed. London: pharmaceutical press; 2007.
9. Tekin A, Tekgul S, Atsu N, Bakkaloglu M, Kendi S. Oral potassium citrate treatment for idiopathic hypocitruria in children with calcium urolithiasis. *J Urol* 2002;168(6):2572-4.
10. Pak CY, Sakhaee K, Fuller C. Successful management of uric acid nephrolithiasis with potassium citrate. *Kidney Int* 1986;30(3):422-8.
11. Pak CY, Peterson RD, Poindexter J. Prevention of spinal bone loss by potassium citrate in cases of calcium urolithiasis. *J Urol* 2002;168(1):31-4.
12. McEvoy GK. AHFS Drug information. Bethesda, MD: American society of health-system pharmacists; 2005.
13. Aulton ME. The science of dosage form design. 2nd ed. New York: Churchil living stone; 2002.
14. United States Pharmacopeia 31/National Formulary 26. Rockville MD USA: United States Pharmacopeial Convention; 2008.
15. Yanze FM, Duru C, Jacob M. A process to produce effervescent tablets: Fluidized bed dryer melt granulation. *Drug Dev Ind Pharm* 2000;26(11):1167-76.
16. Brich GG, Green LF, Coulson CB. Sweetness and sweetners. London: Applied science publisher LTD; 1981.
17. Prabhakar CH, Krishna KB. A review on effervescent tablet. *Int J Pharm Technol 2011*; 3(1): 704-12.
18. Agrawal R, Naveen Y. Pharmaceutical processing – A review on wet granulation technology. *Int J Pharm Front Res 2011*; 1(1): 65-83.
19. Amela J, Salazar R, Cemeli J. Methods for the determination of the carbon dioxide released from effervescent pharmaceuticals. *J pharm bely 2000*; 55(2): 53-6.

In Vitro Antioxidant and Anticancer Activity Studies on *Drosera Indica* L. (Droseraceae)

Raju Asirvatham[1]*, Arockiasamy Josphin Maria Christina[2], Anita Murali[3]

[1] *Department of Pharmacology, Shri Rawatpura Sarkar Institute of Pharmacy, Datia, Mathya Pradesh, India.*

[2] *Department of Pharmacology, AIMST University, Malaysia.*

[3] *MS Ramaiah College of Pharmacy, Banglore, India.*

ARTICLEINFO

Keywords:
Drosera indica L
In vitro antioxidant activity
Anticancer activity
Dalton's Ascitic Lymphoma (DAL)
Ehrlich Ascitic Carcinoma (EAC)

ABSTRACT

Purpose: The aim of present *in vitro* studies was performed to examine the antioxidant and anticancer activities of ethanol and aqueous extracts of *Drosera indica* L. ***Methods***: Different concentrations (5 – 640mcg/ml) of the ethanol (EEDI) and aqueous (AEDI) extracts of *D.indica* L were used in various antioxidant assay methods such as hydroxyl radicals, DPPH, super oxide radical scavenging activity, chelating ability of ferrous ion, nitric oxide radical inhibition, ABTS and reducing power. Ascorbic acid (AA) was used as the standard antioxidant for the free radical scavenging assays. Dalton's Ascitic Lymphoma (DAL) and Ehrlich Ascitic Carcinoma (EAC) cell lines were used as the *in vitro* cancer models for the tryphan blue dye and LDH leakage assays, where 5 to 250mcg /ml of both EEDI and AEDI were tested. ***Results***: EEDI showed antioxidant activities with the minimum IC_{50} values of 34.8±0.43 mcg/ml in scavenging of hydroxyl radical and moreover AEDI showed minimum IC_{50} values of 94.51±0.84 mcg/ml in Fe^{2+}chelating assay. EEDI on the reducing power assay and ABTS showed higher IC_{50} than standard AA. IC_{50} values of AEDI on Fe^{2+} chelating assay and super oxide radical assay was lesser than IC_{50} value of AA. Both extracts at 250mcg/ml dose showed remarkable increase in the percentage of dead cancer cells (90% by EEDI and 86% by AEDI in DAL model and 89% by EEDI and 80% by AEDI in EAC model). ***Conclusion***: It is concluded from this study that *D.indica* L exhibited excellent antioxidant activity against the different *in vitro* antioxidant models and anticancer activity against the two different cell lines tested.

Introduction

Humans are exposed to free radicals in the environment through radiation and pollution. Free radicals are also produced naturally in the body through various metabolic reactions. These free radicals cause severe damage to cells, which can lead to degenerative diseases as well as premature ageing.[1] Antioxidants scavenge these free radicals and enable cells to rejuvenate or stabilize for the process of life.[2] Natural antioxidants increase the antioxidant capacity of the plasma and reduce the risk of certain diseases such as cancer, heart diseases and stroke.[3] The secondary metabolites like phenolics and flavonoids from plants have been reported to be potent free radical scavengers. Various species under Drosera belong to this category because of the presence of flavonoids in them.[4]

Drosera is a cosmopolitan genus of insectivorous plants and consists of approximately 170 species. In India, *Drosera indica* L., *Drosera burmannii* Vahl and *Drosera peltata* J.E.Sm.ex Wild have been reported to be present at different location. These species are used as vital components in the Ayurvedic preparation 'Swarnabhasma'(Golden ash). Swarnabhasma (gold ash) is used in several clinical manifestations including loss of memory, defective eyesight, infertility, overall body weakness and incidence of early aging. It is also used for the treatment of diseases like bronchial asthma, rheumatoid arthritis, diabetes mellitus and nervous disorders.[5] The aim of the present work was to evaluate *in vitro* antioxidant and anticancer potentials of the (EEDI) and aqueous (AEDI) extracts of *D. indica* L.

Material and Methods

Plant material

The whole plant of *D. indica* L was collected from the forests of Savanadurga, Karnataka, India during November 2010. The plant material was identified and authenticated by Dr. S.N.Yoganarasimhan, Taxonomist and Research Coordinator at M. S. Ramaiah College of Pharmacy, Bangalore, Karnataka,India (Herbarium

***Corresponding author:** Raju Asirvatham, Associate Professor, Department of Pharmacology, Shri Rawatpura Sarkar Institute of Pharmacy, Datia, Mathya Pradesh, India. Email: rajuasirvatham@gmail.com

specimen no: SRIP/COGNOSY/2011-04). The material was washed, shade dried, powdered, passed through sieve no. 60 and stored in air tight containers for further experiments.

Preparation of the extracts

Alcohol extract

A weighed quantity of the air-dried powdered drug was extracted with ethanol (90 %v/v) in a soxhlet apparatus. The extract was concentrated in a rotary flash evaporator at a temperature not exceeding 50°C. The ethanol extract (EEDI) was suspended in distilled water for experimental use.

Aqueous extract

The marc from the ethanol extract was macerated with chloroform- water for 24h to obtain the aqueous extract (AEDI). AEDI was concentrated under vacuum and dissolved in distilled water for experimental studies. Both the extracts were stored in air tight containers.

In vitro *antioxidant methods*

All the assays were performed in triplicate.

DPPH (1, 1 diphenyl 2, picrylhydrazyl) Method

To the methanol solution of DPPH (1mM), an equal volume of the extracts dissolved in alcohol was added at various concentrations from 5 to 640mcg/ml to obtain a final volume of 1.0 ml. An equal amount of alcohol was added to the control. After 20 min, absorbance was recorded at 517nm.[6]

Inhibition (%) = $(A_0 - A_1 / A_0) \times 100$

Where A_0 is the absorbance of control and A_1 is the absorbance of test.

Hydroxyl radical scavenging activity

Hydroxyl radical scavenging capacity of an extract is directly related to its antioxidant activity. This method involves *in vitro* generation of hydroxyl radicals using Fe^{3+}/ ascorbate/ EDTA/ H_2O_2 system by Fenton reaction. The hydroxyl radicals formed by the oxidation are made to react with DMSO (dimethyl sulphoxide) to yield formaldehyde. Formaldehyde formed produces intense yellow color with Nash reagent (2M ammonium acetate with 0.05M acetic acid and 0.02M acetyl acetone in distilled water), the intensity of which was measured at 412nm spectrophotometrically against reagent blank.[7]

HRSA (%) = 1-(Differences in absorbance of sample/Difference in absorbance of blank) X100

Nitric oxide radical scavenging

Sodium nitroprusside 5 mM was prepared in phosphate buffer pH 7.4. To 1 ml of various concentrations of test extracts, sodium nitroprusside 0.3 ml was added. The test tubes were incubated at 25 °C for 5 hours after which, 0.5 ml of Griess reagent was added. The absorbance of the chromophore was read at 546nm.[8]

Inhibition (%) = $(A_0 - A_1 / A_0) \times 100$

Where A_0 is the absorbance of control and A_1 is the absorbance of test.

Metal chelating activity

Various concentrations of EEDI and AEDI were added with 1 ml of 2mM $FeCl_2$ separately. The reaction was initiated by the addition of 5 mM ferrozine (1 ml). Absorbance was measured at 562nm after 10min.[9]

Inhibition (%) = $(A_0 - A_1 / A_0) \times 100$

Where A_0 is the absorbance of control and A_1 is the absorbance of test.

Reducing power Assay

1ml of the extracts were mixed with 2.5 ml of phosphate buffer (200 mM, pH 6.6) and 2.5 ml of potassium ferric cyanide (30 mM) and incubated at 50°C for 20 min. Thereafter, 2.5 ml of trichloroacetic acid (600 mM) was added to the reaction mixture, centrifuged for 10 min at 3000 rpm. The upper layer of solution (2.5 ml) was mixed with 2.5 ml of distilled water and 0.5 ml of $FeCl_3$ (6 mM) and absorbance was measured at 700nm.[10]

Inhibition (%) = $(A_0 - A_1 / A_0) \times 100$

Where A_0 is the absorbance of control and A_1 is the absorbance of test.

Superoxide scavenging

The superoxide anion radicals were generated in a mixture containing 0.5 ml of NBT (0.3mM), 0.5 ml NADH (0.936 mM) solution, 1.0 ml extract and 0.5 ml Tris-HCl buffer (16 mM, pH 8.0). The reaction was started by the addition of 0.5 ml PMS (Phenazine methosulphate) solution (0.12 mM) to the mixture, which was then incubated at 25°C for 5 min and the absorbance was measured at 560 nm against a blank sample.[8]

Inhibition (%) = $(A_0 - A_1 / A_0) \times 100$

Where A_0 is the absorbance of control and A_1 is the absorbance of test.

ABTS radical scavenging assay

To the reaction mixture containing 0.3 ml of ABTS radical, 1.7 ml phosphate buffer and 0.5 ml extract was added at various concentrations from 2 to 500mcg/ml. Blank was carried out without drug. Absorbance was recorded at 734nm.[11]

Inhibition (%) = $(A_0 - A_1 / A_0) \times 100$

Where A_0 is the absorbance of control and A_1 is the absorbance of test.

In Vitro *anticancer activity*

Short term cytotoxicity was assessed by Trypan blue exclusion method and Lactate dehydrogenase (LDH) leakage assay.[12]

Trypan blue exclusion method

Trypan blue dye assay method[13, 14] was carried out to evaluate the in vitro cytotoxicity potentials of both alcohol and aqueous extracts of *D. indica* L. EEDI and

AEDI were dissolved in distilled water. Different concentrations (5, 10, 50, 100, 150 and 250mcg/ml) of both extracts were prepared. In a test tube, 100µl of plant extract was mixed with 800µl of phosphate buffer saline and 100µl ($1X10^6$ in 1ml) of Dalton's Ascitic Lymphoma (DAL) was added. Similar method was followed with Ehrlich Ascitic Carcinoma (EAC) cell line also. Each concentration of the extracts was tested in triplicate. All the samples were incubated at 37°C in an incubator for 30min. About 100µl of tryphan blue dye was added to all the test tubes and the number of dead cells was counted in a haemocytometer under a compound microscope. Percentage of cytotoxicity was calculated by the following formula.
% dead cells = Number of dead cells/Sum of dead cells and living cell × 100.

Lactate Dehydrogenase (LDH) leakage assay
LDH leakage assay was carried out using LDH cytotoxicity detection kit by Sigma Aldrich Inc., USA, according to protocol in the user's manual. To determine IC_{50}, different concentrations of herbal extracts were incubated with 100 µl of DAL and EAC cell suspensions having 1x 10^6 cell /ml in 96 well plates and incubated at 37°C for 4 hrs in 5% CO_2 atmosphere. All the control and test substances were tested in triplicates and mean ± SEM of the absorbance values were recorded to calculate the cytotoxicity.
LDH leakage (%) related to control wells containing cell culture medium without extracts was calculated by [A] test / [A] control X100. Where [A]test is the absorbance of the test sample and[A]control is the absorbance of the control sample.

Statistical Analysis
All the assays coming under in vitro antioxidant and anticancer assay were performed in triplicate and the results were expressed as mean± standard deviation.

Results
Concentrations ranging from 5 to 640 mcg/ml of the ethanol and aqueous extracts of *D.indica* L were tested for their antioxidant properties in different *in vitro* models. The percentage of inhibition was observed that free radicals were scavenged by the test compounds in a concentration dependent manner up to the given concentration in all the models (Table 1).

Table 1. *In vitro* Antioxidant assay of EEDI and AEDI

S no.	*In vitro* Model	Extract Concentration Used (mcg/ml)	IC_{50} Concentration of EEDI (mcg)	IC_{50} Concentration of AEDI (mcg)	IC_{50} Concentration of AA (mcg)
1	DPPH Assay		112.5±0.54	264.21±1.57	170±1.42
2	Hydroxyl Scavenging Activity		34.8±0.43	112.71±0.82	76.8±0.35
3	NO Scavenging Assay		58.41±1.3	180.59±0.46	85.71±0.82
4	Fe2+ Chelating Assay	5,10,20,40,80,160,320,640	96.32±0.45	94.51±0.84	110.03±1.02
5	Reducing Power Assay		152.8±0.98	418.32±0.88	95.56±0.78
6	Super Oxide Radical Assay		88.76±0.79	105.37±0.72	160.78±0.26
7.	Radical Scavenging of ABTS		122.7±0.13	321.8±0.62	110.12±0.18

The percentage of scavenging effect on DPPH radical was increased with an increase in concentration of EEDI and AEDI. The percentage inhibition of EEDI was varying from 10% with 5mcg/ml of the extract to 85% with 640 mcg/ml of extract. Similarly the percentage inhibition of AEDI was varying from 6% with 5mcg/ml of the extract to72% with 640mcg/ml of extract. The IC_{50} value of the EEDI and AEDI was calculated to be 112.5±0.54mcg/ml and 264.21±1.57mcg/ml while for the standard ascorbic acid was 170±1.42mcg/ml.
The hydroxyl radical scavenging activity also increased with increase in the concentrations of both extracts. The IC_{50} values of EEDI and AEDI were calculated to be 112.5±0.54 and 264.21±1.57mcg/ml, while that for ascorbic acid was 170±1.42mcg/ml.
The percentage of inhibition in nitric oxide scavenging assay was maximum (94% and 72%) at 640mcg/ml of EEDI and AEDI respectively. The IC_{50} value of the EEDI and AEDI was calculated to be 58.41±1.3 and 180.59±0.46mcg/ml while that for standard ascorbic acid was 85.71±0.82mcg/ml.
In reducing power assay, antioxidant compound forms a colored complex with potassium ferricyanide, trichloro acetic acid and ferric chloride, which is measured at 700nm, where in presence of reductants (antioxidants) in the plant extracts, causes the reduction of Fe^{3+}/ Ferricyanide complex to the ferrous form. The IC_{50} values of EED1 (152.8±0.98) was found to be lesser than that of AEDI (418.32±0.88), indicating that EEDI has more reducing power than AEDI.
In metal chelating assay, ferrozine quantitatively forms complexes with Fe^{2+}. The absorbance of ferrozine-Fe^{2+} complex decreased linearly in a dose-dependent manner. Chelating agents that forms bonds with a metal are effective as secondary antioxidants because they reduce the redox potential, and thereby stabilize the oxidized form of the metal ion. In the present work, EEDI was found to reduce inhibitory concentration (96.32±0.45) as compared to AEDI (94.51±0.84),

whereas standard ascorbic acid showed at a concentration of 110.03±1.02.

Superoxide free radicals were scavenged with the increase in the concentration of EEDI and AEDI. The IC_{50} were calculated to be 88.76±0.79mcg/ml and 105.37±0.72mcg/ml where the standard ascorbic acid was 160.78±0.26mcg/ml.

The principle behind the ABTS assay technique involves the reaction between ABTS and potassium persulphate to produce the ABTS radical cation ($ABTS^+$), a blue green chromogen. In the presence of extracts, the colored radical is converted back to colorless ABTS, the absorbance of which is measured at 734nm. The free radical scavenging activity by this method, showed significant inhibitory concentration with EEDI (122.7±0.13) comparable with that of ascorbic acid (110.12±0.18) whereas AEDI showed an inhibitory concentration of 321.8±0.62.

Anticancer activity of EEDI and AEDI against the test cells DAL and EAC by trypan blue exclusion and LDH leakage assay methods are shown in Figures 1 and 2 respectively. In trypan blue exclusion method, 250, 150,100 mcg/ml of EEDI showed more significant effect against DAL than AEDI towards both the cell lines, whereas 50, 10 and 5 mcg/ml EEDB and AEDB showed less significant effects on DAL and EAC. The inhibition concentration was compared with that of control. A dose dependent increase in the % of LDH leakage was observed. A maximum leakage of LDH was observed at a concentration of 250mcg/ml. From figure 2, the % of LDH release was increased with increasing concentration of EEDI which is in direct proportion to the cell death. Maximum cell death after incubation was observed at 250 mcg/ml concentration.

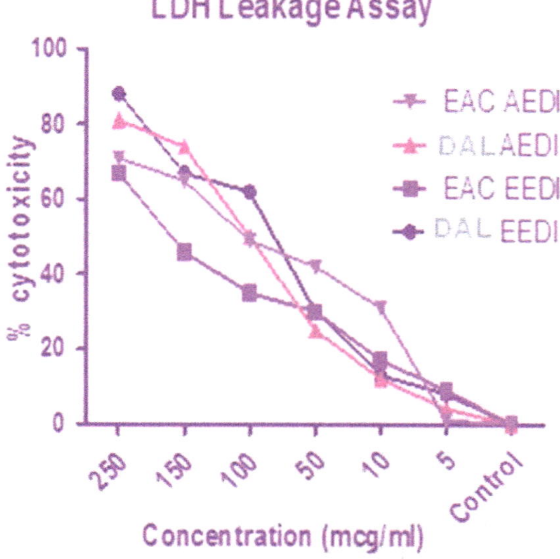

Figure 1. Anticancer activity of EEDI and AEDI against the DAL and EAC cells by LDH leakage assay

Discussion

Traditional Indian and Chinese medicinal herbs have been used in the treatment of different diseases in the country for centuries. There have been claims that some traditional healers can successfully treat cancer using herbal drugs.[15]

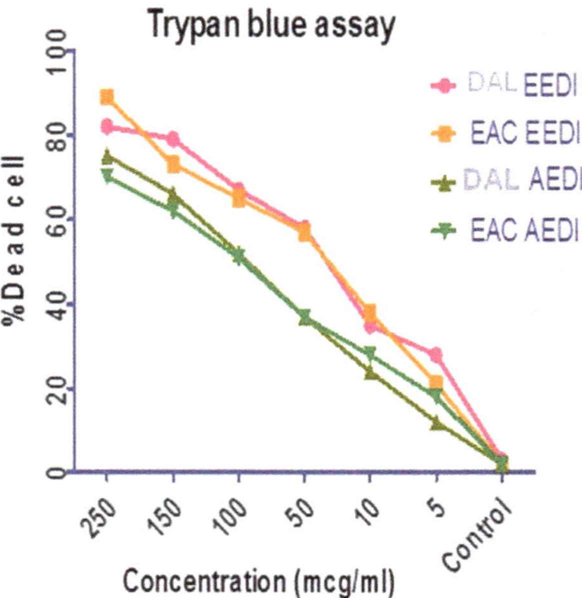

Figure 2. Anticancer activity of EEDI and AEDI against DAL and EAC cells by trypan blue exclusion method

In this study, it is evident that the extracts of *D.indica* L possess effective antioxidant and anticancer activities. This is due to the presence of phytochemicals like naphthoquinones, Quercetin etc. in this species.[16] In vitro antioxidant activity of the ethanol and aqueous extracts of *D.indica* L was investigated in the present study by DPPH, hydroxyl, ABTS, nitric oxide, superoxide radical scavenging assays, reducing power and metal chelating assay. These methods have proved the antioxidant potential of the extracts in comparison with the reference antioxidant, ascorbic acid.

DPPH assay, which is based on the reduction of DPPH in methanol solution, is converted into DPPHH (non radical) in the presence of a hydrogen–donating antioxidant. This transformation results in a color change from purple to yellow, which is measured spectrophotometrically. The disappearance of the purple color is monitored at 517nm. The DPPH, is a stable free radical and is widely used to assess the radical scavenging activity of antioxidant compounds.[9] In the present study, the scavenging effect of different concentrations of the extracts from 5 to 640mcg/ml, on the DPPH radical is illustrated. The extracts had increasing significant scavenging effect with increase in the concentration of both extracts EEDI and AEDI.

EEDI and AEDI showed significant scavenging effects on the hydroxyl radical, which increased with the increase in concentrations from 5-650 mcg/ml. The model used was ascorbic acid-iron-EDTA model of $HO^{\cdot}$ generating system. This is a totally aqueous system in which ascorbic acid, iron and EDTA conspire with each other to generate hydroxyl radicals. It reacts with polyunsaturated fatty acid moieties of cell membrane phospholipids and causes damage to cell. The formed hydroxyl radicals (HO˙) ions chelate with the antioxidants, which results in the suppression of OH generation and inhibition of peroxidation processes of biological molecules.[7, 9]

In nitric oxide scavenging assay, the radicals generated from sodium nitroprusside in aqueous solution at physiological pH interact with oxygen to produce nitrite ions which is estimated with Griess reagent.[17]

The metal ion scavenging effect was increasing with an increase in the concentrations of extracts from 5-640mcg/ml. The high metal ion scavenging activity of the EEDI and AEDI was probably due to the chelating agents, which form sigma bonds with the metal and are effective as secondary antioxidants because they reduce the redox potential, thereby oxidized form of the metal ion.[18]

Reducing power assay is serving as a significant reflection of the antioxidant activity.[19] Compounds with reducing power indicate that they are electron donors and can reduce the oxidized intermediates of lipid peroxidation processes, so that they can act as primary and secondary antioxidants.[20]

Super oxide is biologically important as it forms singlet oxygen and hydroxyl radical. Overproduction of super oxide anion radical contributes to redox imbalance and is associated with harmful physiological consequences. Numerous biological reactions generate superoxide anions which are highly toxic. In the PMS/NADH-NBT system, superoxide anion derived from dissolved oxygen from PMS/NADH coupling reaction reduces NBT.[8] The decrease of absorbance at 560 nm with antioxidants thus indicates the consumption of superoxide anion in the reaction mixture. From the results, it was found that the EEDI and AEDI showed potent free radical scavenging activity compared to the ascorbic acid (standard) at low IC_{50}.

LDH is a more reliable and accurate marker of cytotoxicity, because damaged cells are fragmented completely during the course of prolonged incubation with substances. In the present study, the LDH leakage increased significantly in high dose of when compared AEDI to the control cells. Extensive reports have documented on medicinal plant extract induced cytotoxicity to cancer cells.[21] Hence, the LDH leakage in both cell lines may be due to the cytotoxic nature of the plant extract which confirms its antitumor activity.

Trypan blue is a vital stain used in the identification of dead tissue or cells. Living cells or tissues with intact cell membrane are not colored, because the dye is not absorbed through the intact cell membrane. However it traverses the membrane of dead cells. Hence dead cells are shown as a distinctive blue color under the microscope. In the trypan blue exclusion assay, there is a dose dependent inhibitory effect on both cancer cell lines treated with the extracts at increasing concentrations (5- 250mcg/ml) for 30min.After incubation with extracts significantly affected with cytotoxic values at the maximum concentration of 250mcg/ml. The % of cytotoxicity was in the following order: EEDI against DLA (90%), EEDI against EAC (89%), AEDI against DLA (86%) and AEDI against EAC (80%).

Conclusion

The results of the present study indicate that the EEDI and AEDI of *D. indica* L possess significant antioxidant and anticancer activities when tested against different in vitro models. The antioxidant ability could be attributed to the phenolic compounds, especially flavonoids which possess antioxidant action.[22] Thus, *D. indica* L extracts as promising natural sources of antioxidants and anticancer agent, can be used in nutritional or pharmaceutical fields for the prevention of free radical mediated diseases.

Conflict of Interest

There is no conflict of interest in this study.

References

1. Patel RP, Cornwell T, Darley-Usmar VM. The biochemistry of nitric oxide and peroxynitrite: implications for mitochondrial function. In: Packer L, Cadenas E, editors. *Understanding the process of aging: the roles of mitochondria, free radicals, and antioxidants.* New York: Marcel Dekker; 1999. P. 39-56.
2. Murali A, Ashok P, Madhavan V. Antioxidant activity of leaf of Hemidesmusindicus (L.) R. Br. var. pubescens (W. A.) Hk.f. (Periplocaceae) - an in vivo analysis. *Spatula DD* 2011; 1(2): 91-100.
3. Prior RL, Cao G. Antioxidant phytochemicals in fruits and vegetables; diet health implications Horticultural. *Science* 2000; 35: 588-92.
4. Asirvatham R, Christina AJM. Drosera indica L: Potential effect on liver enzyme, lipid profile and hormone change in Dalton's lymphoma ascites (DLA) bearing mice. *J Intercult Ethnopharmacol* 2012; 1(2): 69-73.
5. Asirvatham R, Christina AJM. Anticancer activity of Drosera indica L., on Dalton's Lymphoma Ascites (DLA) bearing mice. *J Intercult Ethnopharmacol* 2012; 1(3).
6. Al-Tahtawy RHM, El-Bastawesy AM, Monem MGA, Zekry ZK, Al-Mehdar HA, El-Merzabani MM. Antioxidant activity of the volatile oils of zingiber officinale (ginger). *Spatula DD* 2011;1(1):1-8.
7. Klein SM, Cohen G, Cederaum AI. Production of formaldehyde during metabolism of dimethyl sulphoxide by hydroxyl radical generating system. *Biochem* 1991; 20: 6006-12.
8. Basniwal PK, Suthar M, Rathore GS, Gupta R, Kumar V, Pareek A, et al. In vitro antioxidant activity of hot aqueous extract of Helicteresisora Linn. Fruits. Nat prod radiance 2009; 8(5): 483-7.

9. Thambiraj J, Paulsamy S, Sevukaperumal R. Evaluation of *in vitro* antioxidant activity in the traditional medicinal shrub of western districts of Tamilnadu, India, Acalypha fruticosa Forssk. (Euphorbiaceae). *Asian Pac J Trop Biomedicine* 2012; 2(1): S127-30.
10. Makari HK, Haraprasad N, Patil H, Ravikumar S. In vitro antioxidant activity of the hexane and methanolic extracts of *Cordiawallichii* and *Celastruspaniculata*. *Internet J Aesthetic Antiaging Med* 2008; 1: 1-10.
11. Weijuan Han, Xican Li. Antioxidant activity of aloeswood tea in vitro. *Spatula DD* 2012; 2(1):43-50.
12. Decker T, Lohaman-Matthes ML. A quick and simple method for the quantitation of lactate dehydrogenase release in measurements of cellular cytotoxicity and tumor necrosis factor (TNF) activity. *J Immunol Methods* 1988; 115(1): 61-9.
13. Gupta SK. Cytotoxicity Assays. In: Talwar GP, Gupta SK, Editors. *A Handbook of practical and Clinical Immunology*. New Delhi: CBS; 2002. P. 299-300.
14. Rajkapoor B, Jayakar B, Murugesh N. Antitumour activity of *bauhinia variegata* on dalton's ascitic lymphoma. *J Ethnopharmacol* 2003;89(1):107-9.
15. Balakrishnan S, Manmeet SS, Ajay Sh, Namita M. Anti-tumor effect of acetone extract of Madhucalongifolia against Ehrlich Ascites Carcinoma (EAC) in mice. *Phytopharmacol* 2012; 3(1): 130-6.
16. Asirvatham R, Christina AJM, Anita M. Antitumor activity of ethanol and aqueous extracts of Drosera burmannii vahl. in EAC bearing mice. *Spatula DD* 2012; 2(2):83-8.
17. Chanda S, Dave R. In vitro models for antioxidant activity evaluation and some medicinal plants possessing antioxidant properties: An overview. *Afr J Microbiol Res* 2009; 3(13): 981-96.
18. Gulcin I, Beydemir S, Alici HA, Elmastas M, Buyukokuroglu ME. In vitro antioxidant properties of morphine. *Pharmacol res* 2004;49(1):59-66.
19. Oktay M, Gulcin I, Kufrevioglu OI. Determination of in vitro antioxidant activity of fennel (Foeniculumvulgare) seed extracts. *Leb-Wissen Technol* 2003; 36: 263-71.
20. Yen GC, Chen HY. Antioxidant activity of various tea extracts in relation to their antimutagenicity. *J Agric Food Chem* 1995; 43: 27-32.
21. Sivalokanathan S, Vijayababu MR, Balasubramanian MP. Effects of terminalia arjuna bark extract on apoptosis of human hepatoma cell line hepG2. *World J Gastroenterol* 2006; 12(7): 1018-24.
22. Anandakumar AM, Paulsamy S, Sathishkumar P, Senthilkumar P. Preliminary phytochemical studies for the quantification of secondary metabolites of medicinal importance in the plant Acalypha fruticosa Forssk. *J Appl Nat Sci* 2009; 1(1): 41-3.

15

Oreganum vulgare Linn. leaf: An Extensive Pharmacognostical and Phytochemical Quality Assessment

Veni Bharti, Neeru Vasudeva*

Department of Pharmaceutical Sciences, Guru Jambheshwer University of Science and Technology, Hisar, Haryana, India.

ARTICLE INFO

Keywords:
Oreganum vulgare Linn.
Phytochemical screening
Standardization
Traditional medicine

ABSTRACT

Purpose: Standardization and detailed pharmacognostical studies of *Oreganum vulgare* Linn. leaf for authentication and commercial utilization. ***Methods:*** *Oreganum vulgare* Linn. leaf was with standardization according to standard procedures described in WHO, 2011 and I.P. 1996. ***Results:*** The physicochemical parameters total ash, acid insoluble ash, water soluble ash and sulphated ash were found to be 11.5%, 11%, 5, 10.5% w/w respectively. Foaming index was found be <100. The trace elements were found to be copper, lead, cadmium, zinc, cobalt, manganese, nickel and copper in ethanol extract and phytochemical screening of aqueous and ethanol extract showed the presence of carbohydrates, flavonoids, anthocyanins, phenolic compounds etc. ***Conclusion:*** The standardization parameters viz. physico-chemical parameters, macroscopy, microscopy, taxonomy, anatomy and preliminary phytochemical screening, microbial and aflatoxin count, HPTLC profile is being reported to help in authentication and development of monograph of this plant.

Introduction

The use of medicines from natural resources is as old as evolutionary history of human being. Primitive man started using these herbs by hit and trial method and distinguished whether which combination of herbs is effective in treating any ailment or which is exerting toxicity. Plants are defined as 'biochemical factories' producing bio-chemicals responsible for therapeutic activity or toxicological effect. 80% of the world's population especially in developing countries is dependent on herbal medicines because of less side effects, easy availability and economic.[1,2] Herbal drugs are still at the risk of quality because sources of raw material of herbal drugs are different and an herb is mixture of multi-constituents, and lack of availability of efficient analytical methods. Hence, it is necessary to set official standards to maintain quality, the first step of which must be identification of entire constituents and physicochemical parameters in herbs.[3]

Oreganum vulgare Linn. (Lamiaceae) commonly known as Oregano, is used traditionally as expectorant and spasmolitic agent, as diuretic and antiseptic agent and in dermatological affections.[4,5] In the present paper an attempt was made to standardize and identify phytochemical profile.

Materials and Methods

Plant material

Oreganum vulgare leaves were procured from Aum Agreefresh Pvt. Ltd. and were identified by the same company. The voucher specimen (Pcog1101) was deposited in Department of Pharmaceutical sciences, Guru Jambheshwar University of Science & Technology for future references. The leaves were powdered with the help of a pulvarizer and used for all the studies.

Pharmacognostical Evaluation

Morphological characters like colour, surface texture, odour were examined according to Trease.[6] Organoleptic evaluation, physicochemical parameters viz; ash values, extractive values, heavy metals, microbial counts, phytochemical screening was performed.[6-11]

Transverse section of leaf was performed by free hand sectioning. The transverse sections and coarsely powdered leaves were cleared with chloral hydrate, stained with phloroglucinol and concentrated HCl, mounted in glycerol and studied under microscope for transverse section and powder studies respectively.

Both ethanol and aqueous extracts were analysed for nine elements by atomic absorption microscopy.[10]

Phytochemical screening

For phytochemical screening, aqueous extract was prepared by soaking 20 g of crude drug with 200 ml of distilled water and kept for 24 h. the extract was filtered and concentrated in rotary vacuum evaporator. Ethanol extract was prepared by soaking 20 g of crude drug with 200 ml of ethanol and kept for 24 h. the extract was filtered and concentrated in rotary vacuum evaporator.

***Corresponding author:** Neeru Vasudeva, Department of Pharmaceutical Sciences, Guru Jambheshwer University of Science and Technology, Hisar-125001, Haryana, India. Email: neeruvasudeva@gmail.com

Both the extracts were tested for presence of different chemical constituents viz. alkaloids, glycosides, carbohydrates, sterols, phenolic compounds, tannins, flavonoids, saponins, proteins and free amino acids (Table 1).[12-14]

Table 1. Preliminary phytochemical screening of ethanol and aqueous extracts

Plant Constituents /Reagent used		Leaf extract Ethanol	Leaf extract Aqueous
Alkaloids	Dragendroff's reagent	-	-
	Wagner's reagent	-	-
	Hager's reagent	-	-
	Mayer's reagent	-	-
Carbohydrates	Molish test	+	-
	Fehling's reagent	+	+
	Bennedict 's reagent	+	+
	Test for Pentose	-	-
	Charring test	+	+
Glycosides	General test	+	+
Anthraquinone	Borntrager test	+	+
	Modified Borntrager's test	-	-
Cardiac Glycosides	Legal test	-	-
	Baljet test	-	-
	Killer killani test	-	-
Steroids	Salkovaski test	+	-
	Libermann Burchard's test	+	-
Coumarins	Ferric chloride test	+	+
	Fluorescence test	-	-
Cynophoric glycosides	Sodium Picrate test	-	-
Phenolic compounds and Tannins	Matchstick test	+	+
	Chlorgenic acid test	+	+
	Ferric chloride test	+	+
	Lead acetate test	+	+
	Gelatin test	-	-
	Bromine water test	-	-
	Vanillin HCl test	+	+
Phlobatannins	HCl test	-	-
Saponins	Foam test	-	-
	RBC Haemolysis test	-	-
Chalcones	Ammonium Hydroxide test	-	-
Flavonoids	Alkaline reagent test	+	+
	Shinoda test	-	-
	Vannilin HCl test	+	+
	Ammonia test	-	-
Flavanonols	Zinc powder test	+	+
Flavonols	Boric acid test	-	-
Flavones, Flavanones, Flavolol	Sulphuric acid test	-	-
Anthocyanins	Sulphuric acid test	+	+
Leucoanthocyanins	Vanillin test	-	-
Gelatin	Solubility test	-	-
	Soda lime test	-	-
	Precipitation test	-	-
Lipids	Solubility test	-	-
	Grease spot test	-	-
	Emulsification test	-	-
Starch	Jelly test	-	-
Lignin	Phloroglucinol test	-	-
Proteins	Trichloroacetic acid	-	-
	Xanthoproteic test	-	-
	Ninhydrin test	-	-
	Lead sulphid test	-	-
	Biuret test	-	-
Free amino acids	Ninhydrin test	-	-
	Phenolic amino acid test	-	-
Resins	Solubility test	-	-
	Hydrochloric test	-	-
	Ferric chloride test	-	-
	Turbidity test	-	-

+ present, - negative

HPTLC profiling

The solvent system used was Toluene: Ethylacetate (5:1.5). After selecting solvent system for each fraction HPTLC studies was done by using 10×10 cm of glass Plates, CAMAG TLC Scanner3 "Scanner3_130716 (1.14.26) attached with UV detector of D2 &W lamp with 281 V, second order optical fibre at 366 nm and controlled by win CATS software.[15]

Results

Pharmacognostic Evaluation

Macroscopic examination

The leaves are dark green in color; oblong ovate in shape; bract hairs are absent; texture is smooth; corolla color is white; calyx is of green color; calyx hairs are sparse; taste: astringent.

Microscopy of leaf powder

Microscopic examination of leaf powder showed the presence of diacytic stomata, glandular and non-glandular trichomes (Figure 1).

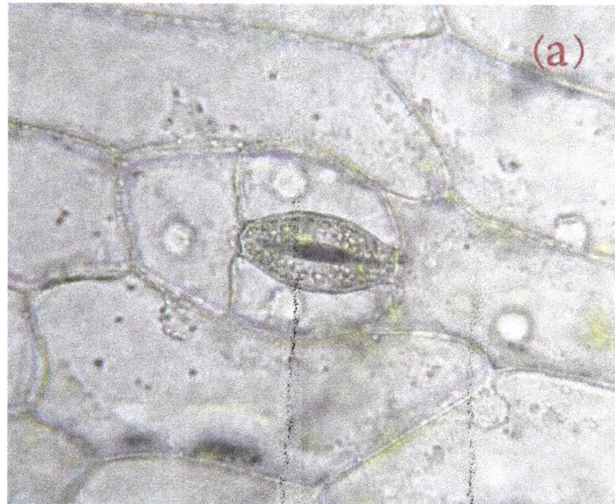

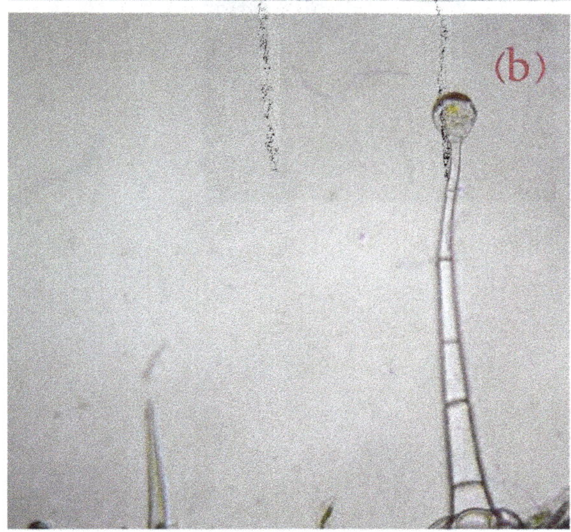

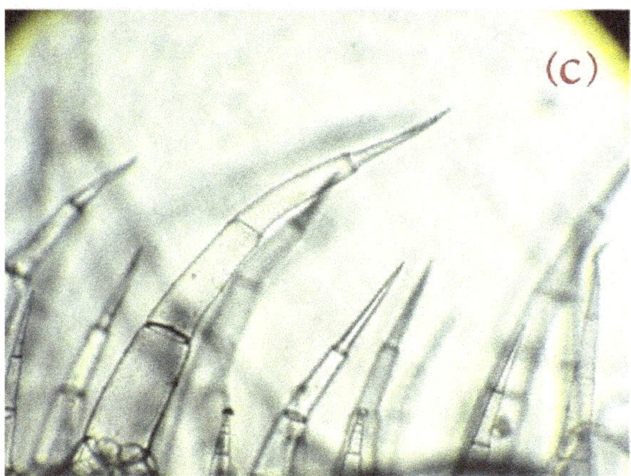

Figure 1. Microscopy of leaf powder (a) diacytic stomata (b) trichomes (c) non-glandular trichomes.

Microscopy (T.S. of leaf)

The transverse section of leaf showed the presence of single layered epidermis with multicellular epidermal hairs, a layer of cuticle and amphistomatic stomata were observed. There was clear cut discrimination between palisade and spongy Parenchymatous cells of Mesophyll. The palisade cells were single layered and columnar. Spongy cells were found to be scattered and loosely arranged. Vascular bundles were conjoint, collateral and closed (Figure 2).

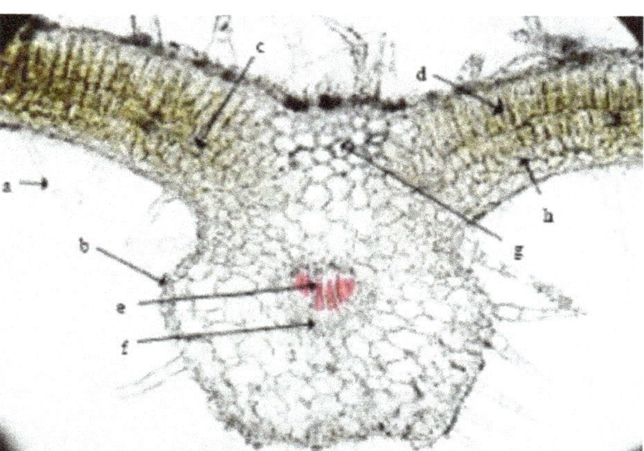

Figure 2. Microscopy T.S. of leaf (a= trichome, b= epidermis, c= mesophyll, d= palisade cells, e= xylem vessel, f= phloem, g= collenchyma).

Determination of physicochemical parameters

The physicochemical parameters total ash, acid insoluble ash, water soluble ash and sulphated ash were found to be 11.5%, 11%, 5, 10.5% w/w respectively. The extractive values of ethanol extract and aqueous extract by hot extraction method were found to be 0.003% and 0.02% w/w respectively and that of by cold extraction method were found to be 0.003%, 0.02% w/w respectively. Swelling index was found to be zero. The drug was not found to be bitter. The foaming index was found to be <100. The % moisture content was found to be 6%. % of volatile oil was found to be 1.67% v/w. crude fiber content was found to be 75% w/w.

Elemental analysis

The Atomic absorption spectroscopy study showed the presence of lead, cadmium, zinc, cobalt, manganese, nickel and copper in ethanol and aqueous extract of leaf but below the permissible limits of WHO and hence are safe to use.

Microbial contamination

The aqueous and ethanol extracts of leaf of *Oreganum vulgare* showed the complete absence of *E.coli, S.typhi, P.aerginosa, S.aureus, Clostridia, Shigella.* Total bacterial count was found to be $<10^3$ and $<10^4$ for ethanol and aqueous extracts respectively.

Preliminary phytochemical screening

The ethanol and aqueous extracts showed the presence of carbohydrates, anthraquinones, coumarins, Phenolic compounds and tannins, flavonoids, flavanonols and anthocyanins. Alkaloids, saponins, cardiac glycosides, lignin, starch, resins, free amino acids and lipids were absent in both ethanol and aqueous extracts.

HPTLC studies

HPTLC profile was developed for ethanol extract of leaf as a preliminary fingerprinting of the extract. Toluene: ethylacetate (5:1.5) was found to be a suitable solvent system for the separation of constituents of leaf extract. Ten spots were observed in HPTLC profiling of ethanol extract of *Oreganum vulgare* at 254 nm with R_f values of 0.15, 0.16, 0.26, 0.51, 0.58, 0.66, 0.71, 0.75, 0.83 and 0.89 respectively while fifteen spots were observed at 366 nm with R_f values of 0.16, 0.18, 0.25, 0.32, 0.36, 0.38, 0.50, 0.56, 0.58, 0.66, 0.71, 0.75, 0.79, 0.83 and 0.93 respectively indicating the presence of different constituents. HPTLC images and data are shown in Figure 3.

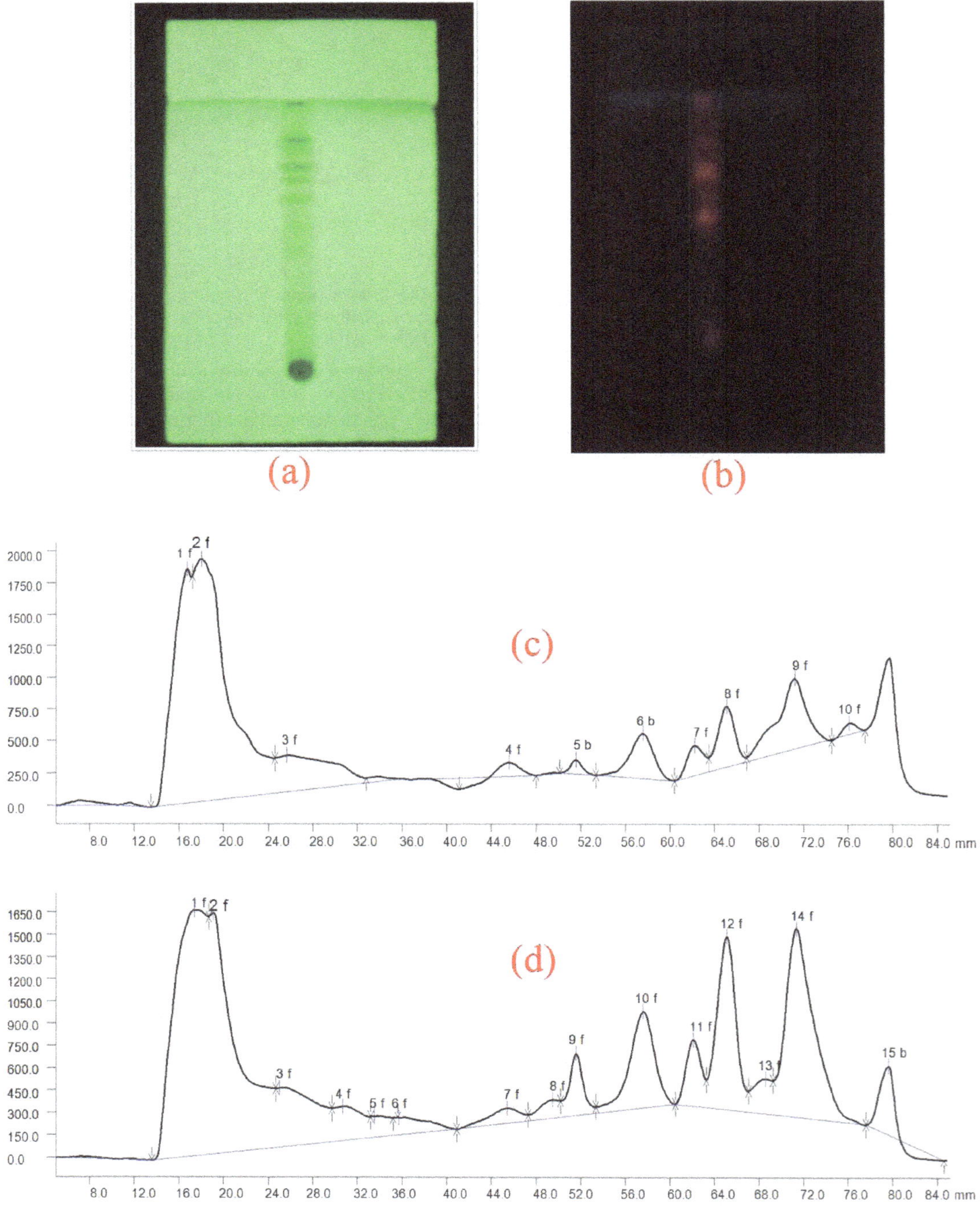

Figure 3. HPTLC profiling of ethanol extract of *Oreganum vulgare* in solvent system Toluene: Ethylacetate (5:1.5) at (a) 254 nm (b) 366 nm (c) R_f value determination at 254 nm (d) R_f value determination at 366 nm.

Discussion

Oreganum vulgare Linn. belonging to family Lamiaceae is commonly known as "Pizza herb" and is commonly served as food material in Lebanese, Italian and Mexican cuisines. It is a perennial herb, distributed among temperate, tropical and subtropical regions. Microscopic analysis and qualitative parameters are carried out in order to establish appropriate data that can be used in identifying crude drug. The phytochemical screening of the test plant was done for their active components present for their medicinal values. Many of the phytochemical tests showed positive results which render the presence of their active compounds. The Total ash, acid insoluble ash, water-soluble ash values and sulfated ash of leaves were observed to be 11.5%, 11%, 5, 10.5% w/w respectively while in a similar study carried out on stem and leaf of *Oreganum vulgare* 10.6%, 5.6%, 0.47% and 9.4% w/w respectively. The microscopic and macroscopic features were found to be same in previous and present study.[16] The present study provides extensive details about microbial count, heavy metal analysis, HPTLC profiling, phytochemical screening, powder studies and physico-chemical features.

Conclusion

Since the plant, *Oreganum vulgare* which is also used for the treatment of various diseases and disorders, it is important to standardize it for use as a drug. The pharmacognostic constants for the leaves of this plant, the diagnostic microscopic features and the numerical standardization parameters reported in this work could be useful for the compilation of a suitable monograph for its proper identification.

Conflict of interest

We declare that we do not have any conflict of interest.

Acknowledgements

We are thankful to Department of Pharmaceutical Sciences, Guru Jambheshwer University of Science & Technology, Hisar, India for providing facilities to conduct this research.

References

1. Mukherjee PK. *Quality Control of Herbal Drugs: An approach to evaluation of botanicals*. 1st ed. New Delhi: Business Horizons; 2002.
2. Bisset NG, Wichtl M. *Herbal Drugs and Phytopharmaceuticals*. 2nd ed. Boca Raton: CRC Press; 1994.
3. Kunle OF, Egharevba HO, Ahmadu PO. Standardization of herbal medicines - A review. *Int J Biodivers Conserv* 2012; 4: 101-12.
4. Blumenthal M, Brusse WR, Goldberg A, Gruenwald J, Hall T, Riggins CW, et al. *The Complete German Commission E Monographs*. Austin TX: American Botanical Council; 1998.
5. Bruneton J. Coumarins. In: Bruneton J, editor. *Pharmacognosy, Phytochemistry, Medicincal Plants*. Paris: Lavoisier Publishing Inc; 1999. P. 263-7.
6. Trease GE, Evans WC. *Pharmacognosy*. 12th ed. East Bourne : Bailliere Tindall; 1983.
7. Kokoski CJ, Kokoski RJ, Slama FJ. Fluorescence of powdered vegetable drugs under ultraviolet radiation. *J Am Pharm Assoc Am Pharm Assoc (Baltim)* 1958;47(10):715-7.
8. Wallis TE. *TextBook of Pharmacognosy*. 5th ed. New Delhi: CBS Publishers and Distributors; 1985.
9. Government of India. Indian Pharmacopoeia. 4th ed. New Delhi, India: Controller of Publication; 1996.
10. Who. Quality control methods for herbal materials. Updated ed. Geneva: World Health Organization; 2011.
11. Brinda PB, Sasikala P, Purusothaman KK. Pharmacognostic studies on Merugan kizhangu. *Bull Med Eth bot Res* 1981; 3: 884-96.
12. Goyal RK, Shah SA, Mehta AA. *Practicals in Biochemistry and Clinical Pathology*. 1st ed. Ahmedabad : Shah prakashan; 1997.
13. Kokate CK. *Practical Pharmacognosy*. 4th ed. New Delhi: Vallabh Prakashan; 1994.
14. Kar A. *Pharmacognosy and Pharmaco-biotechnology*. New Delhi: New Age International (P) Ltd.; 2003.
15. Sethi PD. *High performance thin layer chromatography: Quantitative analysis of pharmaceutical formulations*. New Delhi: CBS Publishers; 1996.
16. Prathyusha P, Subramanian MS, Nisha MC, Santhanakrishnan R, Seena MS. Pharmacognostical and phytochemical studies on Origanum vulgare L.(Laminaceae). *Anc sci life* 2009;29(2):17-23.

Protective Effect against Hydroxyl-induced DNA Damage and Antioxidant Activity of Radix Glycyrrhizae (Liquorice Root)

Xican Li[1]*, Weikang Chen[1], Dongfeng Chen[2]

[1] *School of Chinese Herbal Medicine, Guangzhou University of Chinese Medicine, Guangzhou, China.*

[2] *School of Basic Medical Science, Guangzhou University of Chinese Medicine, Guangzhou, China.*

ARTICLEINFO

Keywords:
Radix *Glycyrrhizae*
Liquorice root
DNA oxidative damage
Total flavonoids
Radical-scavenging

ABSTRACT

Purpose: As a typical Chinese herbal medicine, Radix *Glycyrrhizae* (RG) possesses various pharmacological effects involved in antioxidant ability. However, its antioxidant has not been explored so far. The aim of the study was to investigate its antioxidant ability, then further discuss the antioxidant mechanism. ***Methods***: RG was extracted by ethanol to obtain ethanolic extract of Radix *Glycyrrhizae* (ERG). ERG was then determined by various antioxidant methods, including DNA damage assay, DPPH assay, ABTS assay, Fe^{3+}-reducing assay and Cu^{2+}-reducing assay. Finally, the contents of total phenolics and total flavonoids were analyzed by spectrophotometric methods. ***Results***: Our results revealed that ERG could effectively protect against hydroxyl-induced DNA damage (IC_{50} 517.28±26.61μg/mL). In addition, ERG could scavenge DPPH· radical (IC_{50}165.18±6.48μg/mL) and $ABTS^{+}$• radical (IC_{50}7.46±0.07μg/mL), reduce Fe^{3+} (IC_{50} 97.23±2.88 μg/mL) and Cu^{2+} (IC_{50} 59.21±0.18 μg/mL). Chemical analysis demonstrated that the contents of total phenolics and flavonoids in ERG were 111.48±0.88 and 218.26±8.57 mg quercetin/g, respectively. ***Conclusion***: Radix *Glycyrrhizae* can effectively protect against hydroxyl-induced DNA damage. One mechanism of protective effect may be radical-scavenging which is via donating hydrogen atom (H·), donating electron (e). Its antioxidant ability can be mainly attributed to the flavonoids or total phenolics.

Introduction

It is well known that reactive oxygen species (ROS) are various forms of activated oxygen including free radicals and non-free-radical species. As an important form of ROS, hydroxyl radical (·OH), for example, can cause oxidative damage to DNA, which leads to severe biological consequences including mutation, cell death, carcinogenesis, and aging.[1]

Therefore, it is critical to search for potential therapeutic agents for DNA oxidative damage. In recent years, medicinal plants especially Chinese medicinal herbals have attracted much attention.

As a typical Chinese herbal medicine, Radix *Glycyrrhizae* (RG) or liquorice root (甘草 in Chinese, Figure 1A) has been used in traditional Chinese medicine (TCM) for about 2000 years.[2,3] RG is the dried radixs of *Glycyrrhiza uralensis* Fisch. (Figure 1B), *Glycyrrhiza inflata* Bat., or *Glycyrrhiza glabra* L. From the viewpoint of traditional Chinese medicine (TCM), RG can invigorate *spleen,* replenish *qi,* clear *heat* and remove toxic substance.[3]

Modern medicine indicated that RG possessed various pharmacological effects. It was reported that RG could be used as an effective detoxifying agent and it exerted its detoxifying activity maybe via effects on the function and expression of P-glycoprotein in Caco-2 Cells;[4] Fu suggested that RG and its bioactive components presented neuroprotective effect;[5] Wang pointed out that RG possessed antiviral activity.[6] In addition, RG also showed anti-inflammatory,[7,8] antitumor and antibiosis effects.[9] Based on free radical biology & medicine,[10] we assumed that these pharmacological effects may be associated with antioxidant ability. However, its antioxidant ability has not been explored so far.

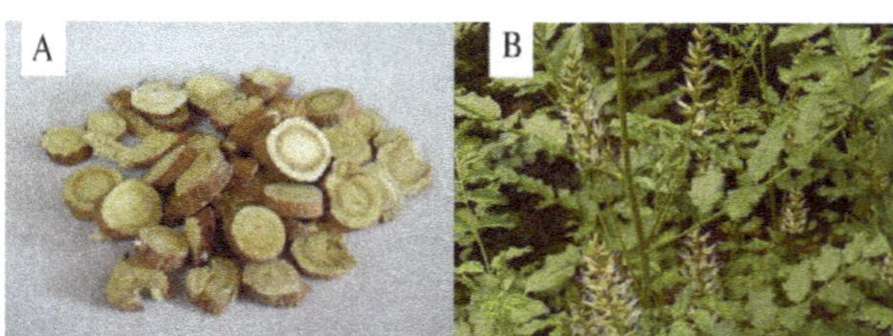

Figure 1. *Rhizoma Glycyrrhizae* (A) and its plant *Glycyrrhiza uralensis* Fisch (B).
Figure 1A was contributed by Weikang Chen, Figure 1B was contributed by www.plantphoto.cn.

Therefore, the aim of the study was to investigate its antioxidant ability, then further discuss the antioxidant mechanism.

***Corresponding author:** Xican Li, School of Chinese Herbal Medicine, Guangzhou University of Chinese Medicine, Guangzhou, China. E-mail: lixican@126.com

Materials and Methods

Plant material

Radix *Glycyrrhizae* was purchased from Caizhilin Pharmacy lacoted in Guangzhou University of Chinese Medicine (Guangzhou, China), and authenticated by Professor Shuhui Tan. A voucher specimen was deposited in our laboratory.

Chemicals

DPPH• (1,1-diphenyl-2-picryl-hydrazl radical), ABTS [2,2′-azino-bis(3-ethylbenzo- thiazoline-6-sulfonic acid diammonium salt)], BHA (butylated hydroxyanisole), Trolox [(±)-6- hydroxyl-2,5,7,8-tetramethlychromane-2-carboxylic acid], DNA sodium salt (fish sperm), neocuproine (2,9-dimethyl-1,10-phenanthroline), and Folin-Ciocalteu reagent were purchased from Sigma Co. (Sigma-Aldrich Shanghai Trading Co., China). Other chemicals used in this study were of analytic grade.

Preparation of extracts from Radix Glycyrrhizae

Radix *Glycyrrhizae* was powdered then extracted by absolute ethanol using a Soxhlet extractor for 6 hr. Extract was filtered using a Buckner funnel and Whatman No 1 filter paper. Filtrate was then concentrated to dryness under reduced pressure to yield ERG (ethanol extract of Radix *Glycyrrhizae*). It was stored at 4°C for analysis.

Protective effect against DNA damage

The experiment was conducted as described in previous report.[11] However, deoxyribose was replaced by DNA sodium. Briefly, sample was dissolved in methanol at 6 mg/mL. Various amounts (20-100 μL) of sample methanolic solutions were then separately taken into mini tubes. After evaporating the sample solutions in tubes to dryness, 400 μL of phosphate buffer (0.2 mol/L, pH 7.4) was added to the sample residue. Subsequently, 50 μL DNA sodium (10.0 mg/mL), 50 μL H_2O_2 (50 mmol/L), 50 μL $FeCl_3$ (3.2 mmol/L) and 50 μL Na_2EDTA (1 mmol/L) were added. The reaction was initiated by adding 50 μL of ascorbic acid (18 mmol/L) and the total volume of the reaction mixture was adjusted to 800 μL with buffer. After incubation in a water bath at 55 °C for 20 min, the reaction was terminated by adding 250 μL of trichloroacetic acid (10g/100mL water). The color was then developed by addition of 150 μL of TBA (2-thiobarbituric acid) (0.4 mol/L, in 1.25% NaOH aqueous solution) and heating in an oven at 105 °C for 15 min. The mixture was cooled and absorbance was measured at 530 nm against the buffer (as blank). The percent of protection against DNA damage is expressed as follows:

$$\text{Protective effect } \% = (1 - A/A_0)\times 100\%$$

Where A_0 is the absorbance of the control without sample, and A is the absorbance of the reaction mixture with sample.

DPPH• radical-scavenging assay

DPPH• radical-scavenging activity was determined as previously described by Li.[12] Briefly, 1 mL DPPH• ethanolic solution (0.1 mmol/L) was mixed with 0.5 mL sample alcoholic solution (4 mg/mL). The mixture was kept at room temperature for 30 min, and then measured with a spectrophotometer (Unico 2100, Shanghai, China) at 519 nm. The DPPH• inhibition percentage was calculated as:

$$\text{Inhibition } \% = (1 - A/A_0)\times 100\%$$

Where A is the absorbance with samples, while A_0 is the absorbance without samples.

$ABTS^{+\bullet}$ radical-scavenging assay

The $ABTS^{\dot{+}}$ -scavenging activity was measured as described[13] with some modifications. The $ABTS^{+}\bullet$ was produced by mixing 0.35 mL ABTS diammonium salt (7.4 mmol/L) with potassium 0.35 mL persulfate (2.6 mmol/L). The mixture was kept in the dark at room temperature for 12 h to allow completion of radical generation, then diluted with 95% ethanol (about 1:50) so that its absorbance at 734 nm was 0.70 ± 0.02. To determine the radical-scavenging activity, 1.2 mL aliquot of diluted $ABTS^{+}\bullet$ reagent was mixed with 0.3 mL of sample ethanolic solution (0.08-0.4 mg/mL). After incubation for 6 min, the absorbance at 734 nm was read on a spectrophotometer (Unico 2100, Shanghai, China). The percentage inhibition was calculated as:

$$\text{Inhibition } \% = (1 - A/A_0)\times 100\%$$

Here, A_0 is the absorbance of the mixture without sample, A is the absorbance of the mixture with sample.

Reducing power (Fe^{3+}) assay

Ferric (Fe^{3+}) reducing power was determined by the method of Oyaizu.[14] In brief, sample solution x μL (2 mg/mL, x = 20, 40, 60, 80, 100 and 120) was mixed with (350-x) μL Na_2HPO_4/KH_2PO_4 buffer (0.2 mol/L, pH 6.6) and 250 μL $K_3Fe(CN)_6$ aqueous solution (1 g/100 mL). After incubation at 50 °C for 20 min, the mixture was added by 250 μL of trichloroacetic acid (10 g/100 mL), then centrifuged at 3500 r/min for 10 min. As soon as 400 μL supernatant was aliquoted into 400 μL $FeCl_3$ (0.1 g/100 mL in distilled water), the timer was started. At 90 s, absorbance of the mixture was read at 700 nm (Unico 2100, Shanghai, China). Samples were analyzed in groups of three, and when the analysis of one group has finished, the next group of three samples was aliquoted into $FeCl_3$ to avoid oxidization by air. The relative reducing ability of the sample was calculated by using the formula:

$$\text{Relative reducing effect } \% = (A-A_{min})/(A_{max}-A_{min})\times 100\%$$

Here, A_{max} is the maximum absorbance and A_{min} is the minimum absorbance in the test. A is the absorbance of sample.

Cu^{2+}-reducing power assay

The Cu^{2+}-reducing capacity was determined by the method,[15] with minor modifications. Briefly, 125 μL

$CuSO_4$ aqueous solution (0.01 mol/L), 125 μL neocuproine ethanolic solution (7.5 mmol/L) and (750-x) μL CH_3COONH_4 buffer solution (0.1 mol/L, pH 7.5) were brought to test tubes with different volumes of samples (2 mg/mL, x = 20 -100 μL). Then, the total volume was adjusted to 1000 μL with the buffer and mixed vigorously. Absorbance against a buffer blank was measured at 450 nm after 30 min (Unico 2100, Shanghai, China). The relative reducing power of the sample as compared with the maximum absorbance, was calculated by the formula:

$$\text{Relative reducing effect } \% = (A-A_{min})/(A_{max}-A_{min})\times 100\%$$

where, A_{max} is the maximum absorbance at 450 nm and A_{min} is the minimum absorbance in the test. A is the absorbance of sample.

Determination of total phenolics

The total phenolics content of ERG was determined using the Folin-Ciocalteu method[16] with a little modifications. In brief, 0.5 mL sample methanolic solution (0.4 mg/mL) was mixed with 0.5 mL Folin-Ciocalteu reagent (2 mol/L). After incubation for 3 min, 1.0 mL of Na_2CO_3 aqueous solution (15 %, w/v) was added. After standing at room temperature for 30 min, the mixture was centrifuged at 3500 r/min for 3 min. The absorbance of the supernatant was measured at 760 nm (Unico 2100, Shanghai, China). The determinations were performed in triplicate, and the calculations were based on a calibration curve obtained with quercetin. The result was expressed as quercetin equivalents in milligrams per gram of extract.

Determination of total flavonoids

The total flavonoid content was measured using the $NaNO_2$ -Al $(NO_3)_3$ method.[17] In brief, 1 mL sample methanolic solution (1 mg/mL) was mixed with 0.15 mL $NaNO_2$ aqueous solution (5%, w/w). The mixture stood for 6 min, followed by the addition of 0.15 mL Al $(NO_3)_3$ aqueous solution (10%, w/w). After incubation at ambient temperature for 6 min, 2 mL NaOH aqueous solution (4%, w/w) was added to the mixture which was then adjusted to 5 mL with distilled water. The absorbance was read at 508 nm on a spectrophotometer (Unico 2100, Shanghai, China). The determinations were performed in triplicate, and the calculations were also based on a calibration curve obtained with quercetin. The result was also expressed as quercetin equivalents in milligrams per gram of extract.

Statistical analysis

Data are given as the mean ± SD of three measurements. The IC_{50} values were calculated by linear regression analysis. All linear regression in this paper was analyzed by Origin 6.0 professional software. Significant differences were performed using the T-test ($p < 0.05$). The analysis was performed using SPSS software (v.12, SPSS, USA).

Results and Discussion

Hydroxyl radical (•OH) is known to be generated in human body via Fenton reaction (Equation 1).

$$Fe^{2+} + H_2O_2 \rightarrow \bullet OH + OH^- + Fe^{3+} \quad \text{Equation 1}$$

Since •OH radical possesses extreme reactivity, it can easily damage DNA to produce malondialdehyde (MDA) and various oxidative lesions[18] (Equation 2 and Figure 2).

P —OCH2 (base pairs) [deoxyribose] —• OH→ $CH_2(OH)COOH$ + $HC(=O)CH_2CH(=O)$ (MDA) + Oxidative lesions Equation **2**

P = Organic phosphate

MDA combines TBA (2-thiobarbituric acid) to yield TBARS (thiobarbituric acid reactive substances) which present a maximum absorbance at 530 nm (Equation 3).[19]

$HC(=O)CH_2CH(=O)$ (MDA) + TBA → TBARS, λmax 530nm Equation 3

On the other hand, as the oxidative lesions mentioned above have not conjugative system in the molecules (Figure 2), they cannot be detected by a spectrophotometer at 530 nm. It means that these oxidative lesions cannot disturb the determination of MDA.

Hence, the value of A_{530nm} can reflect the amount of MDA, and ultimately reflect the extent of DNA damage. In terms of the formula "protective effect % = $(1 - A/A_0)\times 100\%$", it can be deduced that the decrease of A_{530nm}value indicates a protective effect against DNA damage. As seen in Figure 3A, ERG showed a protective effect against DNA damage in a dose dependent manner and its IC_{50} value was 517.28±26.61µg/mL (Table 1).

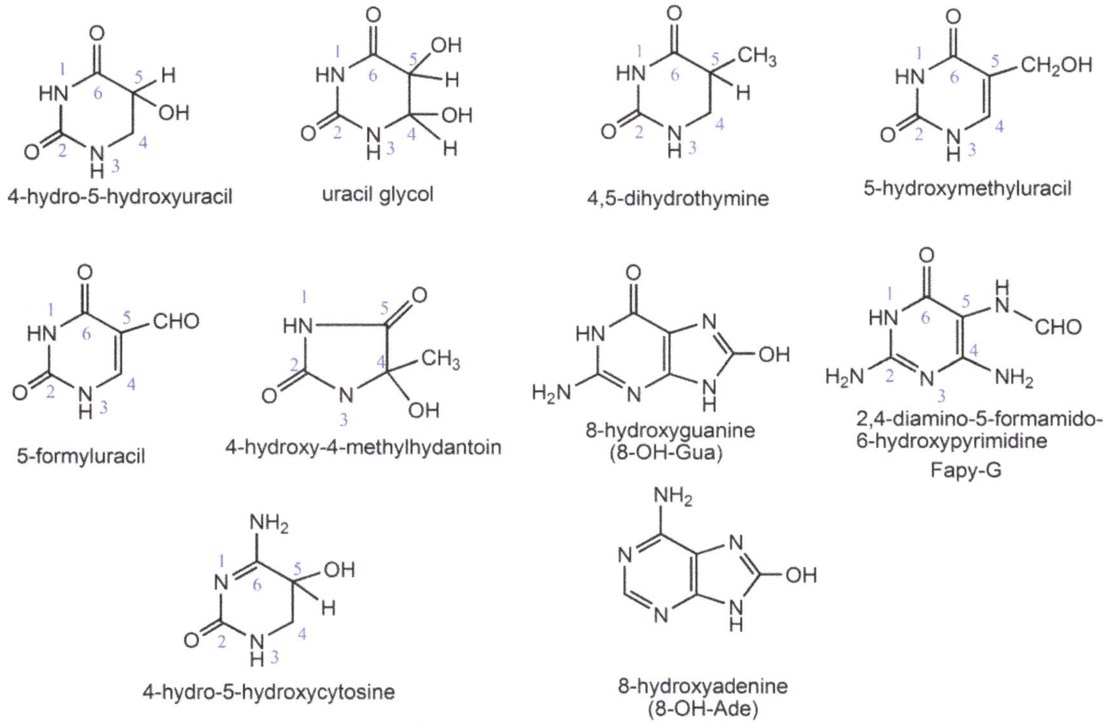

Figure 2. The structures of some oxidative lesions.

Previous reports have shown that there were two approaches for natural phenolic antioxidant to protect DNA oxidative damage: one was to scavenge the •OH radicals then to reduce its attack; one was to fast repair the deoxynucleotide radical cations which were damaged by •OH radicals.[20] In order to further confirm whether the protective effect of ERG against DNA oxidative damage was relevant to its radical-scavenging ability, we then determined the DPPH· and $ABTS^{+\cdot}$ radical-scavenging abilities.

The DPPH assay revealed that ERG can effectively eliminate DPPH• radical (Figure 3B) and its IC_{50} was 165.18±6.48 µg/mL (Table 1). The previous studies suggested that DPPH· may be scavenged by an antioxidant through donation of hydrogen atom (H·) to form a stable DPPH-H molecule which does not absorb at 519 nm.[21] For example, liquifitigenin which occurred in Radix *Glycyrrhizae*,[22] may scavenge DPPH• via the following proposed mechanism[23,24] (Equation 4 and 5)

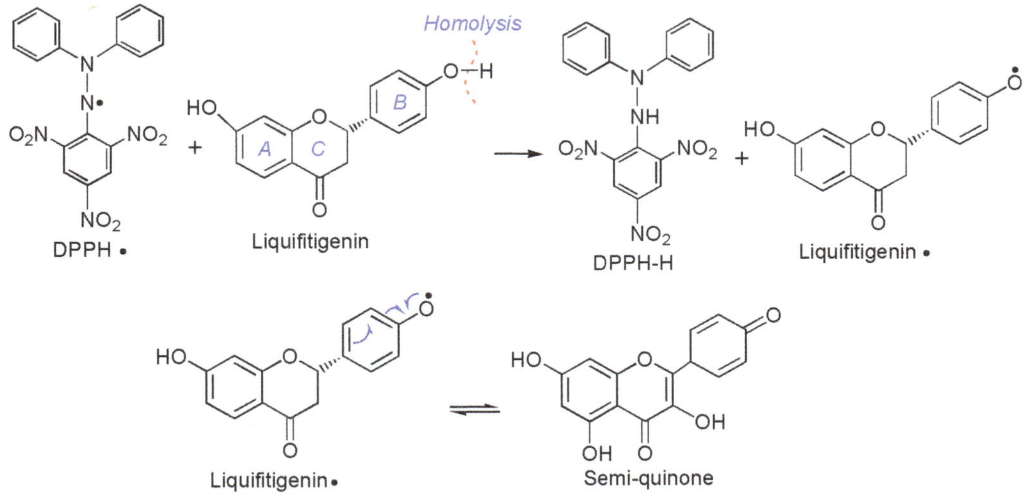

Equation **4**

Equation **5**

Table 1. The IC_{50} values of ethanol extract from Radix *Glycyrrhizae* (ERG) (μg/mL)

		Positive controls	
	ERG	Trolox	BHA
Protecting DNAdamage	517.28±26.61	306.13±26.11	344.89±30.28
DPPH· scavenging	165.18±6.49	9.75±0.06	22.35±0.58
$ABTS^{+}$· scavenging	7.46±0.07	5.09±0.02	5.21±0.25
Fe^{3+}-reducing	97.23±2.88	34.58±1.45	22.88±1.03
Cu^{2+}-reducing	59.21±0.18	13.82±0.30	16.09±0.47

IC_{50} value is defined as the concentration of 50% effect percentage and expressed as Mean±SD (n=3). Means values with different superscripts in the same row are significantly different (p<0.05), while with same superscripts are not signifiacntly different (p<0.05). BHA, butylated hydroxyanisole.

Figure 3C indicated that ERG could also scavenge $ABTS^{+}$· in a dose-dependent manner and its IC_{50} was 7.46±0.07 μg/mL (Table 1). However, $ABTS·^{+}$ scavenging is considered as an electron (e) transfer reaction.[25]

The fact that ERG can effectively scavenge both DPPH· and $ABTS^{+}$· radicals, suggests that: (1) the protective effect of ERG against DNA oxidative damage was relevant to its radical-scavenging ability; (2) ERG exerted radical-scavenging action by donating hydrogen atom (H·) and electron (e).

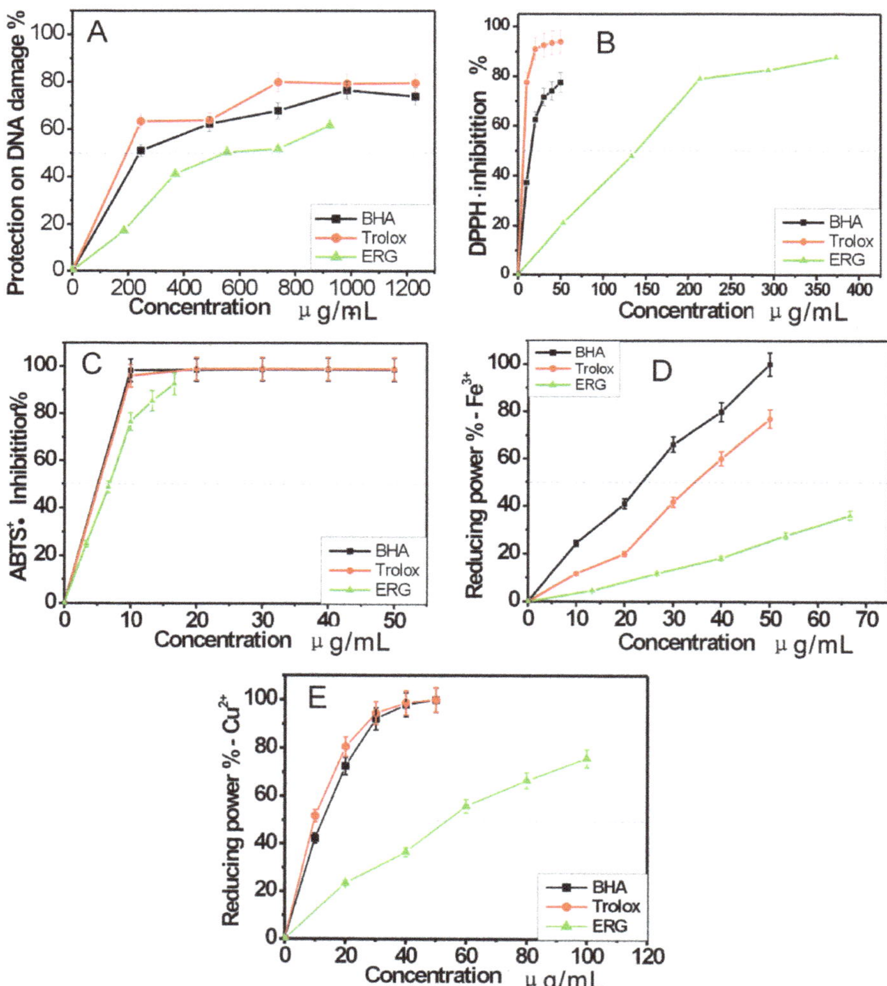

Figure 3. The dose response curves of ERG in the antioxidant assays: (A) protective effect on DNA damage; (B) DPPH· scavenging; (C) $ABTS^{+}$· scavenging (D) Fe^{3+}-reducing; (E) Cu^{2+}-reducing. ERG, absolute ethanol extract of Radix *Glycyrrhizae*. Trolox and BHA (butylated hydroxyanisole) were used as the positive controls. Each value is expressed as Mean±SD (n=3).

Although a reductant is not necessarily an antioxidant, an antioxidant is commonly a reductant.[26] The reducing power of an antioxidant may therefore serve as a significant indicator of its potential antioxidant activity.[27] Figure 3D and 3E showed that ERG exhibited its reducing powers on Fe^{3+} and Cu^{2+} in a concentration dependent manner. The IC_{50} values were 97.23±2.88 μg/mL & 59.21±0.18 μg/mL, respectively for Fe^{3+}-reducing and Cu^{2+}-reducing) (Table 1). Obviously, these data further support the findings mentioned above.

Phytochemical studies suggested that total phenolics and total flavonoids can be responsible for the antioxidant ability in plants, we then determined the total phenolics and total flavonoids contents in ERG. The data showed that ERG contained high amounts of total phenolics and flavonoids (111.48±0.88 mg quercetin/g and 218.26±8.57 mg quercetin/g, respetively). In fact, at least 5 flavonoids have been isolated from Radix *Glycyrrhizae*, including liquiritigenin, isoliquiritigenin, liquiritin, isoliquiritin, neoliquiritin, and so on[22] (Figure 4).

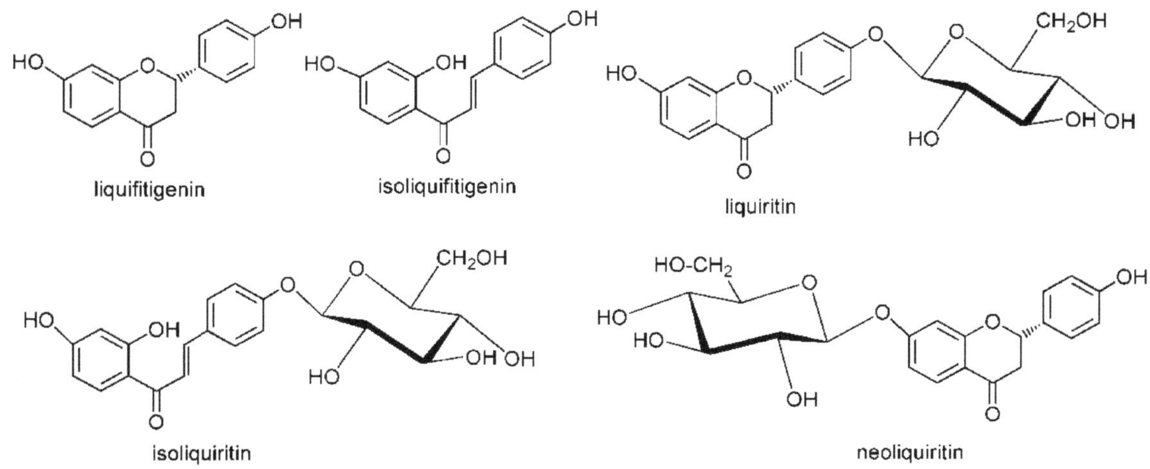

liquifitigenin

isoliquifitigenin

liquiritin

isoliquiritin

neoliquiritin

Figure 4. The structures of flavonoids in Radix *Glycyrrhizae*.

Conclusion

As a typical Chinese herbal medicine, Radix *Glycyrrhizae* can effectively protect against hydroxyl-induced DNA damage. One mechanism of protective effect may be radical-scavenging which is via donating hydrogen atom (H·), donating electron (e). Its antioxidant ability can be mainly attributed to the existence of flavonoids or total phenolics.

Conflict of interest

The authors report no conflicts of interest.

References

1. Bhattacharjee S, Deterding LJ, Chatterjee S, Jiang J, Ehrenshaft M, Lardinois O, et al. Site-specific radical formation in DNA induced by Cu(II)-H_2O_2 oxidizing system, using ESR, immuno-spin trapping, LC-MS, and MS/MS. *Free Radic Biol Med* 2011;50(11):1536-45.
2. Yang SZ, Bob F. The Divine Farmer's Materia Medica: A Translation of the Shen Nong Ben Cao Jing. Boulder, Co: Blue Poppy Press; 1998.
3. China Pharmacopoeia Committee. Pharmacopoeia of The People's Republic of China. Beijing: Chemical Industry Press; 2010.
4. He D, Yan M, Li HD, Liu FQ, Yu DY, Yang CC, et al. Effects of Radix Glycyrrhiza and Its Main Components on the Function and Expression of P-glycoprotein in Caco-2 Cells. *Chin pharm j* 2010;45:751-5.
5. Fu YJ, Li ZY. Each Effective Ingredients of Glycyrrhiza on the Research Progress of the Effect of Nerve Protection. *J Int Neurology Neurosurgery* 2012;3:298-300.
6. Wang XQ, Li HY, Liu XY, Zhang FM, Li X, Piao YA, et al. The anti-respiratory syncytial virus effect of active compound of Glycyrrhiza GD4 in vitro. *Zhong Yao Cai* 2006;29(7):692-4.
7. Jin WW, Li YJ. Recent Studies on Anticancer Constituents in Glycyrrhiza Uralensis Fisch. *Journal of Liaoning university of TCM* 2011;4:163-5.
8. Zhang MF, Shen YQ. Advances in studies on Glycyrrhizae Radix et Rhizoma and its active components in anti-inflammation and mechanism. *Drugs & Clinic* 2011;4:261-8.
9. Wang WQ, Wei SL, Li WD. Review of pharmacological effects of Radix *Glycyrrhiza* and its bioactive compounds. *China Journal of Chinese Materia Medica* 2009;21:2695-700.
10. Zheng RL, Huang ZY. Free radical biology. 3rd Ed. China: Higher Education Press; 2007.
11. Wang X, Li X, Chen D. Evaluation of antioxidant activity of isoferulic acid *in vitro*. *Nat Prod Commun* 2011;6(9):1285-8.
12. Li X, Chen C. Systematic evaluation on antioxidant of magnolol *in vitro*. *Int Res J Pure Appl Chem* 2012;2(1):68-76.

13. Gao Y, Hu Q, Li X. Chemical composition and antioxidant activity of essential oil from *Syzygium samarangense* (BL.) Merr.et Perry flower-bud. *Spatula DD* 2012; 2(1): 23-33.
14. Oyaizu M. Studies on product of browning reaction prepared from glucoseamine. *Jpn J Nutr* 1986; 44:307-15.
15. Li XC, Wang XZ, Chen DF, Chen SZ. Antioxidant activity and mechanism of protocatechuic acid *in vitro. Functional Foods in Health and Disease* 2011;1(7):232-44.
16. Li XC, Wu XT, Huang L. Correlation between antioxidant activities and phenolic contents of Radix *Angelicae Sinensis* (Danggui). *Molecules* 2009;14:5349-61.
17. Li X, Chen D, Mai Y, Wen B, Wang X. Concordance between antioxidant activities in vitro and chemical components of Radix *Astragali* (Huangqi). *Nat Prod Res* 2012; 26(11):1050-3.
18. Cooke MS, Evans MD, Dizdaroglu M, Lunec J. Oxidative DNA damage: Mechanisms, mutation, and disease. *FASEB J* 2003;17(10):1195-214.
19. Cheeseman KH, Beavis A, Esterbauer H. Hydroxyl-radical-induced iron-catalysed degradation of 2-deoxyribose. Quantitative determination of malondialdehyde. *Biochem J* 1988;252(3):649-53.
20. Fang YZ, Zheng RL. Theory and application of free radical biology. China: Science Press; 2002.
21. Bondet V, Brand-Williams W, Berset C. Kinetics and mechanisms of antioxidant activity using the DPPH• free radical method. *LWT-Food Sci Technol* 1997; 30(6):609-15.
22. Tao B, Liu XQ, Qu ZG. Research Progress on the Chemical Constituents of Licorice Root. *J Hebei Agric Sci* 2009;3:77-9.
23. Dimitrios IT, Vassiliki O. The contribution of flavonoid C-ring on the DPPH free radical scavenging efficiency. A kinetic approach for the 3′,4′-hydroxy substituted members. *Innov Food Sci Emerg Technol* 2006;7(1-2):140-6.
24. Khanduja KL, Bhardwaj A. Stable free radical scavenging and antiperoxidative properties of resveratrol compared in vitro with some other bioflavonoids. *Indian J Biochem Biophys* 2003;40(6):416-22.
25. Aliaga C, Lissi EA. Reaction of 2, 2′-azinobis (3-ethylbenzothiazoline-6-sulfonic acid (ABTS) derived radicals with hydroperoxides: Kinetics and mechanism. *Int J Chem Kinet* 1998;30(8):565-70.
26. Prior RL, Cao G. In vivo total antioxidant capacity: Comparison of different analytical methods. *Free Radic Biol Med* 1999;27(11-12):1173-81.
27. Jung MJ, Heo SI, Wang MH. Free radical scavenging and total phenolic contents from methanolic extracts of Ulmus davidiana. *Food Chem* 2008;108(2):482-7.

Rhizomes of *Eremostachys laciniata*: Isolation and Structure Elucidation of Chemical Constituents and a Clinical Trial on Inflammatory Diseases

Abbas Delazar[1]*, Satyajit D. Sarker[2], Lutfun Nahar[3], Shahriar Barzegar Jalali[1], Masoud Modaresi[4], Sanaz Hamedeyazdan[1], Hossein Babaei[1], Yousef Javadzadeh[1], Solmaz Asnaashari[1], Sadeighe Bamdad Moghadam[1]

[1] *Drug Applied Research Centre and School of Pharmacy, Tabriz University of Medical Sciences, Tabriz 51664, Iran.*

[2] *Department of Pharmacy, School of Applied Sciences, University of Wolverhampton, MM Building, Molineux Street, Wolverhampton WV1 SB, UK.*

[3] *Drug Discovery and Design Research Division, Department of Pharmacy, School of Applied Sciences, University of Wolverhampton, City Campus, MA Building, Wulfruna Street, Wolverhampton WV1 1LY, UK.*

[4] *School of Pharmacy, Kermanshah University of Medical Sciences, Kermanshah, Kermanshah 67346, Iran.*

ARTICLEINFO

Keywords:
Eremostachys laciniata
Lamiaceae
Iridoid
Phenylethanoid
Phytosterol
Inflammatory diseases

ABSTRACT

Purpose: The purpose of this study was the isolation and structure elucidation of chemical compounds from the rhizomes of *Eremostachys laciniata (L)* Bunge (EL), an Iranian traditional medicinal herb with a thick root and pale purple or white flowers as well as the clinical studies on the therapeutic efficacy and safety of topical application of the EL extract in the management of some inflammatory conditions, e.g., arthritis, rheumatoid arthritis and septic arthritis (Riter's syndrome). ***Methods:*** The structures of the isolated compounds were elucidated unequivocally on the basis of one and two dimensional NMR, UV and HR-FABMS spectroscopic data analyses. A single-blinded randomized clinical trial was carried out with the extract of the rhizomes of E. laciniata (EL) to determine the efficacy and safety of the traditional uses of EL compared to that of piroxicam in treatment of inflammatory diseases, e.g., osteoarthritis, rheumatoid arthritis and Reiter's syndrome. ***Results:*** Eleven iridoid glycosides, two phenylethanoids and two phytosterols were isolated and identified for the first time from the rhizomes of EL. After 14 days of treatment with the EL and piroxicam ointments, all groups showed significant improvements compared to the control groups. EL (5%) ointment induced better initial therapeutic response than piroxicam (5%) onitment. ***Conclusion:*** This clinical trial established that EL was suitable for topical applications as a safe and effective complementary therapy for inflammatory diseases.

Introduction

Eremostachys laciniata (L) Bunge (family: Lamiaceae alt, Labiatae; sub-family: Lamioideae) is a perennial medicinal herb with a thick root and pale purple or white flowers. It is one of the fifteen endemic Iranian species of the genus *Eremostachys*, and is also grown in other countries of the Middle-East Asia, Western Asia, and Caucasus.[1,2] Traditionally, a decoction of the roots and flowers of E. laciniata (EL) has been used to treat allergies, headache and liver diseases.[3-5] This plant is also used to alleviate inflammatory conditions. It is usually given as a remedy in the form of herbal teas, or tisanes of the roots and flowers. The merit of the traditional uses of EL has been supported by some previous phytochemical studies on the genus *Eremostachys*, providing the isolation and identification of several bioactive compounds. Previous phytochemical study on EL established the presence of mono- and sesqui-tepenes in its essential oils.[6] The crude extract of this plant was reported to possess free-radical-scavenging property.[7] As a part of our on-going studies on plants of Iranian flora,[4,5,8-17] we now report on the isolation and structure elucidation of 11 iridoid glucosides, two phenylethanoids and two phytosterols from the rhizomes of EL as well as the clinical studies on the therapeutic efficacy and safety of topical application of the EL extract in the management of some inflammatory conditions, *e.g.*, arthritis, rheumatoid arthritis and septic arthritis (Riter's syndrome).

***Corresponding author:** Abbas Delazar, Drug Applied Research Centre and School of Pharmacy, Tabriz University of Medical Sciences, Tabriz 51664, Iran, E-mails: delazara@hotmail.com and delazara@tbzmed.ac.ir

Materials and Methods

General experimental procedures

UV spectra were obtained in MeOH using a Shimadzu UV-160A spectrometer. NMR spectra were recorded in CD_3OD on a Bruker DRX 500 MHz NMR spectrometer (500 MHz for ^1H and 125 MHz for ^{13}C) using the residual solvent peaks as an internal standard. HMBC spectra were optimized for a long range J_{H-C} of 9 Hz and a NOSEY experiment was carried out with a mixing time of 0.8 s. MS analyses were performed on a Finnigan MAT95 spectrometer. HPLC separation was performed on a Shimadzu HPLC system coupled with a photo-diode-array detector (SPD-M20A). A Supelco Sep-Pak C_{18} 10 g cartridge was used for pre-HPLC fractionation.

Plant material

The rhizomes of *Eremostachys laciniata* (L) Bunge, were collected during September-October 2005 from Ajabshir county in East Azarbaijan province in Iran (37° 36' 46.7''North latitude, 46° 11' 15.6''East longitude and altitude 1900 m over sea level). A voucher specimen (TUM-ADE 0204) for this collection has been retained in the herbarium of the School of Pharmacy, Tabriz University of Medical science, Iran.

Extraction and isolation

The dried and ground rhizomes of EL (100 g) were Soxhlet-extracted, successively, with *n*-hexane, dichloromethane (DCM) and MeOH (1.1 L each). All these extracts were separately concentrated using a rotary evaporator at a maximum temperature of 45 °C to yield 1.52 g, 0.92 g and 14.72 g of dried *n*-hexane, DCM and MeOH extracts, respectively. The MeOH extract (2 g) was subjected to Sep-Pack fractionation (Sep-Pak, C_{18} cartridge; 10 g) using a step gradient of MeOH-water mixture (10:90, 20:80, 40:60, 60:40, 80:20 and 100:0). The preparative reversed-phase HPLC analysis of the 10% methanolic Sep-Pak fraction afforded eight iridoid glycosides (compounds **1-8**) and the 20% methanolic Sep-Pak fraction of afforded two iridoid glycosides (compounds **9** and **10**). Similar HPLC purification of the 40% methanolic Sep-Pak fraction provided an iridoid glycoside and two phenyl ethanoids (compounds **11**, **12** and **13**, respectively). The *n*-hexane extract (1.28 g) was subjected to vacuum liquid chromatography (VLC) on silica gel 60H using a step gradient of *n*-hexane: ethyl acetate (100:0, 90:10, 80:20, 60:40, 40:60, 20:80, 100:0). Further purification of the 10% ethyl acetate fraction was carried out by preparative thin layer chromatography on silica gel GF_{254} using chloroform:acetone (92:8) resulted in the isolation of the compounds **14** and **15** (R_f = 0.51 and 0.54, respectively). The relative physical characteristics, retention times and weights of the compounds **1-15** are outlined in Table 1. The chemical structures of these compounds were elucidated by spectroscopic means.

Table 1. Appearance, molecular formula, retention time and weights of the compounds (1-15) isolated from *Eremostachys laciniata*

Compound name	Physical characteristic	Molecular formula	Retention Time (min) /R_f value	Weight (mg)
9-*epi*-Phlomiol (**1**)	Pale yellow amorphous solid	$C_{17}H_{26}O_{13}$	12.8	16.2
9-*epi*-pulchelloside II (**2**)	White amorphous solid	$C_{17}H_{26}O_{12}$	17.9	8.3
6-β-Hydroxy-7-*epi*-loganin (**3**)	Pale yellow amorphous solid	$C_{17}H_{26}O_{11}$	19.1	10.0
Lamalbide (**4**)	Pale yellow amorphous solid	$C_{17}H_{26}O_{12}$	23.8	98.9
Sesamoside (**5**)	Pale yellow amorphous solid	$C_{17}H_{24}O_{12}$	32.2	78.9
6'-*O*-β-D-Glucopyranosyl-sesamoside (**6**)	White amorphous solid	$C_{23}H_{34}O_{17}$	38.9	1.8
Shanzhiside methyl ester (**7**)	Pale yellow amorphous solid	$C_{17}H_{26}O_{11}$	47.1	13.9
5, 9-*epi*-Phlomiol (**8**)	White amorphous solid	$C_{17}H_{26}O_{13}$	13.6	9.5
Phloyoside II (**9**)	White amorphous solid	$C_{17}H_{25}O_{12}Cl$	29.6	5.1
5,9-*epi*-Penstemoside (**10**)	Pale yellow amorphous solid	$C_{17}H_{26}O_{11}$	40.3	2.0
6,9-*epi*-8-*O*-Acetyl-shanzhiside metyl ester (**11**)	Brown amorphous solid	$C_{19}H_{27}O_{12}$	25.9	6.5
Forsythoside B (**12**)	Brown amorphous solid	$C_{34}H_{44}O_{19}$	41.1	15.0
Verbascoside (**13**)	Brown amorphous solid	$C_{29}H_{36}O_{15}$	48.6	7.9
Stigmasterol (**14**)	White crystalline solid	$C_{29}H_{48}O$	0.51*	2.3
?-Sistosterol (**15**)	White crystalline solid	$C_{29}H_{50}O$	0.54*	2.8

* R_f value on silica gel GF_{254} using chloroform: acetone (92:8) as the mobile phase

Clinical study

Efficiency of the dried MeOH extract of EL in topical management of inflammatory diseases was studied in patients suffering from osteoarthritis, rheumatoid arthritis and Reiter's syndrome. A single-blinded randomized clinical trial was designed to evaluate the therapeutic efficiency of EL alone and also in comparison with piroxicam. Ethics Committee of Tabriz University of Medical Sciences approved this study. Written informed consent was obtained from each participant before the commencement of the project. One hundred and thirty seven patients with an age range of 18-80 years of either sex (female 60% and male 40%) were randomly divided into two major groups. One group (67 patients) received EL and the other (70 patients) was treated with topical piroxicam. Both the EL extract and piroxicam were applied in the form of topical ointments with 5% of active ingredient. Each major group was divided into three minor groups according to the type of disease (osteoarthritis, rheumatoid arthritis and reiter's syndrome). Medications which were administered along with our treatment protocol were cartigene, indomethacin and methotrexate, in the case of osteoarthritis, rheumatoid arthritis and reiter's syndrome, respectively. Furthermore, the piroxicam and EL ointments were well matched for colour, smell, and consistency. Neither the nurse nor the patient could distinguish the differences between preparations. The ointments (piroxicam and EL) were gently massaged around the affected joint, mostly knee joints, for 2 to 3 minutes, two times a day, for a consecutive 14 days. Massaging for several minutes was used to facilitate penetration of the cream by increasing local blood supply and encouraging local movement. After application, the area was covered with a cotton cloth. The patients were personally examined by a physician every week during the course of the study. During these visits, the patients were asked about compliance, correctness of the ointment application and the level of pain they had, as well as the size of inflammated joint. Patients were instructed to record the level of their pain on a 10 cm visual analogue scale (VAS) labelled as "no pain" at one side and "worst pain ever" at the other side. The amount of inflammation for each joint was measured by nurses using a centimetre. As a control, inflammation of the joints and the associated pain for each group was recorded at the beginning of the study before application of the ointments. Additionally, any irritations or possible side effects in the patients were assessed to evaluate the safety of the EL in topical application. All nondrug modalities of treatment and all adjunctive drug treatments remained constant during the study for the parallel groups with the same types of diseases.

Statistical analysis

All data were statistically analysed by the analysis of variance or Tukey's multiple comparison tests. A probability level of $P<0.05$ was taken to be statistically significant in the analysis.

Results and Discussion

A combination of solid-phase extraction and preparative reversed-phase HPLC of the MeOH extract of the rhizomes of EL afforded a total of 13 compounds (**1-13**), 11 of which were iridoid glycosides (**1-11**), and two other were phenylethanoids (**12** and **13**) (Table 1; Figure 1). The VLC followed by prep-TLC of the *n*-hexane extract of this plant yielded two phytosterols (**14** and **15**) (Table 1). The chemical structures of these compounds were elucidated unambiguously on the basis of one and two dimensional NMR, UV and HR-FABMS spectroscopic data analyses, and also by comparing experimental data with literature data. The ^1H and ^{13}C NMR data of all iridoids (**1-11**) are presented in Tables 2-4. The identified compounds were: 9-*epi*-phlomiol (**1**),[18] 9-*epi*-pulchelloside II (**2**),[18,19] 6-β-hydroxy-7-*epi*-loganin (**3**) [20-22], lamalbide (lamiridoside, **4**),[23] sesamoside (**5**),[18,24-26] 6'-O-β-D-glucopyranosyl sesamoside (**6**),[5,6, 27-30] shanzhiside methyl ester (**7**),[31] 5,9-*epi*-phlomiol (**8**),[28,29] phloyoside II (**9**),[18] 5,9-*epi*-penstemoside (**10**),[4] 6,9-*epi*-8-O-acetyl shanzhiside methyl ester (**11**),[4,32] forsythoside B (**12**) and verbascoside (**13**),[16] stigmasterol (**14**) and □-sitosterol (**15**).[16]

To the best of our knowledge, this is the first report on the thorough phytochemical investigation on the rhizomes of EL growing in Iran as well as the presence of 6'-O-β-D-glucopyranosyl sesamoside (**6**) in the genus *Eremostachys*. This compound was first reported in *Lamiophlomis rotata*, another plant from the family Lamiaceae.[30] Most of these iridoid glycosides were, however, previously reported from the aerial parts of this plant growing in Turkey,[29] and phloyoside I, pulchelloside I and phlomiol exhibiting anti-bacterial activities also were reported before from this plant.[17] Iridoid glycosides also occur in other species of the genus *Eremostachys*[4,28,29] which is taxonomically close to the genus *Phlomis*. Interestingly, the *Phlomis* is also well known for producing variety of iridoid glycosides.[4] Both the genera, *Eremostachys* and *Phlomis*, belong to the subtribe Lamieae of the family Lamiaceae[4,33] and they are morphologically similar. Anatomical and cytological studies on the species of these genera also established this close affinity between these two genera. During the preliminary chemotaxonomic studies on the family Lamiaceae using flavonoids as the markers, some degrees of similarities between these genera were also identified.[4] Iridoids have been considered as valuable chemotaxonomic markers,[33] and in fact, they have been employed successfully to describe chemotaxonomic relationships among the taxa within various families, e.g. Acanthaceae, Bigoniaceae, Cornaceae, Oleaceae, and Rubiaceae. Within the family Lamiaceae, iridoid glycosides have recently been employed as chemotaxonomic markers for the species of the genus *Lamium*.[25] Therefore, the co-occurrence of iridoid glycosides, in the closely related genera *Eremostachys* and *Phlomis* could be significant chemotaxonomically. It is also worth-mentioning that the iridoid profiles in the aerial parts and the rhizomes were found to be similar, and so is within the plant samples collected from two different geographical locations, one from Turkey[28] and the other from Iran.

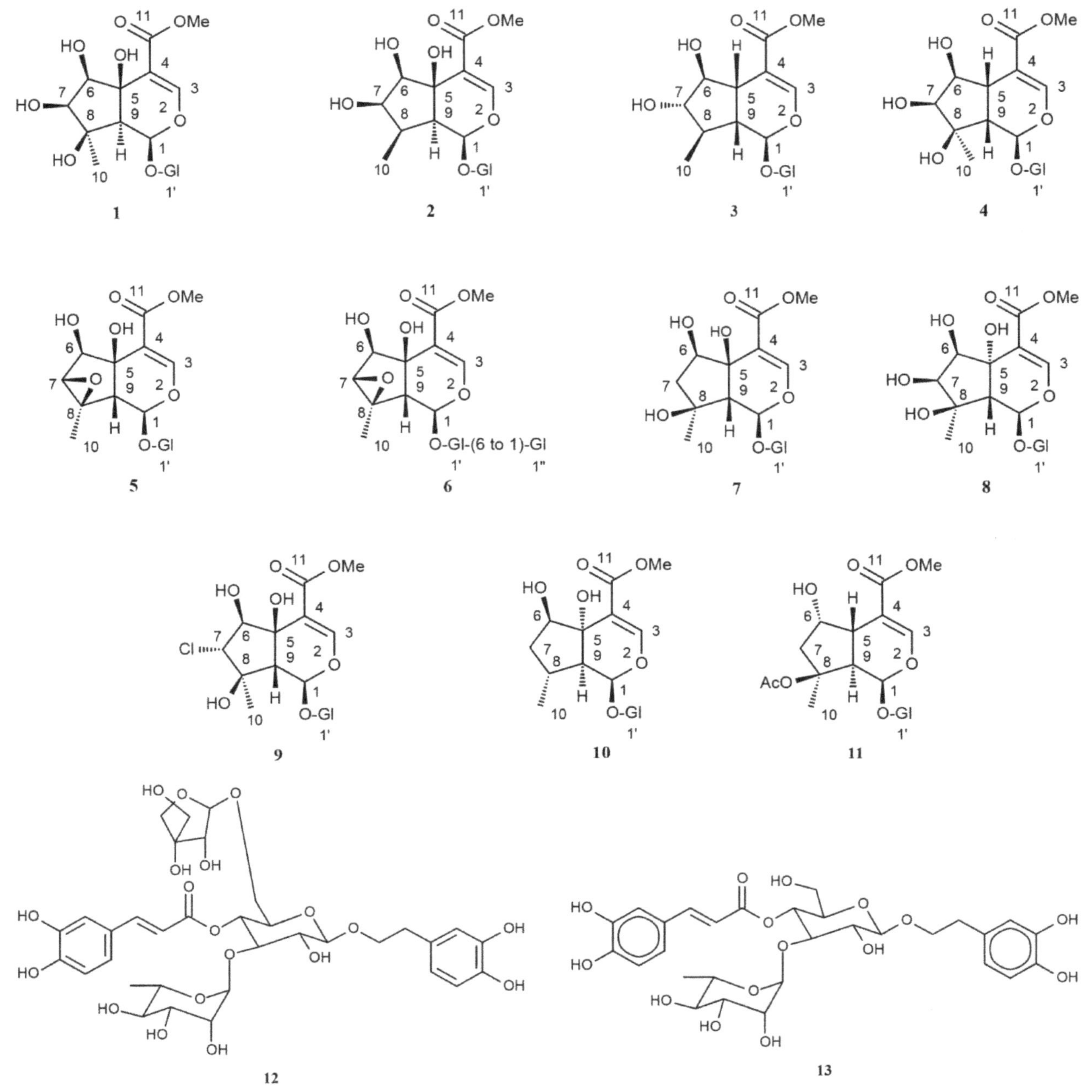

Figure 1. Structures of iridoids (**1-11**) and phenylethanoidsisolated (**12** and **13**) from *Eremostachys laciniata*.

In order to evaluate the efficacy and safety of topical treatment of EL extract containing ointment (EL) in patients with inflammatory complications, a total of 137 patients were screened during 14 days of the study. Data from patients were analyzed, and the demographics are presented in Figures 2 and 3. Figure 2 illustrates the pain scores (VAS) before and after treatment in both groups treated with EL and piroxicam. In terms of VAS values for EL, the mean score in patients suffering from arthritis, rheumatoid arthritis and Reiter's syndrome fell from 5.9, 6.6 and 8.1 to 3.5, 3.5 and 4.4 points after 14 days, respectively. In treatment with piroxicam, the values showed a decrease from 6.3, 7.0 and 8.1 to 3.7, 3.7 and 4.8 for the patients with arthritis, rheumatoid arthritis and Reiter's syndrome correspondingly. After 14 days of treatment with the EL and piroxicam ointments, all groups showed significant improvement when compared with their control groups ($p<0.001$) consequently, both ointments were effective in relieving patients' pains. Nevertheless, EL induced much better initial therapeutic response than piroxicam. In the cases of osteoarthritis and rheumatoid arthritis, notable differences between the two groups (piroxicam and EL) were observed in the first week of treatment (Figure 2), indicating enhanced onset of drug action for EL.

Table 2. ^{13}C NMR (125 MHz, CD_3OD) data of iridoids 1-11

	Chemical shift δ_c in ppm										
Position	**1**	**2**	**3**	**4**	**5**	**6**	**7**	**8**	**9**	**10**	**11**
1	93.1	95.0	95.1	93.9	95.9	96.5	93.8	93.9	92.0	94.8	94.7
2	-	-	-	-	-	-	-	-	-	-	-
3	153.7	153.6	152.0	151.9	154.6	154.4	151.8	154.2	152.8	154.3	152.7
4	115.0	114.9	110.2	110.7	112.0	112.0	110.4	114.4	113.6	112.5	108.8
5	64.9	68.7	40.1	36.6	74.0	74.2	40.4	70.1	65.1	72.5	41.3
6	79.7	83.3	83.4	77.7	76.5	76.8	77.0	77.2	79.7	75.7	74.9
7	83.7	83.0	84.8	76.9	65.0	65.0	48.2	80.5	72.1	39.6	46.6
8	74.9	37.8	38.4	78.0	62.8	62.6	78.0	78.4	73.6	30.5	88.8
9	57.6	53.9	43.5	48.2	53.4	53.4	50.7	56.9	57.4	49.6	48.9
10	17.2	16.0	16.2	21.2	16.8	17.0	23.7	22.3	17.5	15.6	21.2
11	168.3	168.5	169.1	168.6	168.1	169.8	168.7	168.8	167.1	167.3	168.0
11-OMe	51.9	51.8	50.9	51.1	51.4	51.3	50.9	51.7	51.0	50.7	50.8
Me-COO	-	-	-	-	-	-	-	-	-	-	21.2, 172.2
1′	99.7	100.0	99.1	98.8	99.0	99.2	98.8	99.5	98.7	98.8	99.4
2′	74.4	74.4	73.7	73.6	73.7	73.8	73.6	74.4	73.3	73.4	73.7
3′	77.4	77.5	77.0	76.9	76.7	76.7	76.5	77.5	76.4	76.4	77.0
4′	71.7	71.6	70.6	70.6	70.8	70.8	70.6	71.6	70.6	70.7	70.6
5′	78.4	78.5	77.4	77.3	77.7	77.2	77.4	78.5	77.4	77.4	77.3
6′	62.8	62.7	61.7	61.8	62.0	71.0	61.9	62.6	61.8	61.8	62.0
1″	-	-	-	-	-	104.7	-	-	-	-	-
2″	-	-	-	-	-	73.6	-	-	-	-	-
3″	-	-	-	-	-	76.7	-	-	-	-	-
4″	-	-	-	-	-	70.7	-	-	-	-	-
5″	-	-	-	-	-	77.0	-	-	-	-	-
6″	-	-	-	-	-	61.8	-	-	-	-	-

Table 3. ^{1}H NMR (500 MHz, coupling constant J in Hz in parentheses, CD_3OD) data of iridoids 1-6

	Chemical shift δ_H in ppm					
Position	**1**	**2**	**3**	**4**	**5**	**6**
1	5.83 s	5.67 d (2.0)	5.44 d (3.9)	5.65 s	5.53 d (8.6)	5.49 d (9.3)
2	-	-	-	-	-	-
3	7.49 s	7.48 s	7.47 s	7.45 s	7.62 s	7.60 s
4	-	-	-	-	-	-
5	-	-	2.78 dd (8.6, 4.8)	2.97 dd (10.7, 2.6)	-	-
6	3.56 d (9.0)	3.67 d (7.0)	3.50 dd (8.7, 5.9)	3.99 t (3.8)	4.36 s	4.45 d (1.4)
7a	3.82 d (9.0)	3.43 dd (7.0, 6.5)	3.72 d (5.2)	3.59 d (4.2)	3.51 s	3.56 s br
7b	-	-	-	-	-	-
8	-	1.35 m	1.73 m	-	-	2.54 d (9.3)
9	2.47 s	1.96 dd (12.0, 1.5)	2.07 dt (9.4, 3.8)	2.84 d (10.9)	2.56 d (8.6)	1.57 s
10	1.02 s	1.14 d (6.5)	1.19 d (6.6)	1.24 s	1.54 s	-
11	-	-	-	-	-	3.78 s
11-OMe	3.74 s	3.73 s	3.77 s	3.77 s	3.78	4.77 d (7.8)
Me-COO	-	-	-	-	-	3.20-3.30*
1′	4.60 d (7.5)	4.58 d (8.0)	4.67 d (7.8)	4.66 d (7.8)	4.77 d (7.8)	3.35-3.52*
2′	3.19 dd (9.5, 8.0)	3.19 dd (9.0, 8.0)	3.21 t (8.2)	3.21 t (8.3)	3.27 dd (8.8, 3.1)	3.26-3.36*
3′	3.38 t (9.0)	3.37 t (8.8)	3.36-3.43*	3.37-3.46*	3.36-3.44*	3.33-3.42*
4′	3.28 t (9.3)	3.27 t (9.3)	3.24-3.36*	3.25-3.34*	3.26-3.36*	3.56-3.78*
5′	3.32-3.35*	3.32-3.35 *	3.30-3.40*	3.34-3.42*	3.33-3.40*	4.23 d br (11.8, 1.5)
6′a	3.66 dd (12.0, 6.0)	3.67 dd (12.0, 5.5)	3.69 dd (12.4, 5.3)	3.70 dd (12.1, 5.1)	3.65 dd (11.8, 6.5)	4.38 d (7.4)
6′b	3.90 dd (11.8, 2.3)	3.90 dd (11,8, 1.8)	3.93 d (12.1)	3.96 d (13.3)	3.96 d (11.7)	3.20-3.30*
1″	-	-	-	-	-	3.35-3.52*
2″	-	-	-	-	-	3.26-3.36*
3″	-	-	-	-	-	3.33-3.42*
4″	-	-	-	-	-	3.56-3.78*
5″	-	-	-	-	-	3.91 dd (12.0, 1.4)
6″a	-	-	-	-	-	7.60 s
6″b	-	-	-	-	-	-

Table 4. ^{1}H NMR (500 MHz, coupling constant *J* in Hz in parentheses, CD_3OD) data of iridoids 7-11

	Chemical shift δ_H in ppm				
Position	**7**	**8**	**9**	**10**	**11**
1	5.61 d (2.6)	5.38 s	5.89 s	5.85 s	5.95 s
2	-	-	-	-	-
3	7.44 d (0.9)	7.46 s	7.54 s	7.59 s	7.48 d (1.3)
4	-	-	-	-	-
5	3.04 dd (10.1, 2.9)	-	-	-	3.11 dd (9.0, 1.4)
6	4.08 m	4.18 d (4.5)	3.78 d (9.7)	4.32 t (4.47)	4.37 m
7a	1.86 dd (13.2, 6.0)	3.66 d (4.5)	4.08 d (9.7)	1.52 m	2.05 dd (14.9, 5.3)
7b	2.06 dd (13.2, 6.4)	-	-	1.83 m	2.24 d (15.0)
8	-	-	-	2.54-2.70*	-
9	2.65 dd (10.2, 2.5)	2.51 s	2.56 s	2.54-2.70*	3.03 dd (9.0, 2.1)
10	1.30 s	1.39 s	1.16 s	0.98 d (6.9)	1.55 s
11	-	-	-	-	-
11-OMe	3.77 s	3.73 s	3.78 s	3.76 s	3.75 s
Me-COO	-	-	-	-	2.05 s
1′	3.67 (d 7.8)	4.61 d (8.0)	4.64 d (7.8)	4.61 d (7.7)	4.67d (7.8)
2′	3.20 t (8.3)	3.20 t (8.5)	3.23 t (8.8)	3.22 dd (8.9, 7.9)	3.21 t (8.4)
3′	3.36-3.44*	3.35-3.38*	3.36-3.47*	.3.36-3.46*	3.36-3.45*
4′	3.25-3.34*	3.22-3.31*	3.27-3.35*	3.22-3.35*	3.25-3.35*
5′	3.33-3.40*	3.31-3.36*	3.32-3.39*	3.33-3.39*	3.33-3.40*
6′a	3.68 dd (12.0, 5.7)	3.66-3.71*	3.70 dd (11.9, 5.5)	3.69 dd (12.0, 5.8)	3.64-3.75*
6′b	3.94 dd (11.9, 1.6)	3.90 d (12.0)	3.94 dd (11.9, 1.6)	3.95 dd (11.9, 1.8)	3.90-3.96*

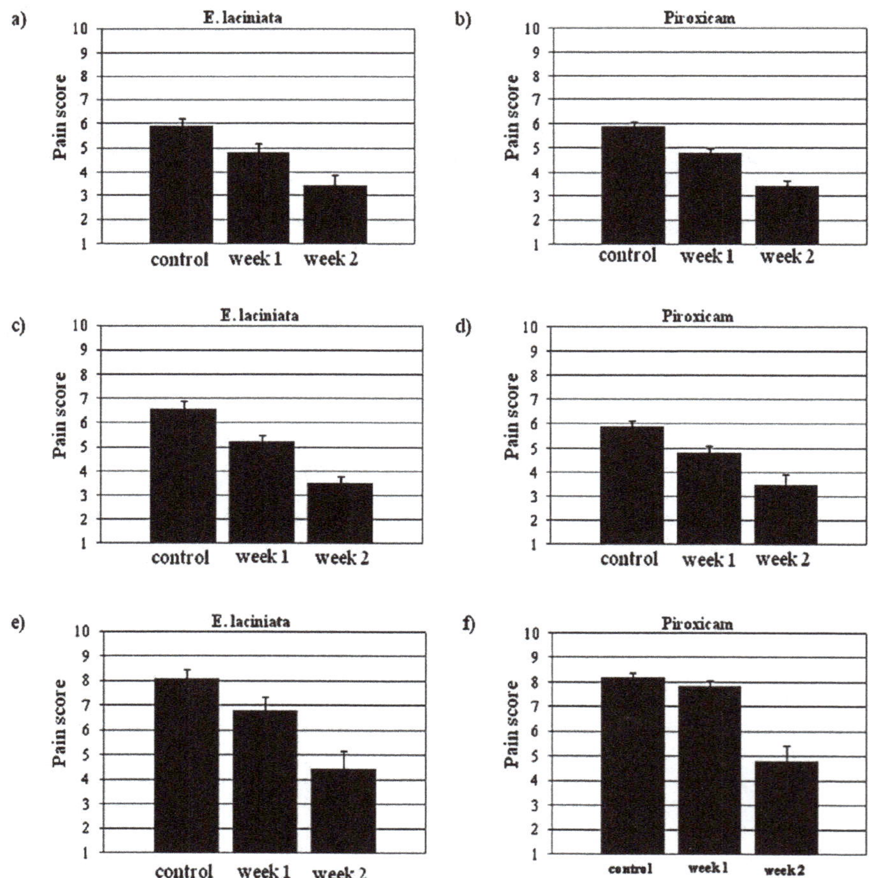

Figure 2. Effects of EL and piroxicam on pain relief in patients; (a/b) arthritis, (c/d) rheumatoid arthritis and (e/f) Reiter's syndrome.

Scatter diagrams were used to determine and compare variations in the size of inflammated joints for patients in different groups, during the 14 days of the study (Figure 3). The profiles for the inflammated joints did not alter significantly within the EL and piroxicam treated groups. However, the results showed a significant difference in efficiency of the ointments between the EL and piroxicam in the arthritis-patients ($p<0.005$; Figure 3a and 3b). Moreover, two of the patients demonstrated dermatitis leading to withdrawal from the study and five patients reported itching after applying the ointment; but no more serious side effects from other patients were recorded.

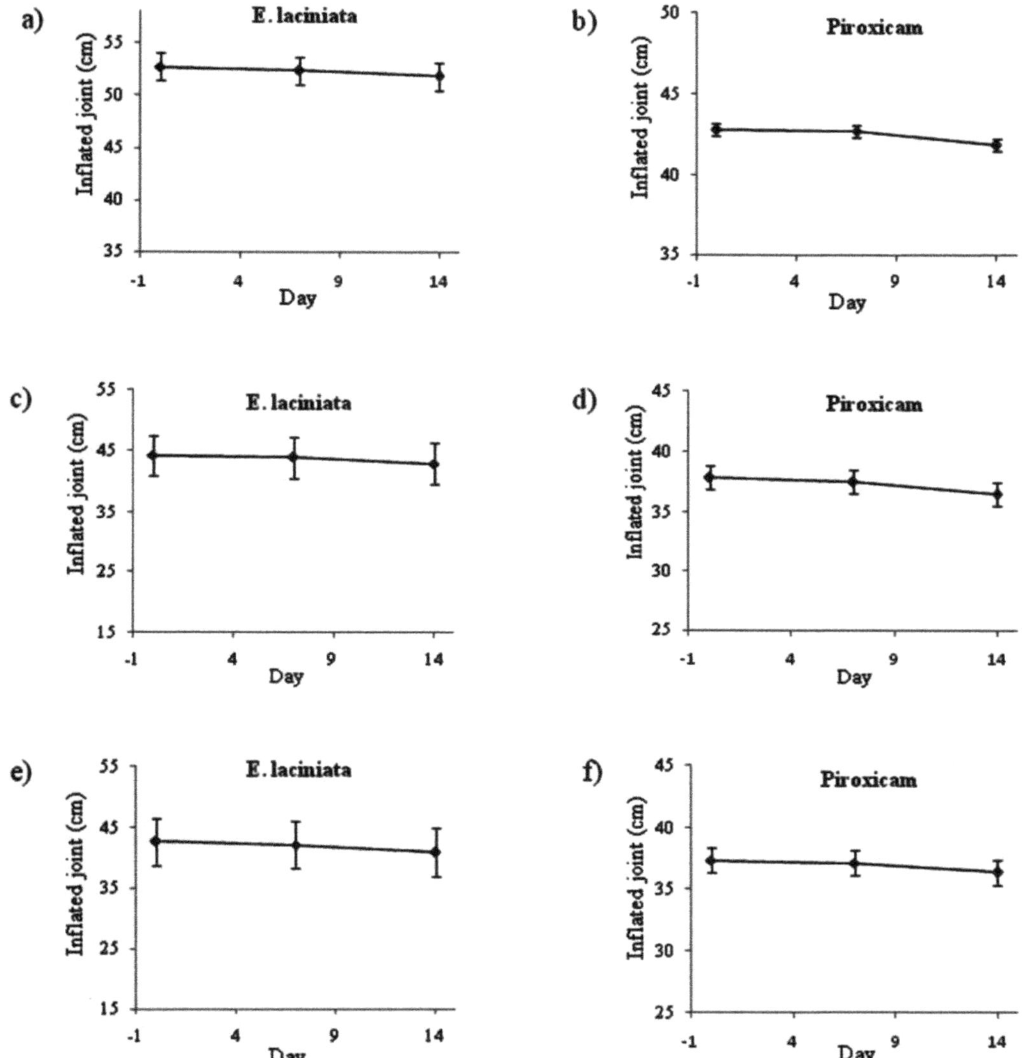

Figure 3. Effects of EA and piroxicam on the size of inflammated joints in patients; (a/b) arthritis, (c/d) rheumatoid arthritis and (e/f) Reiter's syndrome.

To the best of our knowledge, this clinical trial is the first attempt to provide evidence-based scientific support for topical application of EL extract containing ointment for the management of inflammatory diseases. Clinical observations in relation to anti-inflammatory property of EL described in this paper are in good agreement with the findings from previous animal study on mice model.[34]

Conclusion

The present study has shown that the rhizomes of EL are rich in irirdoid glycosides. Since the analgesic, anti-inflammatory and anti-arthritic properties of iridoid glycosides have previously been demonstrated by several researchers in animal models,[35] it is therefore reasonable to infer that the clinical effects of EL on managing inflammation in arthritic patients, as demonstrated in the present study, is probably owing to the presence iridoids in this plant. Some of the anti-inflammatory effects may also be partially due to the phenylethanoids (**12**, **13**), as these compounds are also known to produce anti-inflammatory and antioxidant effects.[36-38]

Acknowledgements

We thank the EPSRC National Mass Spectrometry Service Centre (Grove Building, Swansea University, Singleton Park, Swansea, SA2 8PP, Wales, UK) for MS analyses. The Medicinal Plants Research Network of the Ministry of Health and Medical Education Iran is thanked for financial support for this study.

Conflict of Interest

The authors report no conflicts of interest.

References

1. Mozaffarian V. A Dictionary of Iranian Plant Names. Tehran: Farhang Moaser; 1996.
2. Germplasm Resources Information Network - (GRIN). USDA, ARS, National Genetic Resources Program. [Online Database] Beltsville, Maryland: National Germplasm Resources Laboratory; 2013 [cited 2013 06 August]; Available from: http://www.ars-grin.gov/cgi-bin/npgs/html/taxon.pl?15378.
3. Said O, Khalil K, Fulder S, Azaizeh H. Ethnopharmacological survey of medicinal herbs in Israel, the Golan Heights and the West Bank region. *J Ethnopharmacol* 2002;83(3):251-65.
4. Delazar A, Byres M, Gibbons S, Kumarasamy Y, Modarresi M, Nahar L, et al. Iridoid glycosides from Eremostachys glabra. *J Nat Prod* 2004;67(9):1584-7.
5. Delazar A, Modarresi M, Shoeb M, Nahar L, Reid RG, Kumarasamy Y, et al. Eremostachiin: a new furanolabdane diterpene glycoside from Eremostachys glabra. *Nat Prod Res* 2006;20(2):167-72.
6. Navaei MN, Mirza M. Chemical composition of the oil of *Eremostachys laciniata* (L.) Bunge from Iran. *Flavour Frag J* 2006;21(4): 645-6.
7. Erdemoglu N, Turan NN, Cakoco I, Sener B, Aydon A. Antioxidant activities of some Lamiaceae plant extracts. *Phytother Res* 2006;20(1):9-13.
8. Delazar A, Reid RG, Sarker SD. GC-MS analysis of essential oil of the oleoresin from *Pistacia atlantica* VAR *mutica*. *Chem Nat Comp* 2004;40(1):24-7.
9. Delazar A, Celik S, Gokturk RS, Unal O, Nahar L, Sarker SD. Two acylated flavonoid glycosides from Stachys bombycina, and their free radical scavenging activity. *Die Pharmazie* 2005;60(11):878-80.
10. Delazar A, Biglari F, Esnaashari S, Nazemiyeh H, Talebpour AH, Nahar L, et al. GC-MS analysis of the essential oils, and the isolation of phenylpropanoid derivatives from the aerial parts of Pimpinella aurea. *Phytochemistry* 2006;67(19):2176-81.
11. Delazar A, Talischi B, Nazemiyeh Z, Rezazadeh H, Nahar L, Sarker SD. Chrozophorin: a new acylated flavone glucoside from Chrozophora tinctoria (Euphorbiaceae). *Braz J Pharmacogn* 2006;16(3):286-90.
12. Delazar A, Gibbons S, Kosari AR, Nazemiyeh H, Modarresi M, Nahar L, et al. Flavonoid C-glycosides and cucurbitacin glycosides from *Citrullus colocynthis*. *DARU* 2006;14(3):109-14.
13. Delazar A, Naseri M, Nazemiyeh H, Talebpour A-H, Imani Y, Nahar L, et al. Flavonol 3-methyl ether glucosides and a tryptophylglycine dipeptide from *Artemisia fragrans* (Asteraceae). *Biochem Syst Ecol* 2007;35(1):52-6.
14. Delazar A, Naseri M, Nahar L, Moghadam SB, Esnaashari S, Nazemiyeh H, et al. GC-MS analysis and antioxidant activities of essential oils of two cultivated *Artemisia* species. *Chem Nat Comp* 2007;43(1):112-4.
15. Nazemiyeh H, Maleki N, Mehmani F, Kumarasamy Y, Shoeb M, Garjani A, et al. Assessment of anti-inflammatory properties of ethyl acetate extract of *Stachys schtschegleevii* Sosn. *DARU* 2007;15(4):174-82.
16. Nazemiyeh H, Delazar A, Ghahramani MA, Talebpour AH, Nahar L, Sarker SD. Phenolic glycosides from *Phlomis lanceolata* (Lamiaceae). *Nat Prod Commun* 2008;3(1):53-6.
17. Modaressi M, Delazar A, Nazemiyeh H, Fathi-Azad F, Smith E, Rahman MM, et al. Antibacterial iridoid glucosides from Eremostachys laciniata. *Phytother Res* 2009;23(1):99-103.
18. Gao YL, Lin RC, Wang GL, Zhao HR, Gao Y, Ciren B. Studies on the chemical constituents of Phlomis younghusbandii. *Zhong Yao Cai* 2007;30(10):1239-42.
19. Franzyk H, Jensen SR, Olsen CE, Quiroga JM. A 9-hydroxyiridoid isolated from Junellia seriphioides (Verbenaceae). *Org Lett* 2000;2(5):699-700.
20. Boros CA, Stermitz FR. Iridoids – An updated review, Part I. *J Nat Prod* 1990;53(5):1055-147.
21. Boros CA, Stermitz FR. Iridoids – An updated review, Part II. *J Nat Prod* 1991;54(5):1173-465.
22. Boros CA, Stermitz FR, McFarland N. Processing of the Iridoid Glycoside Antirrinoside from *Maurandya antirrhiniflora* (Scrophulariaceae) by Meris paradoxa (Geometridae) and *Lepipolys* Species (Noctuidae). *J Chem Ecol* 1991;17(6):1123-33.
23. Li C, Gu D, Tao B. Iridoid glycosides from Pedicula dicora Franch. *Zhongguo Zhong Yao Za Zhi* 1999;24(1):40-1, 64.
24. Kang J, Jia Z. Chemical constituents of Pedicularis muscicola Maxim. *Zhongguo Zhong Yao Za Zhi* 1997;22(3):167-8, 91-2.
25. Alipieva KI, Taskova RM, Evstatieva LN, Handjieva NV, Popov SS. Benzoxazinoids and iridoid glucosides from four Lamium species. *Phytochemistry* 2003;64(8):1413-7.
26. Liu P, Teng J, Zhang YW, Takaishi Y, Duan HQ. Chemical constituents from rhizome of Phlomis umbrosa. *Yao Xue Xue Bao* 2007;42(4):401-4.

27. Eigtved P, Jensen SR, Nielsen B. A novel iridoid glucoside isolated from *Lamium album* L. *Acta Chem Scand B* 1974;28:85-91.
28. Calis I, Guvenc A, Armagan M, Koyuncu M, Gotfredsen CH, Jensen SR. Iridoid glucosides from *Eremostachys molucelloides* Bunge. *Helv Chim Acta* 2007;90:1461-66.
29. Calis I, Guvenc A, Armagan M, Koyuncu M, Gotfredsen CH, Jensen SR. Secondary metabolites from *Eremostachys laciniata. Nat Prod Commun* 2007;3:117-24.
30. Tan JJ, Tan CH, Jiang SH, Zhu DY. Iridoid glycosides from *Lamiophlomis rotata. Helv Chim Acta* 2007;90(1):143-8.
31. Yu ZX, Wang GL, Bianba C, Lin RC. Studies on chemical constituents in root of Phlomis medicinalis I. Zhongguo Zhong Yao Za Zhi 2006;31(8):656-8.
32. Jensen SR, Calis I, Gotfredsen CH, Sotofte I. Structural revision of some recently published iridoid glucosides. *J Nat Prod* 2007;70(1):29-32.
33. Azizian D, Cutler DF. Anatomical, cytological and phytochemical studies on *Phlomis* L and *Eremostachys* Bunge (Labiatae). *Bot J Linn Soc* 1988;85:249-81.
34. Delazar A, Habibi Asl H, Mohammadi O, Afshar FH, Nahar L, Modarresi M, et al. Evaluation of analgesic activity of *Eremostachys laciniata* in mice. *J Nat Remedies* 2009;9:1-7.
35. Dinda B, Debnath S, Harigaya Y. Naturally occurring secoiridoids and bioactivity of naturally occurring iridoids and secoiridoids. A review, part 2. *Chem Pharm Bull (Tokyo)* 2007;55(5):689-728.
36. Backhouse N, Delporte C, Apablaza C, Farias M, Goity L, Arraus S, et al. Antinociceptive activity of *Buddleja globosa* (matico) in several models of pain. *J Ethnopharmacol* 2009;119:160-5.
37. Asnaashari S, Delazar A, Alipour SS, Nahar L, Williams AS, Pasdaran A, et al. Chemical composition, free-radical-scavenging and insecticidal activities of the aerial parts of *Stachys byzantina. Arch Biol Sci* 2010;62:653-62.
38. Speranza L, Franceschelli S, Pesce M, Reale M, Menghini L, Vinciguerra I, et al. Antiinflammatory effects in THP-1 cells treated with verbascoside. *Phytother Res* 2010;24(9):1398-404.

18

Formulation and Quality Determination of Indapamide Matrix Tablet: A Thiazide Type Antihypertensive Drug

Jannatun Tazri[1], Md. Mizanur Rahman Moghal[1]*, Syed Masudur Rahman Dewan[1], Wahiduzzaman Noor[1], Nor Mohammad[2]

[1] *Department of Pharmacy, Noakhali Science and Technology University, Sonapur, Noakhali-3814, Bangladesh.*

[2] *Department of Chemistry, University of Chittagong, Chittagong-4331, Bangladesh.*

ARTICLEINFO

Keywords:
Higuchi equation
Hypertension
Indapamide
Polymer
Sustained Release Tablet

ABSTRACT

Purpose: The present study was explored to develop a sustained release matrix tablet of Indapamide, a low-dose thiazide-type diuretic, using hydroxylpropyl methylcellulose (Methocel K15MCR) in various proportions as release controlling factor.
Methods: The tablets were formulated using direct compression method. The powers for tableting were evaluated for angle of response, loose bulk density, tapped bulk density, compressibility index, total porosity and drug content etc. The tablets were subjected to thickness, weight variation test, drug content, hardness, friability, and *in vitro* dissolution studies.
Results: The granules showed satisfactory flow properties, compressibility index, and drug content. All the formulated tablets complies pharmacopoeia specifications. The release kinetics of the drug decreased exponentially with the addition of polymer concentration. Indapamide release rate was observed to be the highest with the lowest concentration of polymer used. The release mechanism was explored with zero order, first order, Higuchi and Krosmeyer equations. Stability tests of the drug showed no notable changes in the rate of drug release, related substances and drug content.
Conclusion: In the context, it can be suggested that this formulation of sustained release Indapamide tablets can be marketed to treat patients with hypertension ensuring proper healthcare.

Introduction

Sustained release matrix dosage forms are designed to achieve a prolonged therapeutic action by continuous releasing medication over an extended period of time after administration of single dose. In order to achieve steady level of medication, biodegradable polymer may play a vital role due to their biodegradability.[1] Sustained drug delivery involves the application of physical and polymer chemistry to produce well characterized and reproducible dosage forms, which control drug entry into the body within the specifications of the required drug delivery profile. A sustained release dosage forms allows a twofold or greater reduction in frequency of administration of the drug in comparison with frequency required by a conventional dosage forms.[2] Typically, sustained release products provide an immediate release of drug that promptly produces the desired therapeutic effect, followed by gradual release of additional amounts of drug to maintain this effect over a predetermined period. In this type of dosage forms, the rate of drug release mainly controlled by the delivery system itself, though it may be influenced by external conditions, like pH, enzymes, ions, motility and physiological conditions.[3] A wide array of polymers has been employed as retarding agents each of which presents a different approach to the matrix concept. Polymers that primarily forming insoluble of skeleton matrices are considered as the first category of retarding materials are classified as plastic matrix systems. The second class represents hydrophobic and water-insoluble materials, which are potentially erodible and the third group behaves hydrophilic properties. Plastic matrix systems, due to their chemical inertness and drug embedding ability, have been widely used for sustaining the release of drug. Liquid penetration into the matrix is the rate limiting step in such systems unless channeling agents are used. The hydrophobic and waxy materials, on the other hand, are potentially erodible and control the release of drug through pore diffusing and erosion.[2] The drug release from matrix tablet depends on other factors such as pore permeability, shape and size of matrix, drug solubility, polymer molecular weight, drug loading, compression force, and hydrodynamic conditions.[4] Previous studies

***Corresponding author:** Md. Mizanur Rahman Moghal, Department of Pharmacy, Noakhali Science and Technology University, Sonapur, Noakhali-3814, Bangladesh. Email: pharmamizan@ymail.com

developed by Williams *et al.*[5] led to the conclusion that the type and level of excipients influence the rate and extension of drug release.

Indapamide is an orally active sulphonamide diuretic agent. Although some evidence appears to indicate that the antihypertensive action of indapamide is primarily a result of its diuretic activity, only a limited diuresis occurs with the usual antihypertensive doses of 2.5 mg daily, and *in vitro* and *in vivo* data suggest that it may also reduce blood pressure by decreasing vascular reactivity and peripheral vascular resistance. In mild to moderate hypertension it is as effective as thiazide diuretics and β -adrenergic blocking agents in lowering blood pressure when used as the sole treatment.[6] Indapamide has been successfully combined with β - adrenergic blocking agents, methyldopa, and other antihypertensive agents. While such findings need confirmation, it appears that indapamide shares the potential with other diuretic agents to induce electrolyte and other metabolic abnormalities, although it may do so with less frequency or severity.[6] The main purpose of our present study was to formulate sustained release matrix tablet of Indapamide using hydroxypropyl methylcellulose (Methocel[1]) and evaluate its quality and release profile as well to justify the formulation.

Materials and Methods

Materials

The ingredients and the equipments used in the formulations are mentioned in Table 1 and Table 2 respectively.

Table 1. List of active ingredient and other excipients used in the preparation of matrix tablets

Name	Category	Source
Indapamide	Active Ingredient	Merck, Germany
Methocel K15M CR	Matrix forming agent	Colorcon, USA
Lactose	Diluent	Colorcon, USA
Talc	Lubricant	Colorcon, USA
Magnesium stearate	Antiadherent	Colorcon, USA
Aerosil	Flow promotor	Colorcon, USA

Table 2. List of equipments used in the method of Indapamide SR tablets

Name	Model	Source	Country
Sieve	-	Endecotts, Test Sieve	UK
Compression Machine	Manesty D type	-	UK
Electronic Balance	AR2140	OHAIS	Switzerland
Digital pH meter	pH 209	HANNA	Romania
Shaker	Power Sonic 505	Hwashin Technology	South Korea
Hardness tester	EH-01P	Electro Lab	India
Fribilator	EF-2	Electro Lab	India
Dissolution Tester	TDT-08L Plus	Electro Lab	India
UV-Spectrophotometer	UV-1800	SHIMADZU Corporation	Japan

Methods

Preparation of Matrix Tablet: Indapamide

The tablets were prepared by direct compression method. In all the formulations (Table 3), the weight of the active is 2.5 mg and the total weight of the tablet is 200 mg. At first all the ingredients along with the active were measured appropriately and carefully. The initial stage of the preparation was mixing. The active ingredient, matrix forming polymer Methocel K15M CR and the filler or diluents lactose were mixed well. The next step was milling of the mixed ingredients. At the last stage of the method, microcrystalline cellulose, magnesium stearate and aerosil were added to the formulation. The tablets were prepared by compressing the tablets in using 5 punch compression machine with a 15.00×7.00 mm round punch and die set. The compression force was 10 ton. Before the compression the face of the die and punch were lubricated with purified talc.

Table 3. Formulation of Indapamide sustained release tablet.

Ingradients	F_1 mg	F_2 mg	F_3 mg	F_4 mg	F_5 mg
Indapamide	2.5	2.5	2.5	2.5	2.5
Methocel K15MCR	20	40	60	80	100
Aerosil	3.0	3.0	3.0	3.0	3.0
Microcrystalline Cellulose	4	4	4	4	4
Magnesium stearate	3.5	3.5	3.5	3.5	3.5
Lactose Monohydrate	167.0	147.0	127.0	107.0	87.0

Physical Characterization of Indapamide Tablets

Length, Width, Size and Shape: The length and width of tablets depends on the die and punches selected for making the tablets. The tablets of various sizes and shapes are prepared but generally they are circular with either flat or biconvex faces. Here we prepared round cylindrical shape tablets.

Thickness: The thickness of a tablet can vary without any change in its weight. This is generally due to the difference of density of granules, pressure applied for compression and the speed of compression. The thickness of the tablets was determined by using a Digital Caliper (range 0-150 mm).

Uniformity of Weight: It is desirable that every individual tablet in a batch should be in uniform weight and weight variation within permissible limits. If any weight variation is there, that should fall within the prescribed limits (generally ±10% for tablets weighing 130 mg or less, ±7.5% for tablets weighing 130 to 324 mg and ±5% for tablets weighing more than 324 mg).[7] The weights of 10 tablets of each batch were taken at individually and calculate the average weight of 10 tablets. The weights were determined by using an electronic balance. Then we determined the percentage of weight variation of each tablet by using following formula.

Percentage of weight variation= [(Average weight – Individual weight)/ Average wt.] ×100

Friability: Friability test was performed to evaluate the ability of the tablets to withstand abrasion in packing, handling and transporting. The instrument used for this test is known as 'Friability Test Apparatus' or 'Friabilator'. Friability of the tablets was determined by using Electrolab, EF-2 friability test apparatus. It consists of a plastic chamber which is divided into two parts and revolves at a speed of 25 rpm. A number of tablets were weighed (W_1) and placed in the tumbling chamber which was rotated for four minutes or for 100 revolutions. During each revolution the tablets fall from a distance of six inches to undergo shock. After 100 revolutions the tablets were again weighed (W_2) and the loss in weight indicates the friability. The acceptable limits of weights loss should not be more than 1 percent.[8]

$$\text{Friability} = \{(W_1 - W_2)/W_1\} \times 100$$

Hardness: The hardness of tablet depends on the weight of the material used, space between the upper and lower punches at the time of compression and pressure applied during compression. The hardness also depends on the nature and quantity of excipients used during compression. The hardness of the tablets was determined by using a hand operated hardness tester apparatus (Electrolab, EH-01P). A tablet hardness of about 6-8 kg-ft was considered for mechanical stability.[7] If the finished tablet is too hard, it may not disintegrate in the required period of time and if the tablet is too soft it may not withstand the handling during packing and transporting. Therefore it is very necessary to check the hardness of tablets when they are being compressed and pressure adjusted accordingly on the tablet machine.

Assay of Indapamide

Preparation of Sample Solution: At first, 10 tablets of indapamide SR tablets from each formulation were weighed accurately and were grinded to a fine powder. Then 20 mg of powder was taken in a 100 ml volumetric flask and diluted with phosphate buffer up to the mark. Then 1ml solution was taken into another 100ml volumetric flask and diluted with buffer up to the mark. Then their absorbance was measured at 242 nm using a UV spectrophotometer (UV- 1800, UV-VIS spectrophotometer, Shimadzu, Japan).

Then the percentage of potency was calculated by the following equation:

$$\%\text{ of Potency} = \frac{Aspl \times Wstd \times Pstd \times \text{Average weight}}{Astd \times Wspl \times \text{Label claimed value}}$$

Where,

A_{spl} =Absorbance of Sample

W_{std} =Weight of Standard

P_{std} =Potency of standard

A_{std} = Absorbance of standard

W_{spl} =Weight of sample

Dissolution Procedure: Dissolution studies were conducted by USP type II test apparatus (Electrolab, TDL-80L Plus, India) at a speed of 50 rpm and the temperature was maintained at 37° ± 0.5°C.

This operation was continued for 8 hours. At every 1-hour interval samples of 6 ml were withdrawn from the dissolution medium and replaced with fresh dissolution medium to maintain the volume constant. After filtration and appropriate dilution, the sample solution was analyzed at 242 nm for indapamide by UV spectrophotometer. The amounts of the drug present in the sample were calculated with the help of straight line equation obtained from the standard curve for the drugs. The dissolution study was continued to get a simulated picture of the drug release in the *in vivo* condition and drug dissolved at specified time periods was plotted as percent release versus time (h) curves. This drug release profile was fitted into several mathematical models to get an idea of the release mechanism of the drug from the dosage form.

Analysis of Release Data

The release data obtained were treated according to zero-order (cumulative amount of drug release versus time), first order (log cumulative percentage of drug remaining versus time), Higuchi (cumulative percentage of drug release versus square root of time), and Korsmeyer-Peppas (log cumulative percentage of drug release versus log time) equation models.

Dissolution data were also fitted according to the well-known exponential equation, which is often used to describe the drug release behavior from polymeric systems introduced by Korsmeyer-Peppas *et al.*[9]

$$M_t / M_\infty = k\, t^n$$

Where, M_t is the amount of drug release at time t, M_∞ is the amount of drug release after infinite time; k is a release rate constant incorporating structural and geometric characteristics of the tablet and n is the diffusion exponent indicative of the mechanism of drug release. A value of $n = 0.45$ indicates Fickian (case I) release, > 0.45 but < 0.89 for non-Fickian (anomalous) release and > 0.89 indicates super case II type of release. Case II generally refers to the erosion of the polymeric chain and anomalous transport (non-Fickian) refers to a combination of both diffusion and erosion controlled-drug release.[2] Mean dissolution time (MDT) was calculated from dissolution data using the following equation.[2]

$$MDT = (n/n+1)\, k^{-1/n}$$

Where, n=release exponent and k= release rate constant

Results and Discussion

Drug Content and Physical Evaluation of Indapamide Matrix Tablets

After preparing the matrix tablets, all the tablets of the proposed formulations were subjected to various evaluation tests such as hardness, thickness, uniformity of weight, drug content and friability (Table 4).

Table 4. Physical properties of Indapamide

Formulations	Weight variations (mg)±SEM	Hardness (kg/cm^2)±SEM	Thickness (mm)	Friability (%)	Drug content (%)
F 1	200.45 ± 0.98	6.5 ± 0.21	4.2 ± 0.05	0.03	99.0 ± 1.2
F 2	200.51 ± 1.1	7.1 ± 0.35	4.3 ± 0.04	0.04	101.12 ± 0.97
F 3	200.43 ±1.3	7.9 ± 0.65	4.5 ± 0.04	0.02	99.23 ± 0.27
F 4	201.3± 0.95	8.1 ± 0.24	4.4 ± 0.03	0.03	100.52 ± 0.86
F 5	201.7 ± 1.12	8.0 ± 0.37	4.2 ± 0.04	0.02	98.33 ± 0.96

Here, n=10; SEM= Standard Error Mean

Polymeric Effect on Formulated Indapamide Tablets

For this study different matrix tablets containing Indapamide as active ingredient and Methocel K15MCR as the rate retarding polymer were prepared. The polymer concentrations were 10%, 20%, 30%, 40%, and 50% of the total tablet weight having the formulation codes F1, F2, F3, F4, and F5 respectively. After preparing the tablets the dissolution studies were conducted in paddle method at a speed of 50 rpm and the temperature was maintained at 37° ± 0.5°C. This operation was continued for 8 hours. Three tablets from each formulation were taken for the test. *In vitro* release kinetics and mechanisms are explained by zero order, first order, higuchi and korsmeyer models. The highest Methocel K15MCR containing formulation F5 showed the highest MDT and t_{50} value which indicates the rate retarding effect of Methocel K15MCR (Table 5). From Figure 1- 4, we can see the zero order, first order, Higuchi and Korsmeyer-Peppas release kinetics of the formulated drugs respectively.

Table 5. MDT and t_{50} value of the drug Indapamide

Formulation	t_{50} (hr)	MDT
F1	5.6663	4.67745
F2	8.6633	6.637662
F3	12.7643	11.63254
F4	15.754	14.76884
F5	23.6574	21.65762

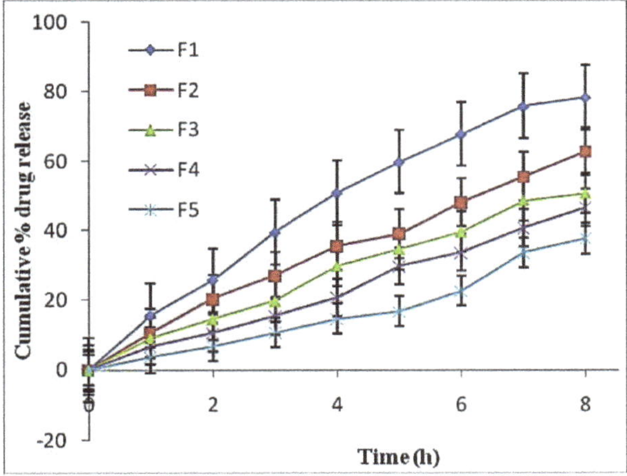

Figure 1. Zero order release kinetics of Indapamide from Methocel K15MCR matrices

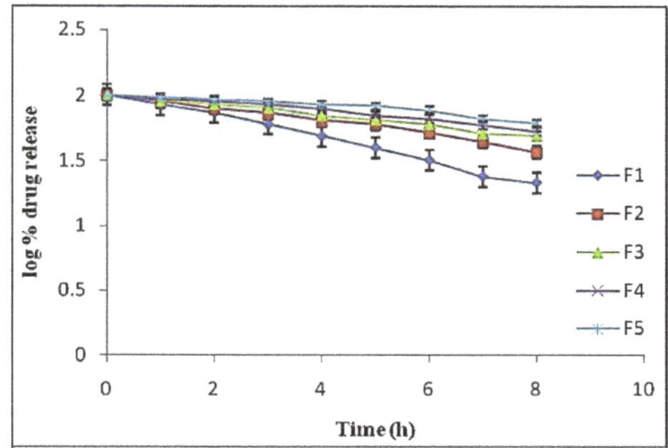

Figure 2. First order release kinetics of Indapamide from Methocel K15MCR matrices

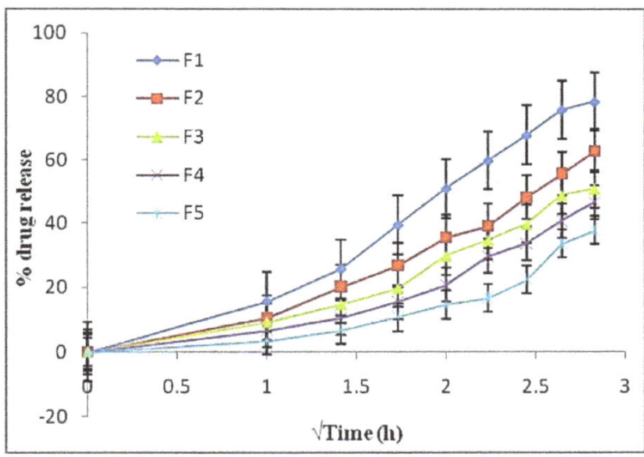

Figure 3. Higuchi release kinetics of Indapamide from Methocel K15MCR matrices

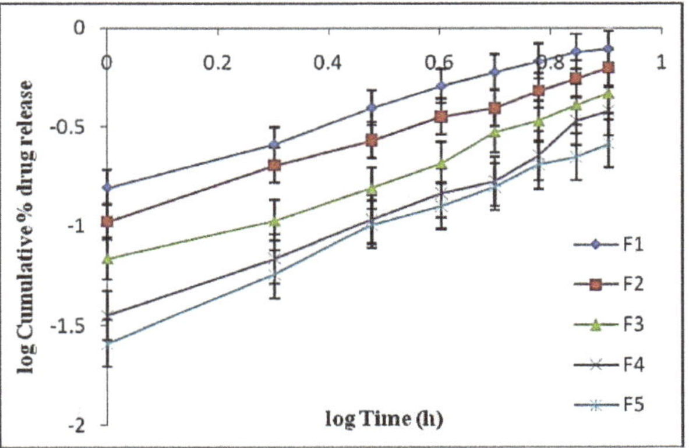

Figure 4. Korsmeyer- Peppas release kinetics of Indapamide from Methocel K15MCR matrices

Conclusion

The study reveals that it is possible to design sustained release solid dosage form with Methocel K15MCR polymer. The polymers which were used in the formulations seem to be satisfactory for sustained release properties. The polymeric effects on the formulated tablets are evident. The MDT and t_{50} value of the formulated tablets were also satisfactory. In fine, further investigation is required to establish *in-vivo-in-vitro* correlation to manifest the exact pattern of drug release *in-vivo* condition from this polymeric system.

Acknowledgements

The authors are thankful to the Silva Pharmaceuticals Ltd., Bangladesh for the generous donation of active ingredient of Indapamide and giving the chance to work in their product development department which was very helpful in accomplishing the project work in time and make it successful. The authors are also thankful the Department of Pharmacy, Noakhali Science and Technology University for giving opportunity to use the laboratory facility.

Conflict of Interest

The authors declare that they have no conflict of interest.

References

1. Ahmed M, Ahamed SK, Dewan SMR, Moghal MMR. Development of sustained release matrix tablets of ramipril and evaluation of polymer effect *on in-vitro* release pattern. *Int J Pharm Sci Res* 2013;4(3):1039-45.
2. Ira IJ, Ahamed SK, Dewan SMR, Moghal MMR, Islam MA. Formulation and *in-vitro* evaluation of theophylline sr matrix tablets and comparison of release rate with marketed products dispensed in Bangladesh. *Int J Pharm Ther* 2013;4(2):91-7.
3. Rahela U, Moghal MMR, Dewan SMR, Amin MN. Formulation and evaluation of polymer effect on *in-vitro* kinetics of sustained release matrix tablets of carvedilol using model dependent methods. *Int J Pharm Life Sci* 2013;2(2):70-9.
4. Ashkari ST, Moghal MMR, Dewan SMR, Amin MN. Development of sustained release matrix tablets of carvedilol and evaluation of polymer effect on *in-vitro* release pattern. *Int J Curr Pharm Clin Res* 2013;3(1):18-22.
5. Williams RO, 3rd, Reynolds TD, Cabelka TD, Sykora MA, Mahaguna V. Investigation of excipient type and level on drug release from controlled release tablets containing HPMC. *Pharm Dev Technol* 2002;7(2):181-93.
6. Chaffman M, Heel RC, Brogden RN, Speight TM, Avery GS. Indapamide. A review of its pharmacodynamic properties and therapeutic efficacy in hypertension. *Drugs* 1984;28(3):189-235.
7. British Pharmacopoeia. London: Her Majesty's Stationary Office; 2000.
8. Gupta AK. *Introduction to Pharmaceutics.* 3rd ed. Delhi: CBS publishers; 1994.
9. Korsmeyer RW, Gurny R, Doelker E, Buri P, Peppas NA. Mechanism of solute release from porous hydrophilic polymers. *Int J Pharm* 1983;15(1):25-35.

Construction of Yeast Recombinant Expression Vector Containing Human Epidermal Growth Factor (hEGF)

Jamal Mohammadian[1], Sima Mansoori-Derakhshan[2], Masood Mohammadian[3], Mahmoud Shekari-Khaniani[2]*

[1] *Department of Clinical Biochemistry, Division of Medical Biotechnology, Faculty of Medicine, Tabriz University of Medical Sciences, Tabriz, Iran.*

[2] *Department of Medical Genetics, Faculty of Medicine, Tabriz University of Medical Sciences, Tabriz, Iran.*

[3] *East Azerbaijan Agriculture and Jahad Organization, Tabriz, Iran.*

ARTICLEINFO

Keywords:
Epidermal Growth Factor
pPIC9
Polymerase Chain Reaction
Cloning
Expression
Sequencing

ABSTRACT

Purpose: The objective of this study was construction of recombinant hEGF-pPIC9 which may be used for expression of recombinant hEGF in following studies. ***Methods:*** EGF cDNA was purchased from Genecopoeia Company and used for PCR amplification. Prior to ligation, the PCR product and pPIC9 vector was digested with EcoRI and XhoI and ligated in pPIC9 vector and subjected to colony PCR screening and sequencing analysis. ***Results:*** PCR amplification of EGF cDNA using recombinant hEGF-pPIC9 vector as template was concluded in amplification of 197bp fragment. Construction of recombinant hEGF-pPIC9 of EGf gene was verified by PCR and sequencing. ***Conclusion:*** Construction of Recombinant hEGF-pPIC9 was the primary stage for production and expression of EFG in the future study.

Introduction

Epidermal growth factor (EGF) is a member of an extensive class of molecules, reffered to as growth factors, that intervenes in cell growth and differentiation.[1] Epidermal growth factor (EGF), a small polypeptide consist of 53 amino acids with molecular weight of about 6.3kDa, is present in copious mammalian species[2-5] There are six cysteine residues in the hEGF sequence that comprised three disulfide band.[6] Human EGF was purified from urine by Cohen & Carpenter; Starkey et al. EFG was first isolated from the parotid gland of male mice and subsequently from human urine as urogastrone.[7] Mouse EGF is derived from a 1217 amino acid precursor protein which contains 7 additional EGF-like domains. Human EGF is come apart from a 1207 amino acid precursor.[8] Studies have demonstrated that EGF can prompt abundant effect on both cells and epithelial tissue. Besides, hEGF has been noticed to have many biological actions both in vivo and in vitro. Studies have focused on the proliferative efficiency of EGF on keratinocytes, fibroblasts and epithelial cells.[9,10] The yeast Pichia pastoris is a practical system for the expression of milligram-to-gram amounts of proteins for both simple laboratory experimentation and industrialized production.[11,12] The aim of this study was construction of recombinant pPIC9/hEGF which will be used for expression of recombinant hEGF in the following studies.

Materials and Methods

Materials

All restriction endonucleases, T4 DNA ligase, Plasmid Miniprep Kit and Gel Extraction Kit were purchased from fermentas company (Vilnius, Lithuania). EGF cDNA was purchased from genecopoeia company (Accession: NM_001963.2). Plasmid pPIC9 which contains AOX1 prompter and E. coli strain DH5-α (F– Φ80lacZΔM15 Δ (lacZYA-argF) U169 recA1 endA1 hsdR17 (rK–, mK+) phoA supE44 λ– thi-1 gyrA96 relA1) were provided from Pasteur Institute of Iran (Tehran). LB medium was purchased from Sigma Aldrich (L7658-1KG).

Amplification of hEGF gene with PCR

Amplification of EFG gene was accomplished by the following primers: Forward primer 5′ATCTGGAGAAAAGAGAGGCTGAAGCTAAT AGTGACTCTCAATGTCCC3′ and reverse primer 5′AATGAATTCTTAGCGCAGTTCCCACCACTTC

***Corresponding author:** Mahmoud Shekari-Khaniani, Department of Medical Genetics, Faculty of Medicine, Tabriz University of Medical Sciences, Tabriz, Iran. Email: Shekarima@tbzmed.ac.ir

AGGTCTC3′ that contain restriction sites for XhoI and EcoRI at 5′terminal respectively (underlined). PCR reaction contain 10 x PCR buffer, 400 µM dNTPs, 50 ng Genomic DNA, primers (EGF-F, EGF-R) 0.2 µM from each primer, 3 mM MgCl2 and 1 unit from Taq DNA polymerase (cinnagen) and following program was accomplished for amplification of desired fragment: Initial denaturation at 94 °C for 5 minute followed with 94 °C for 1 minute, 52 °C for 20 second for annealing and 72 °C for 45 second for extention that repeated for 35 cycles.

Constructing of recombinant vector and sequencing

The PCR product was purified with GeneJET PCR Purification Kit (Fermentas) and digested by EcoRI and XhoI restriction enzymes. Then this fragment with pPIC9 vector that previously digested by mentioned enzymes subjected to ligation reaction and its product was transformed to DH5-α by heat shock method.Various clone screened by colony PCR method and the positive clones analyzed by sequencing using EGF-F primer.

Results

Amplification of EGF gene

For this purpose thermal gradient PCR (50-54) was carried out to optimized temperature of primer annealing. As seen in Figure 1, PCR in annealing temperature over than 52 °C give rise to specific amplification of 197bp fragment. (Figure 1)

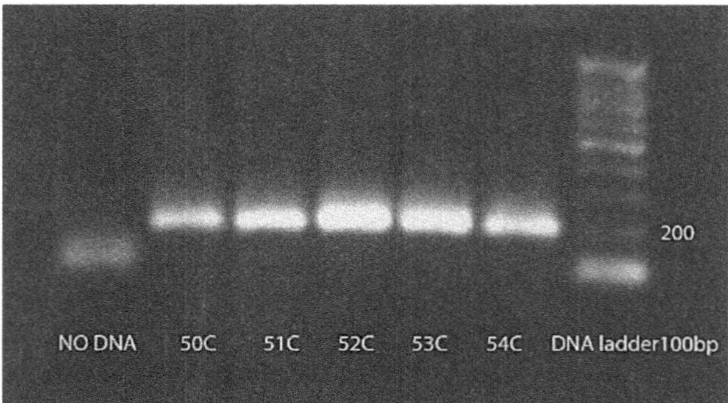

Figure 1. Optimization of PCR reaction for amplification of *EGF* gene.PCR in annealing temperature in 52 °C gives rise to specific amplification of 197bp fragment.

Cloning and sequencing of EGF gene

The double-digested PCR products were mixed with predigested pPIC9 vector (Figure 2) and introduced in ligation reaction. Then ligation product was transformed to DH5-α *E.coli* bacteria and recombinant plasmid extracted. The colony PCR was carried out on transformant using the mentioned primers and desired 197bp fragment was observed on 1% Agarose by UV transilluminator (Figure 3). In the next step, recombinant pPIC9 was analyzed by sequencing. Comparison of hEGF sequence with available sequences in Gene bank showed that obtained sequence has 100% homology with Homo sapiens epidermal growth factor (hEGF), transcript variant 3 (NM_001178131.1).

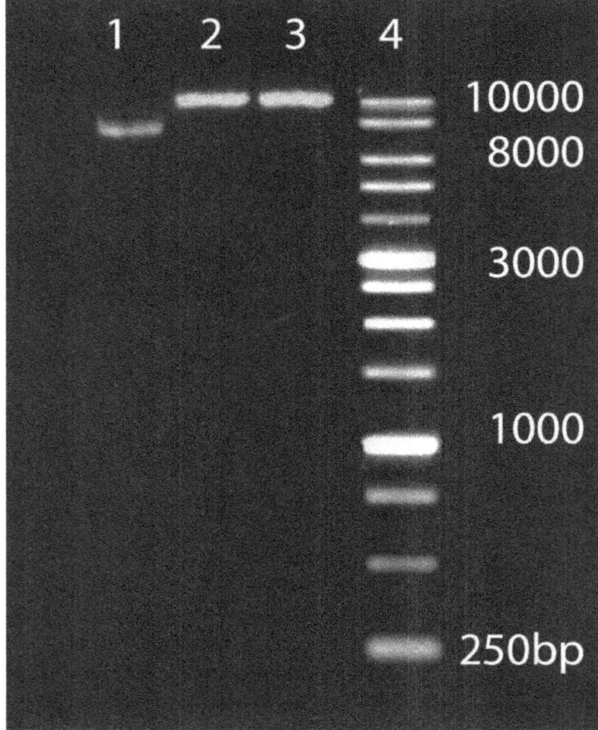

Figure 2. Digestion of pPIC9 vector: line 1; undigested pPIC9 vector line 2 and 3; digested pPIC9 vector line 4; DNA ladder (1kb).

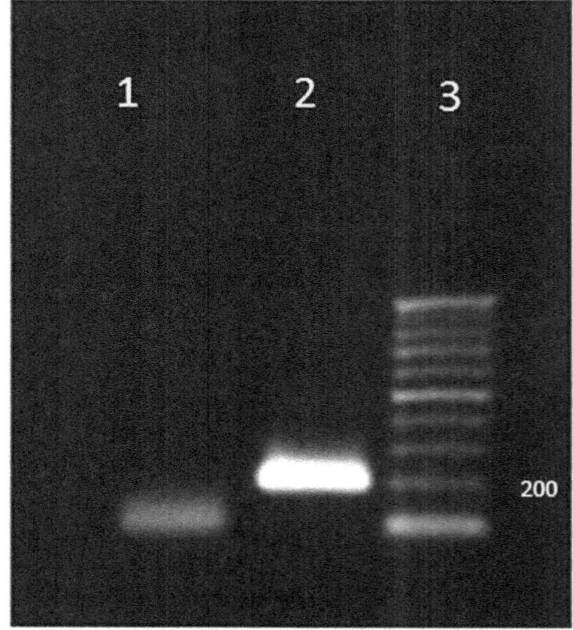

Figure 3. PCR assay for detection of desired 197bp fragment in recombinant pPIC9/hEGF vector: line 1; no DNA line 2; EGF gene (197bp) line 3; DNA ladder (100bp).

Discussion

The application of P.pastoris for the production of heterologous proteins is highly successful[13] Essential to the production of heterologous proteins in P.pastoris is construction of expression vector. This necessitates the selection of both proper expression vector and related strain.[14-16] In the present study recombinant pPIC9/hEGF was constructed. This expression vector rely on the AOX1 promoter and contains α-mating factor secretion signal for secretion of recombinant protein into extracellular environment.[17] A more superiority of Pichia is that it is remarkably suitable for fermentation and can reach high cell densities that may improve overall protein yields.[13,18,19] Also pichia has a secretory system that enable to secrete desired protein and conformation of disulfide bind was performed easily.[20] For soluble secretory proteins, undoubtedly, it is the most simple and the most trustworthy expression system with possible to yield grams of the favorite protein.[21,22]

The construction of recombinant hEGF has been conducted by many researchers in a variety of vector for many applications.[23,24] In construction of pPIC9/hEGF, the important point which should be considered is insertion of correct ORF of gene. At this stage of this research, the correction of insert ORF was confirmed by PCR and sequencing analysis. In the future study, the construction of recombinant vector pPIC9/hEGF should be more characterized for expression of recombinant protein.

Acknowledgements

We thank laboratory of genetics, laboratory of school of advanced medical science and all staffs that collaborated in this project. This work was supported by staff development and application of stem cell research grant.

Conflict of Interest

The authors report no conflicts of interest.

References

1. Bell GI, Fong NM, Stempien MM, Wormsted MA, Caput D, Ku LL, et al. Human epidermal growth factor precursor: cDNA sequence, expression in vitro and gene organization. *Nucleic Acids Res* 1986;14(21):8427-46.
2. Fisher DA, Lakshmanan J. Metabolism and effects of epidermal growth factor and related growth factors in mammals. *Endocr Rev* 1990;11(3):418-42.
3. Parries Gregory, Chen K, Misono KS, Cohen S. The human urinarrry epidermal growyh factor (EGF) precursor. *J Biol Chem* 1995;270(46):27954-60.
4. Valcarce C, Bjork I, Stenflo J. The epidermal growth factor precursor. A calcium-binding, beta-hydroxyasparagine containing modular protein present on the surface of platelets. *Eur J Biochem* 1999;260(1):200-7.
5. Fisher DA, Salido EC, Barajas L. Epidermal growth factor and the kidney. *Annu Rev Physiol* 1989;51:67-80.
6. Lee DN, Kuo TY, Chen MC, Tang TY, Liu FH, Weng CF. Expression of porcine epidermal growth factor in Pichia pastoris and its biology activity in early-weaned piglets. *Life Sci* 2006;78(6):649-54.
7. Razis AFA, Ismail EN, Hambali Z, Abdullah MNH, Ali AM, Lila MAM. The Periplasmic Expression of Recombinant Human Epidermal Growth Factor (hEGF) in Escherichia coli. *AsPac J Mol Biol Biotechnol* 2006;14(2):41-5.
8. Mroczkowski B, Reich M, Chen K, Bell GI, Cohen S. Recombinant human epidermal growth factor precursor is a glycosylated membrane protein with biological activity. *Mol Cell Biol* 1989;9(7):2771-8.
9. Milani S, Calabro A. Role of growth factors and their receptors in gastric ulcer healing. *Microsc Res Tech* 2001;53(5):360-71.
10. Chairmandurai AR, Kanappa SV, Vadrevu KM, Putcha UK, Venkatesan V. Recombinant Human Epidermal Growth Factor Alleviates Gastric Antral Ulcer Induced by Naproxen: A Non-steroidal Anti Inflammatory Drug. *Gastroenterol Res* 2010;3(3):125-33.
11. Hamilton SR, Bobrowicz P, Bobrowicz B, Davidson RC, Li H, Mitchell T, et al. Production of complex human glycoproteins in yeast. *Science* 2003;301(5637):1244-6.
12. Faber KN, Harder W, Ab G, Veenhuis M. Review: methylotrophic yeasts as factories for the production of foreign proteins. *Yeast* 1995;11(14):1331-44.
13. Boze H, Celine L, Patrick C, Fabien R, Christine V, Yves C, et al. High-level secretory production of recombinant porcine follicle-stimulating hormone by Pichia pastoris. *Process Biochem* 2001;36:907-13.
14. Cereghino GPL, Sunga AJ, Cereghino JL, Cregg JM. Expression of foreign genes in the yeast Pichia pastoris. In: Setlow JK, editor. Genetic Engineering: Principles and Methods. London: Kluwer Academic/Plenum; 2001. P. 157-69.
15. Cereghino GP, Cereghino JL, Ilgen C, Cregg JM. Production of recombinant proteins in fermenter cultures of the yeast Pichia pastoris. *Curr Opin Biotechnol* 2002;13(4):329-32.
16. Cregg JM, Madden KR. Development of the methylotrophic yeast, Pichia pastoris, as a host system for the production of foreign proteins. *Dev Ind Microbiol* 1988;29:33-41.
17. Wegner GH. Emerging applications of the methylotrophic yeasts. *FEMS Microbiol Rev* 1990;7(3-4):279-83.
18. Brankamp RG, Sreekrishna K, Smith PL, Blankenship DT, Cardin AD. Expression of a synthetic gene encoding the anticoagulant-antimetastatic protein ghilanten by the

methylotropic yeast Pichia pastoris. *Protein Expr Purif* 1995;6(6):813-20.

19. Brocca S, Schmidt-Dannert C, Lotti M, Alberghina L, Schmid RD. Design, total synthesis, and functional overexpression of the Candida rugosa lip1 gene coding for a major industrial lipase. *Protein Sci* 1998;7(6):1415-22.
20. Vad R, Nafstad E, Dahl LA, Gabrielsen OS. Engineering of a Pichia pastoris expression system for secretion of high amounts of intact human parathyroid hormone. *J Biotechnol* 2005;116(3):251-60.
21. Magherini F, Tani C, Gamberi T, Caselli A, Bianchi L, Bini L, et al. Protein expression profiles in Saccharomyces cerevisiae during apoptosis induced by H2O2. *Proteomics* 2007;7(9):1434-45.
22. Baneyx F. Recombinant protein expression in Escherichia coli. *Curr Opin Biotechnol* 1999;10(5):411-21.
23. Elloumi I, Kobayashi R, Funabashi H, Mie M, Kobatake E. Construction of epidermal growth factor fusion protein with cell adhesive activity. *Biomaterials* 2006;27(18):3451-8.
24. Li X, Sui X, Zhang Y, Sun Y, Zhao Y, Zhai Y, et al. An improved calcium chloride method preparation and transformation of competent cells. *Afr J Biotechnol* 2010;9(50):8549-54.

Isolation and Antimicrobial and Antioxidant Evaluation of Bio-Active Compounds from *Eriobotrya Japonica* Stems

Khaled Nabih Rashed[1*], **Monica Butnariu**[2]

[1] *Pharmacognosy Department, National Research Centre, Dokki, Giza, Egypt.*

[2] *Chemistry and Vegetal Biochemistry, Banat's University of Agricultural Sciences and Veterinary Medicine from Timisoara, Calea Aradului, Timisoara 300645, Romania.*

ARTICLEINFO

Keywords:
Eriobotrya japonica
Stems
Antimicrobial
Antioxidant
Chemical constituents

ABSTRACT

Purpose: The present study was carried out to evaluate antimicrobial and antioxidant activities from *Eriobotrya japonica* stems as well investigation of its chemical composition.
Methods: Methanol 80% extract of *Eriobotrya japonica* stems was tested for antimicrobial activity against bacterial and fungal strains and for antioxidant activity using oxygen radical absorbance capacity (ORAC) and the trolox equivalent antioxidant capacity (TEAC) assays and also total content of polyphenols with phytochemical analysis of the extract were determined.
Results: The results showed that the extract has a significant antimicrobial activity, it inhibited significantly the growth of *Candida albicans* suggesting that it can be used in the treatment of fungal infections, and it showed no effect on the other bacterial and fungal strains, the extract has a good antioxidant activity, it has shown high values of oxygen radical absorbance capacity and trolox equivalent antioxidant capacity, while it showed a low value of polyphenol content. Phytochemical analysis of the extract showed the presence of carbohydrates, terpenes, tannins and flavonoids, further phytochemical analysis resulted in the isolation and identification of three triterpenic acids, oleanolic, ursolic and corosolic acids and four flavonoids, naringenin, quercetin, kaempferol 3-*O*-*β*-glucoside and quercetin 3-O-α-rhamnoside.
Conclusion: These results may help to discover new chemical classes of natural antimicrobial antioxidant substances.

Introduction

Medicinal plants represent a rich source of antimicrobial agents. A wide range of medicinal plant parts is used for extract as a raw drugs and they possess varied medicinal properties. Natural products are known to play an important role in both drug discovery and chemical biology. Infectious diseases account for approximately one-half of all death in tropical countries, approximately 5 million people in Africa. Bacterial and fungal infection have been a major problem considered for decades that causes spoilage of food products and various diseases in plants and humans, which leads to significant losses in the crop productivity and health problems worldwide. The World Health Organization estimates that plant extracts or their active constituents are used as folk medicine in traditional therapies of 80% of the worlds population.[1] The effect of plant extracts on microorganism have been studied by a very large number of researchers in different parts of the world.[2-5] *Eriobotrya japonica* Lindl (Rosaceae family) is a well known medicinal plant in Japan and China. In folk medicine, *E. Japonica* leaves have beneficial effects in numerous diseases including asthma, gastroenteric discorders, diabetes mellitus and chronic bronchitis.[6] Previous phytochemical studies on *E. Japonica* proved the presence of various triterpenes, sesquiterpenes, flavonoids, tannins and megastigmane glycosides in the leaves and some of these compounds have been found to possess antiviral, antitumor, hypoglycemic and anti-inflammatory activities.[7-10] The present study were undertaken to evaluate antimicrobial and antioxidant activities from stems of *E. Japonica* as well investigation of its chemical composition.

Materials and Methods

UV/VIS: Shimadzu UV-visible recording spectrophotometer model-UV 240 (NRC, Egypt). ^{1}H-NMR spectra and ^{13}C-NMR spectra: Varian Unity Inova 400 Varian Unity (Graz University, Austria). MS (Finnigan MAT SSQ 7000, 70 ev). Silica gel (0.063-

***Corresponding author:** Khaled Nabih Rashed, Pharmacognosy Department, National Research Centre, Dokki, Giza, Egypt.
Email: khalednabih2015@yahoo.co.uk

0.200 mm for column chromatography) and Sephadex LH-20 (Pharmacia Fine Chemicals). Paper Chromatography (PC) Whatman No.1 (Whatman Led. Maid Stone, Kent, England) sheets.

Plant material

Finely ground stems of *Eriobotrya japonica* were collected from the Agricultural Research Centre, Giza, Egypt in May 2011 and the plant was identified by Dr. Mohammed El-Gebaly, Department of Botany, National Research Centre (NRC). A voucher specimen is deposited in the herbarium of Agricultural Research Centre, Giza, Egypt.

Preparation of Plant Extract

Air dried powder from the stems of *Eriobotrya japonica* (840 g) was extracted with methanol 80% at room temperature several times until exhaustion by maceration method. The extract was concentrated under reduced pressure to give 45 g of crude extract. The extract was tested for the presence of bioactive compounds according to following standard tests (Molisch 's test for carbohydrates, Shinoda test for flavonoids, forth test for saponins, Salkowski 's for terpenes and sterols, $FeCl_3$ and Mayer's reagents for detecting of tannins and alkaloids, respectively.[11-13]

Isolation of bio-active compounds from methanol extract of *E. japonica stems:* Methanol extract 42 g was subjected to silica gel column chromatography eluting with n-hexane, dichloromethane, ethyl acetate and methanol gradually. The fractions that showed similar thin layer chromatography (TLC) were collected and according to that four fractions were collected. Fraction 1 (930 mg) eluted with dichloromethane: ethyl acetate (60:40) gave compound 1 (oleanolic acid, 16 mg). Fraction 2 (1.12 g) eluted with dichloromethane: ethyl acetate (50:50) gave compound 2 (ursolic acid, 21 mg) and compound 3 (corosolic acid, 18 mg). Fraction 3 (835 mg) eluted with ethyl acetate: dichloromethane: (70:30) gave compound 4 (naringenin, 12 mg) and further elution with ethyl acetate gave compound 5 (quercetin, 8 mg). Compound 6 (kaempferol 3-*O*-*β*-glucoside, 25 mg) and compound 7 (Quercetin 3-O-α-rhamnoside, 19 mg) were obtained from fraction 4 (840 mg) with further elution of ethyl acetate and methanol. All the compounds were purified on sephadex LH–20 column using methanol and water as eluents.

Acid hydrolysis of flavonoids

Solutions of 5 mg of compounds 6 and 7 in 5 ml 10% HCl was heated for 5 h. The aglycones were extracted with ethyl acetate and identified by co-TLC with authentic standards. The sugars in the aqueous layer were identified by co-paper chromatography (co-PC) with authentic markers on Whatman No. 1 sheets in solvent system (n-BuOH-AcOH-H_2O 4:1:5 upper layer).

Antimicrobial Assays

The quantitative assay of the antimicrobial activity was performed by broth microdilution method[14,15] in 96–well microplates in order to establish the minimal inhibitory concentration (MIC). The antimicrobial activity was tested against Gram–positive strains (*Staphylococcus aureus, Bacillus subtilis*), Gram–negative (*Escherichia coli, Pseudomonas aeruginosa, Klebsiella pneumoniae*) and fungal strain (*Candida albicans*). The methanol extract of *E. japonica* was tested for its antimicrobial activity using a qualitative screening assay of the antimicrobial properties by the adapted disk diffusion method, Kirby–Bauer method.[16] The quantitative assay of the antimicrobial activity was performed by binary microdilution method,[14] in order to establish the minimal inhibitory concentration (MIC). The antimicrobial activity of the investigated extract was tested against bacterial and fungal strains: Gram positive (*Staphylococcus aureus, Bacillus subtilis*), Gram–negative (*Escherichia coli, Pseudomonas aeruginosa, Klebsiella pneumoniae*) and fungal strains (*Candida albicans*). The microbial strains were identified using a VITEK I automatic system. VITEK cards for the identification and the susceptibility testing (GNS–522) were inoculated and incubated according to the manufacturer's recommendations. In our experiments there were used bacterial suspensions of $1.5x10^8$ UFC/ mL or 0.5 McFarland density obtained from 15–18 h bacterial cultures developed on solid media. The antimicrobial activity was tested on Mueller–Hinton medium recommended for the bacterial strains and Yeast Peptone Glucose (YPG) medium for *Candida albicans*. Solutions of the extract in DMSO (dimethyl sulfoxide) having 2048 μg/ mL concentration were used.

Qualitative screening of the antimicrobial properties of the extract

The antimicrobial activity of the extract was investigated by qualitative screening of the susceptibility spectrum of different microbial strains to the tested extract solubilised in DMSO (1 mg/mL) using adapted variants of the diffusion method. In the 1st variant, 10 μL of the extract solution were equally distributed on the paper filter disks placed on Petri dishes previously seeded "in layer" with the tested bacterial strain inoculums. In the 2nd variant, 10 μL of the tested extract solutions were placed in the agar wells cut in the solid culture medium seeded with the microbial inoculum. In the 3rd variant of the qualitative antimicrobial activity assay, 10 μL of the extract solutions were spotted on Petri dishes seeded with bacterial/yeast inoculum. In all the three variants, the Petri dishes were left at room temperature to ensure the equal diffusion of the compound in the medium or to allow the drop of solution to be adsorbed in the medium and afterwards the dishes were incubated at 37°C for 24 hours. The solvent used was also tested in order to evaluate a potential antimicrobial activity.

Quantitative assay of the antimicrobial activity

For the quantitative assay of the antimicrobial activity of the extract by the microdilution method[14,17] in liquid medium distributed in 96–well plates, binary serial dilutions of the tested extract solutions were performed. There were obtained concentrations from 1000 µg/mL to 0.97 µg/mL in a 200 µL culture medium final volume, afterwards each well was seeded with a 50 µL microbial suspension of 0.5 MacFarland density. In each test a microbial culture control (a series of wells containing exclusively culture medium with the microbial suspension) and a sterility control (a series of wells containing exclusively culture medium) were performed. The plates were incubated for 24 hours at 37°C.

Antioxidant assays: Extraction: 0.2 g of extract with 10 mL Millipore water boiled was sonic, centrifuged and filtered. Evaluation of antioxidant activity of the extract, using methods Oxygen Radical Absorbance Capacity (ORAC), Trolox equivalent antioxidant capacity (TEAC) and determination of total polyphenols content:

Oxygen Radical Absorbance Capacity (ORAC)

This method determines peroxil radical inhibition capacity, inducing oxidation highlighting the classical radical release; H atom transfer ORAC values were reported as Trolox equivalents, is expressed as micromol TE/DW. The intensity was monitored at 485 nm and 525 nm for 35 min.

Trolox equivalent antioxidant capacity method (TEAC)

This method is based the neutralizing capacity the radical anion $ABTS^+$ [2,2'–azino–bis (3–ethylbenzothiazoline–6–sulphonic acid)] by antioxidants. ABTS is oxidized by radicals peroxil or other oxidants to its radical cation $ABTS^+$, intensely colored (λmax = 734 nm). Antioxidant capacity is expressed compounds tested as potential, to discoloration by direct reaction with it radical $ABTS^+$.

The total content of polyphenols

The blue compounds formed between phenols and Folin–Ciocalteu reagent phenolic compounds are independent of structure, thus developing complex between metal center and phenolic compounds. Absorption was recorded at a wavelength of 765 nm. Total phenol content was expressed as gallic acid equivalents.[18]

Results

The present investigation was focused to evaluate the antimicrobial activity (expressed in µg/ mL) and antioxidant capacity (expressed as Trolox equivalents and total polyphenol content) as can be seen in Figures 1 and 2, as well investigation of the presence of phytochemicals, where phytochemical analysis revealed that carbohydrates, triterpenes, tannins and flavonoids are present in the extract Table 1, estimation of the main bioactive constituents of *Eriobotrya japonica* stems MeOH extract has shown that the bioactive components of *Eriobotrya japonica* stems were three triterpenic acids, Oleanolic, Ursolic and corosolic acids and four flavonoids,, quercetin, naringenin, kaempferol 3-*O*-*β*-glucoside and quercetin 3-O-α-rhamnoside. The chemical structures of the isolated compounds as in Figure 3.

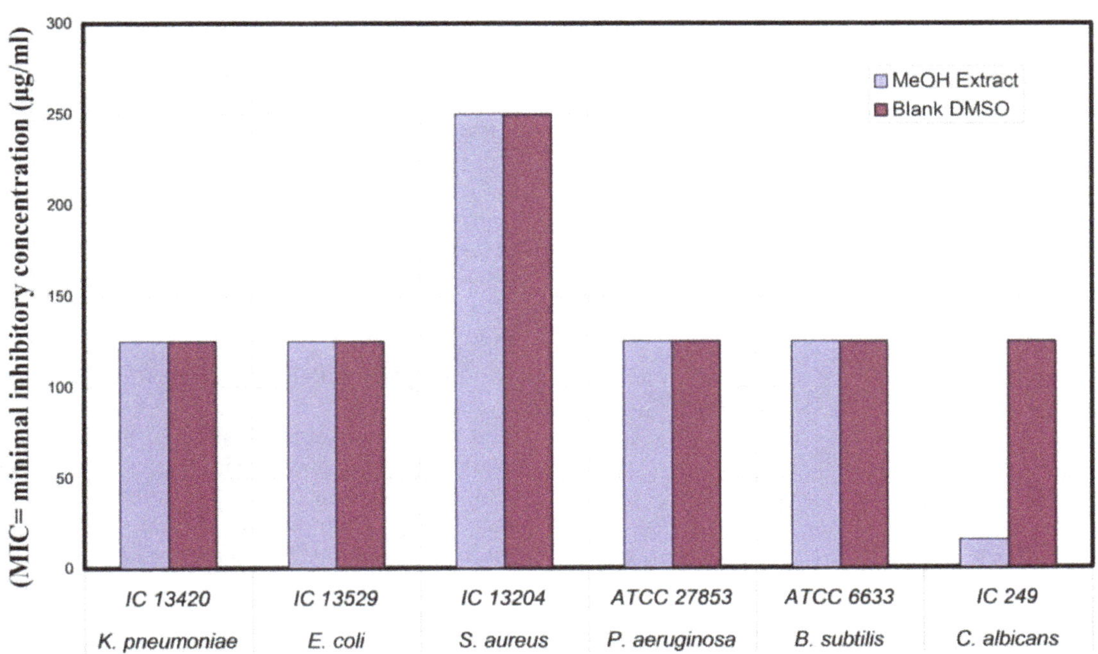

Figure 1. Antimicrobial activity of *Eriobotrya japonica* methanol extract

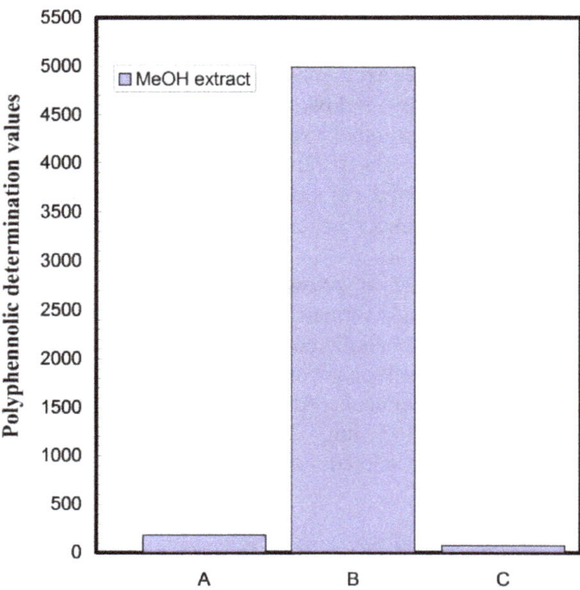

Figure 2. Antioxidant capacity of *Eriobotrya japonica* methanol extract was expressed as Trolox equivalents. **(A):** Total polyphenol content (gallic acid mg/g DW), (**B**): Oxygen radical absorbance capacity (ORAC) assay values, (**C**): Trolox equivalent antioxidant capacity (TEAC) assay values.

Table 1. Phytochemical Analysis of the *Eriobotrya japonica* methanol extract

Constituents	Methanol extract
Triterpenes and /or Sterols	+
Carbohydrates and/or glycosides	+
Flavonoids	+
Coumarins	-
Alkaloids and/or nitrogenous compounds	-
Tannins	+
Saponins	-
(+) presence of constituents, (-) absence of constituents	

Structure Elucidation of the isolated compounds

Oleanolic acid (1): White amorphous powder. ^{1}H-NMR ($CDCl_3$, 400 MHz): δ 5.23 (IH, t, J=3.4, H-12), 3.17 (1H, dd, J=10, 4.2 Hz, H-3), 2.74 (1H, dd, J=12.5, 4 Hz, H-18), 0.95 (3H, s, Me-23), 0.76 (3H, s, Me-24), 0.85 (3H, s, Me-25), 0.77 (3H, s, Me-26), 1.23 (3H, s, Me-27), 0.89 (3H, s, Me-29), 0.95 (3H, s, Me-30). (+) ESI-MS: m/z 455 $[M-H]^+$.

Ursolic acid (2): White powder. ^{1}H-NMR ($CDCl_3$, 400 MHz):δ 5.26 (IH, t, J=3.5, H-12), 3.17 (1H, dd, J=10, 4.2 Hz, H-3), 2.15 (1H, d, J=11.5 Hz, H-18), 1.92 (1H, dd, J=12.8, 4.2 Hz, H_b-22), 1.12 (1H, m, H_a-22), 1. 22 (3H, s, Me-23), 0.94 (3H, s, Me-24), 0.75 (3H, s, Me-25), 1.04 (3H, s, Me-26), 1.12 (3H, s, Me-27), 0.92 (3H, d, J= 6.4 Hz, Me-29), 0.89 (3H, d, *J*=5.8Hz, Me-30). (+) ESI-MS: m/z 455 $[M-H]^+$.

Corosolic acid (3): White amorphous powder. ^{1}H-NMR (pyridine-d_5, 500 MHz): δ 4.07 (1H, ddd, *J* = 3.8, 9.4, 11.0 Hz, H-2), 3.41 (1H, d, *J* = 9.5 Hz, H-3), 5.42 (1H, br s, H-12), 2.61 (1H, d, *J* = 10.9 Hz, H-18), 1.36 (3H, s, H-23), 1.12 (3H, s, H-24), 1.09 (3H, s, H-25), 1.04 (3H, s, H-26), 1.21 (3H, s, H-27), 1.03 (3H, d, *J* =6 Hz, H-29), 0.96 (3H, d, *J* = 6.0 Hz, H-30). (^{13}C-NMR, pyridine-d_5) δ 48.58 (C-1), 69.14 (C-2), 84.35 (C-3), 40.39 (C-4), 56.46 (C-5), 19.35 (C-6), 34.9 (C-7), 41.2 (C-8), 49.5 (C-9), 39.2 (C-10), 23.7 (C-11), 126.28 (C-12), 139.85 (C-13), 43.8 (C-14), 29.5 (C-15), 25.9 (C-16), 48.65 (C-17), 54.28 (C-18), 40.22 (C-19), 40.45 (C-20), 31.58 (C-21), 38.4 (C-22), 29.7 (C-23), 19.1 (C-24), 18.6 (C-25), 17.95 (C-26), 25.2 (C-27), 181.2 (C-28), 18.24 (C-29), 21.95 (C-30). EI-MS: *m/z* 472.

Naringenin (4): Pale yellow needles, ^{1}HNMR (CD_3OD, 500 MHz,) δ 7.25 (2H, d, *J* = 8.2 Hz, H-2', 6'), 6.89 (2H, d, *J* = 8.2 Hz, H-3', 5'), 5.82 (1H, d, *J* = 2.4 Hz, H-8), 5.8 (1H, d, *J* = 2.4 Hz, H-6), 5.28 (1H, dd, *J* = 13 3.5 Hz, H-2), 3.12 (1H, dd, *J* = 17.3, 13.1 Hz, H-3a), 2.72 (1H, dd, *J* = 17.3, 3.5 Hz, H-3b). EI-MS: m/z :272.

Quercetin (5): Yellow powder. ^{1}H-NMR (DMSO-d_6, 400 MHz): δ 7.74 (1H, d, J = 8, 2 Hz, H-2'), 7.55 (1H, d, J = 2 Hz, H-6'), 6.92 (1H, d, J = 8 Hz, H-5'), 6.42 (1H, d, *J* = 1.2 Hz, H-8), 6.15 (1H, d, *J* = 1.2 Hz, H-6). (+) ESI-MS: m/z 303 $[M+H]^+$.

Kaempferol 3-*O*-*β*-glucoside (6): Yellow powder. UV λmax (MeOH): 266, 344; (NaOMe): 274, 327sh, 401; ($AlCl_3$): 274, 302, 349, 396; ($AlCl_3$/HCl): 274, 347, 394; (NaOAc): 274, 307, 391; (NaOAc/H_3BO_3): 267, 352. 1H–NMR (DMSO–d_6, 500 MHz): δ 8.1 (2H, d, J = 8.5 Hz, H–2',6'), 6.92 (2H, d, J=8.5 Hz, H–3',5'), 6.54 (1H, d, J = 2 Hz, H–8), 6.22 (1H, d, J = 2 Hz, H–6), 5.35 (1H,d, J=7.5, H–1``), 4–3.1 (5H,m, other sugar protons).

Quercetin 3-O-α-rhamnoside (7): Yellow crystals. ^{1}H–NMR (DMSO–d_6, 400 MHz,) δ ppm 7.26 (2H, m, H–2`/6`), 6.83 (1H, d, J=9 Hz, H–5'), 6.49 (1H,d, *J*=2.5 Hz, H–8),6.14 (1H, d, J=2.5Hz, H–6), 5.25 (1H, br s, H–1") 0.78 (3H, d, *J*=6Hz). ^{13}C–NMR (DMSO–d_6,100 MHz): δ ppm 177.42 (C–4), 167.45 (C–7), 161.40 (C–5), 157.01 (C–2), 157 (C–9), 149.19 (C–4`), 145.57 (C–3`), 134.12 (C–3), 131.97 (C–6`), 121.40 (C–1`), 115.71 (C–2`), 115.40 (C–5`), 103.10 (C–10), 101.97 (C–1``), 99.98 (C–6), 94.47 (C–8), 71.47 (C–4"), 70.94, 70.85, 70.62 (C–2``, C–5``, C–3"), 17.78 (C6").

Discussion

***Antimicrobial activity of E. japonica* stems methanol extract**

For the antimicrobial qualitative methods, i.e. paper filter disks impregnated with the tested extract solution and disposal of the respective solutions in agar wells, the reading of the results was performed by measuring the microbial growth inhibition zones around the filter disks impregnated with the testing extract and around the wells, respectively. The most efficient qualitative method proved to be the direct spotting of the tested solutions on the seeded medium, the results being very well correlated with the results of the (minimal inhibitory concentration) MIC quantitative assay. For the quantitative methods of the antimicrobial activity of the tested extract by the microdilution method in liquid medium, the MIC was read by wells observation: in the first wells containing high concentrations of extract, the culture growth was not visible, the microbial cells being killed or inhibited by the tested extract. At lower concentrations of the tested extract, the microbial culture becomes visible. The lowest concentration which inhibited the visible microbial growth was considered the MIC (μg/mL) value for the extract. In the next wells, including the standard culture growth control wells, the medium become muddy as a result of the microbial growth. In the sterility control wells series, the medium had to remain clear. From the last well without any visible microbial growth and from the first one that presented microbial growth, Gram stained smears were performed for the results confirmation. In Figure 1, there are the results of the quantitative assay of the antimicrobial activity of the *E. japonica* stems methanol extract. Our results have shown that the extract was highly active against *C. albicans,* suggesting its possible use in the treatment of fungal infections, but it *was* not active on other bacterial strains.

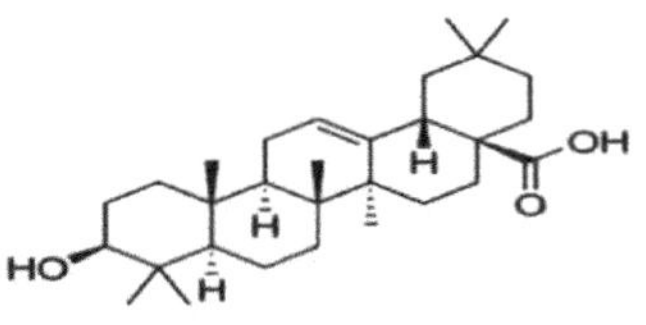

1: (Oleanolic acid) 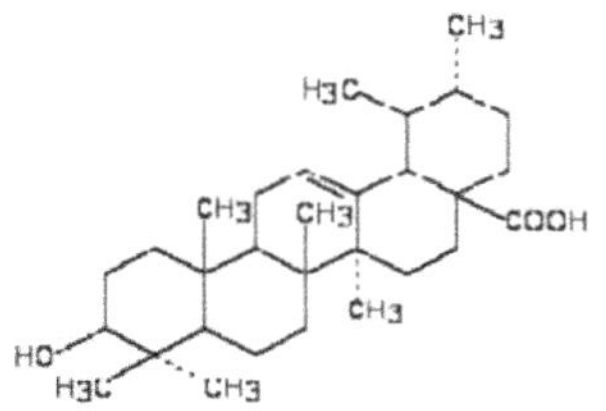 **2: (Ursolic acid)** 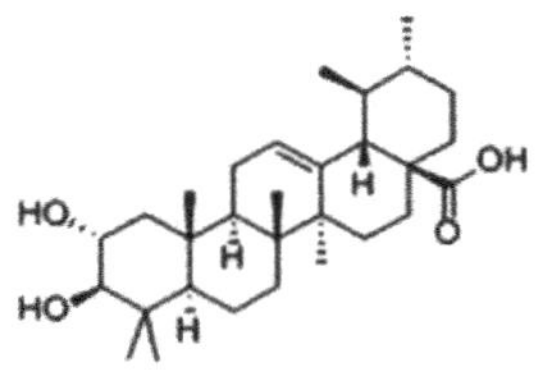 **3: (Corosolic acid)**

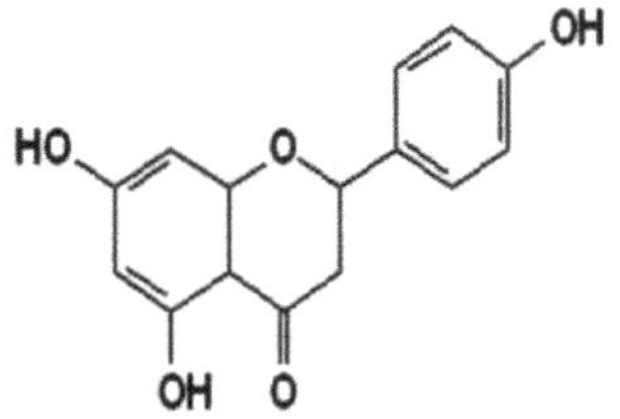

4: (Naringenin) 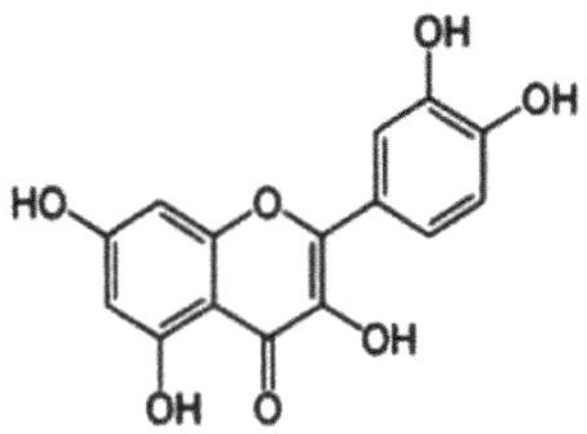 **5: (Quercetin)** 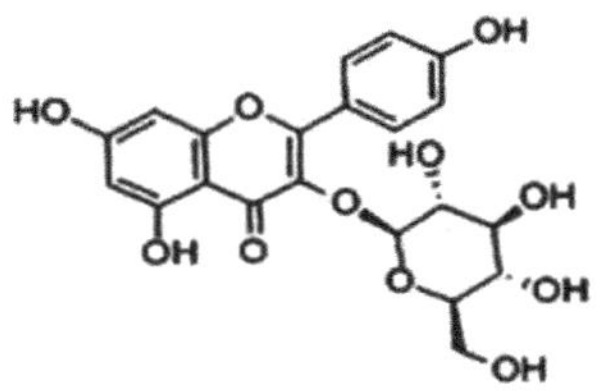 **6: (Kaempferol 3-*O*-*β*-glucoside)**

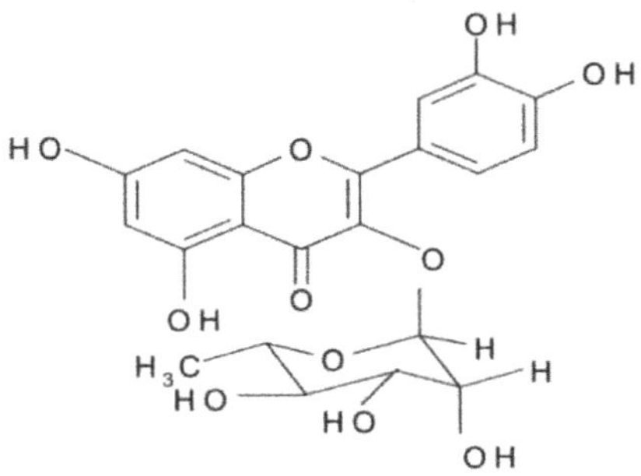

7: (Quercetin 3-O-α-rhamnoside)

Figure 3. Compounds isolated from *Eriobotrya japonica* stems methanol extract

Antioxidant activity E. japonica* stems methanol extract *and Total polyphenol content

Antioxidant activity was evaluated by Oxygen Radical Absorbance Capacity (ORAC) and Trolox equivalent antioxidant capacity method (TEAC) assays. In (TEAC) assay, *E. japonica* methanol extract showed high TEAC value 179±6.6 mM TE/g, and also in (ORAC) assay, it showed a high ORAC value (4988 mM TE/g) (Figure 2), while it showed a low total polyphenol content 74.43 ±1.60 mg/g (Figure 2) which was expressed as gallic acid equivalents and these results suggest the antioxidant activity of *E. japonica* extract and the activity can be proved by phytochemical analysis of the extract which has shown the presence of triterpenes, flavonoids, tannins and carbohydrates (Table 1).

Identification of the isolated compounds

Chromatographic separation of *Eriobotrya japonica* stems Methanol extract resulted in the isolation and identification of compound 1 (Oleanolic acid), compound 2 (ursolic acid) and compound 3 (corosolic acid) were monitored by TLC, and the spot of each compound was detected by heating the plates at 110°C after spraying with p-anisaldehyde–sulfuric acid, also spectral data were in agreement with published data.[19] Compound 4 (naringenin) is obtained as a deep purple spot on TLC and it gave yellow colour with AlCl3 reagent, the molecular formula, $C_{15}H_{12}O_5$, was obtained of the [M+] ion at m/z 272 in EI-MS is in agreement with naringenin chemical structure and the spectral data showed basically agreement with the reported literature of naringenin.[20] Compound 5 (quercetin) gave as yellow spot on paper chromatography (PC) under UV light and its spectral data very similar to that of Lawrence et al., 2005.[21] Compound 6 (kaempferol 3-O-β-glucoside) and 6 (quercetin 3-O-α-rhamnoside) were obtained as deep purple spots under UV light and each gave yellow colour with $AlCl_3$ reagent, Complete acid hydrolysis of compounds 6 and 7 revealed the presence of kaempferol as an aglycone and glucose as the sugar moiety for compound 6 and the presence of quercetin as an aglycone and rhamnose as the sugar moiety for compound 7. UV spectral data and NMR signals for both compounds 6 and 7 are very similar to that of compound 6 (kaempferol 3-O-β-glucoside) and compound 7 (quercetin 3-O-α-rhamnoside.[21] Antimicrobial and antioxidant activity of *Eriobotrya japonica* stems methanol extract is due to the presence of flavonoids which have shown a significant antimicrobial activity,[22,23] as well for tannins which have shown a significant antimicrobial and antioxidant activities,[24] also some isolated compounds from the extract has shown a good antioxidant activity as ursolic acid which proved a significant antioxidant activity, it has a significant DPPH radical scavenging activity at various degrees,[25] and kaempferol 3-*O*-*β*-glucoside has shown a significant antimicrobial and antioxidant activity.[26]

Conclusion

Based on our results and discussion, it can be concluded that *E. japonica* stems methanol extract possess a significant antimicrobial and antioxidant activity due to the presence of bioactive compounds as flavonoids and triterpenes and also for the isolated and identified compounds from the extract. These results also suggest that the extract could serve as potential source of bioactive compounds. Further research is needed in which the extract could possibly be exploited for pharmaceutical use.

Conflict of interest

There is no conflict of interest associated with the authors of this paper.

References

1. World Health Organisation. Summary of WHO guidelines for the assessment of herbal medicines. *Herbal Gram* 1993;28:13-4.
2. Kivcak B, Mert T, Ozturk HT. Antimicrobial and cytotoxic activities of Cerratonia siliqua L extracts. *Turk J Biol* 2002;26:197-200.
3. Ates A, Erdogrul OT. Antimicrobial activities of various medicinal and commercial plant extracts. *Turk J Biol* 2003;27:157-62.
4. Nair R, Kalariye T, Chanda S. Antimicrobial activity of some selected Indian medicinal flora. *Turk J Biol* 2005;29:41-7.
5. Kumar VP, Chauhan NS, Padh H, Rajani M. Search for antibacterial and antifungal agents from selected Indian medicinal plants. *J Ethnopharmacol* 2006;107(2):182-8.
6. Ito H, Kobayashi E, Takamatsu Y, Li SH, Hatano T, Sakagami H, et al. Polyphenols from Eriobotrya japonica and their cytotoxicity against human oral tumor cell lines. *Chem Pharm Bull (Tokyo)* 2000;48(5):687-93.
7. Shimizu M, Fukumaura H, Tsuji H, Tanaami S, Hayashi T, Morita N. Antiinflammatory constituents of tropically applied crude drugs. I. Constituents and anti-inflammatory effect of *Eriobotrya japonica* LINDL. *Chem Pharm Bull (Tokyo)* 1986;34(6):2614-17.
8. De Tommasi N, De Simone F, Cirino G, Cicala C, Pizza C. Hypoglycemic effects of sesquiterpene glycosides and polyhydroxylated triterpenoids of Eriobotrya japonica. *Planta Med* 1991;57(5):414-6.
9. Taniguchi S, Imayoshi Y, Kobayashi E, Takamatsu Y, Ito H, Hatano T, et al. Production of bioactive triterpenes by Eriobotrya japonica calli. *Phytochemistry* 2002;59(3):315-23.
10. Kim SH, Shin TY. Antiinflammatory effect of leaves of *Eriobotrya japonica* correlating with attenuation of p38 MAPK, ERK and NF-kappaB activation in mast cells. *Toxicol In Vitro* 2009;23(7):1215-9.
11. Sofowra A. Medicinal Plants And traditional Medicine in Africa. Ibadan, Nigeria: Spectrum Books Ltd; 1993.
12. Trease GE, Evans WC. Pharmacology. 11th ed. London: Bailliere Tindall; 1989.
13. Harborne JB. Phytochemical Methods. London: Chapman and Hall Ltd; 1973.
14. Luber P, Bartelt E, Genschow E, Wagner J, Hahn H. Comparison of broth microdilution, E Test, and agar dilution methods for antibiotic susceptibility testing of Campylobacter jejuni and Campylobacter coli. *J Clin Microbiol* 2003;41(3):1062-8.
15. Bagiu RV, Vlaicu B, Butnariu M. Chemical Composition and in Vitro Antifungal Activity Screening of the Allium ursinum L. (Liliaceae). *Int J Mol Sci* 2012;13(2):1426-36.
16. Das K, Tiwari RKS, Shrivastava DK. Techniques for evalauation of medicinal plant products as antimicrobial agent: Current methods and future trends. *J Med Plants Res* 2010;4(2):104-11.
17. Zuo GY, An J, Han J, Zhang YL, Wang GC, Hao XY, et al. Isojacareubin from the Chinese Herb

Hypericum japonicum: Potent Antibacterial and Synergistic Effects on Clinical Methicillin-Resistant Staphylococcus aureus (MRSA). *Int J Mol Sci* 2012;13(7):8210-8.
18. Folin O, Ciocalteu V. On tyrosine and tryptophan determination in proteins. *J Biol Chem* 1927;73:627-50.
19. Seebacher W, Simic N, Weis R, Saf R, Kunert O. Complete assignments of 1H and 13C NMR resonances of oleanolic acid, 18α-oleanolic acid, ursolic acid and their 11-oxo derivatives. *Mag Reson Chem* 2003;41(8):636-8.
20. Wilcox LJ, Borradaile NM, Huff MW. Antiatherogenic properties of naringenin, a citrus flavonoid. *Cardiovasc Drug Rev* 1999;17(2):160-78.
21. Lawrence O, Arot M, Ivar U, Peter L. Flavonol Glycosides from the Leaves of *Embelia keniensis. J Chin Chem Soc* 2005;52(1):201-8
22. Cushnie TP, Lamb AJ. Antimicrobial activity of flavonoids. *Int J Antimicrob Agents* 2005;26(5):343-56.
23. Tapas AR, Sakarkar DM, Kakde RB. Flavonoids as Nutraceuticals: A review. *Trop J Pharm Res* 2008;7(3):1089-99.
24. Reddy MK, Gupta SK, Jacob MR, Khan SI, Ferreira D. Antioxidant, antimalarial and antimicrobial activities of tannin-rich fractions, ellagitannins and phenolic acids from Punica granatum L. *Planta Med* 2007;73(5):461-7.
25. Özgen U, Mavi A, Terzi Z, Kazaz C, Aşçı A, Kaya Y, et al. Relationship Between Chemical Structure and Antioxidant Activity of Luteolin and Its Glycosides Isolated from *Thymus sipyleus* subsp. *sipyleus* var. *sipyleus*. *Rec Nat Prod* 2011;5(1):12-21.
26. Skalicka-Wozniak K, Melliou E, Gortzi O, Glowniak K, Chinou IB. Chemical constituents of Lavatera trimestris L.--antioxidant and antimicrobial activities. *Z Naturforsch C* 2007;62(11-12):797-800.

21

DNA Protective Effect of Mangosteen Xanthones: an in Vitro Study on Possible Mechanisms

Jing Lin, Yaoxiang Gao, Haiming Li, Lulu Zhang, Xican Li*

School of Chinese Herbal Medicine, Guangzhou University of Chinese Medicine, Guangzhou, 510006, China.

ARTICLEINFO

Keywords:
Mangosteen shell
Hydroxyl-induced
DNA oxidative damage
Antioxidant
Mechanism
Xanthones

ABSTRACT

Purpose: The aim of this study was to evaluate antioxidant ability of mangosteen shell and explore the non-enzymatic repair reaction and possible mechanism of xanthones in mangosteen shell.

Methods: Mangosteen shell was extracted by methanol to obtain the extract of mangosteen shell. The extract was then determined by various antioxidant assays in vitro, including protection against DNA damage, •OH scavenging,DPPH• (1,1-diphenyl-2-picryl-hydrazl radical) scavenging, $ABTS^{+}$• (2,2′-azino-bis(3-ethylbenzo- thiazoline-6-sulfonic acid diammonium) scavenging, Cu^{2+}-chelating, Fe^{2+}-chelating and Fe^{3+} reducing assays.

Results: Mangosteen shell extract increased dose-dependently its percentages in all assays. Its IC_{50} values were calculated as 727.85±2.21,176.94±19.25, 453.91±6.47, 84.60±2.47, 6.81±0.28, 1.55±0.10, 3.93±0.17, and 9.52±0.53μg/mL, respectively for DNA damage assay, •OH scavenging assay, Fe^{2+}-Chelating assay, Cu^{2+}-Chelating assay, DPPH• scavenging assay, $ABTS^{+}$• scavenging assay, Fe^{3+} reducing assay and Cu^{2+} reducing assay.

Conclusion: On the mechanistic analysis, it can be concluded that mangosteen shell can effectively protect against hydroxyl-induced DNA oxidative damage. The protective effect can be attributed to the xanthones. One approach for xanthones to protect against hydroxyl-induced DNA oxidative damage may be ROS scavenging. ROS scavenging may be mediated via metal-chelating, and direct radical-scavenging which is through donating hydrogen atom (H·) and electron (*e*). However, both donating hydrogen atom (H·) and electron (*e*) can result in the oxidation of xanthone to stable quinone form.

Introduction

As we know, reactive oxygen species (ROS) are various forms of activated oxygen including free radicals and non-free-radical species. ROS, particularly hydroxyl radical (·OH) with high reactivity, can attack DNA to cause its transient damage. If the transient damage cannot be repaired in time, it may be developed to permanent damage which causes severe biological consequences including mutation, cell death, carcinogenesis, and aging.[1,2] It is well known that the transient DNA damage can be repaired via enzymatic or non-enzymatic mechanisms.[2] Although the non-enzymatic repair reaction is faster than the enzymatic one, however, it is not well-known yet.[2] In general, non-enzymatic repair is finished by phenolics from plants.

Recent study has indicated a potent antigenotoxic effect of xanthones in mangosteens shell (山竹壳 in Chinese).[3] Hence, we used mangosteen shell as a reference to explore the non-enzymatic repair reaction and its possible mechanism.

Materials and Methods

Plant materials

Mangosteen (*Garcinia mangostana* L.) was purchased from Changzhou fruit market, Guangzhou, China. It was peeled off to obtain mangosteen shell. The voucher specimens were deposited in our laboratory.

Chemicals

DPPH• (1,1-diphenyl-2-picryl-hydrazl), ABTS [2,2′-azino-bis(3-ethylbenzo- thiazoline-6-sulfonic acid diammonium salt)], neocuproine, BHA (butylated hydroxyanisole), Trolox [(±)-6- hydroxyl-2,5,7,8-tetramethlychromane-2-carboxylic acid] were purchased from Sigma Co. (Sigma-Aldrich Shanghai Trading Co., China). Other chemicals used in this study were of analytical grade.

***Corresponding author:** Xican Li, School of Chinese Herbal Medicine, Guangzhou University of Chinese Medicine, Guangzhou, China.
Email: lixican@126.com

Preparation of methanol extract from mangosteen shell

The dried mangosteen shell was coarsely powder then extracted with methanol by Soxhlet extractor for 12 hours. The extract was concentrated under reduced pressure to a constant weight. Then the dried extract was stored at 4°C until used.

Total phenol content determination

Total phenol contents of methanol extract from mangosteen shell was determined using the Folin-Ciocalteu method[4] with slight modifications. Briefly, 0.5 mL sample methanolic solution (1 mg/mL) was mixed with 0.5 mL Folin-Ciocalteu reagent (0.25 M). The mixture was kept for 3 min, followed by the addition of 1.0 mL Na_2CO_3 aqueous solution (15 %, w/w). After incubation at ambient temperature for 30 min, the mixture was centrifuged at 3500 rpm for 3 min. The supernatant was measured using a spectrophotometer (Unico 2100, Shanghai, China) at 760 nm. The results were expressed as pyrogallol equivalents (Pyr.) in milligrams per gram extract.

Protective effect against hydroxyl-induced DNA damage

The experiment was conducted using our method.[5] Briefly, sample was dissolved in methanol to prepare the sample solution. Various amounts (50 – 250 μL) of sample solutions (4 mg/mL) were then separately taken into mini tubes. After evaporating the sample solution in tube to dryness, 300 μL phosphate buffer (0.2 M, pH 7.4) was brought to the sample residue. Then, 50 μL DNA (10.0 mg/mL), 75 μL H_2O_2 (33.6 mM), 50 μL $FeCl_3$ (0.3 mM) and 100 μL Na_2EDTA solutions (0.5 mM) were added. The reaction was initiated by mixing 75 μL ascorbic acid (1.2 mM). After incubation in a water bath at 50 °C for 20 min, the reaction was terminated by 250 μL trichloroacetic acid (0.6 M). The color was then developed by addition of 150 μL 2-thiobarbituric acid (TBA) (0.4 M, in 1.25% NaOH aqueous solution) and heated in an oven at 105 °C for 15 min. The mixture was cooled and absorbance was measured at 530 nm against the buffer (as blank). The percent of protection of DNA is expressed as follows:

$$\text{Protective effect \%} = (1-A/A_0)\times 100\%$$

Where A is the absorbance with samples, while A_0 is the absorbance without samples.

Hydroxyl (•OH) radical-scavenging assay

The hydroxyl radical-scavenging activity was investigated by the deoxyribose method improved by our laboratory.[6] In brief, the sample was dissolved in methanol, and then the sample solution was aliquoted into mini tubes. After evaporating the sample solutions in the tubes to dryness (64-192 μg), 300 μL of phosphate buffer (0.2 M, pH 7.4) was added to the sample residue. Subsequently, 50 μL deoxyribose (2.8 mM), 50 μL H_2O_2 (2.8 mM), 50 μL $FeCl_3$ (25 μM), and 100 μL Na_2EDTA (0.8 mM) were added. The reaction was initiated by mixing 50 μL ascorbic acid (1.2 mM) and the total volume of the reaction mixture was adjusted to 600 μL with buffer. After incubation in a water bath at 50 °C for 20 min, the reaction was terminated by addition of 500 μL trichloroacetic acid (5%, w/w). The color was then developed by addition of 500 μL TBA (1g/100 mL, in 1.25% NaOH aqueous solution) and heated in an oven at 105 °C for 15 min. The mixture was cooled and the absorbance was measured at 532 nm against the buffer (as a blank control). The inhibition percentage on ·OH was expressed as follows:

$$\text{Inhibition \%} = (1-A/A_0)\times 100\%$$

Where A is the absorbance containing samples, while A_0 is the absorbance without samples.

Fe^{2+}-chelating activity

The Fe^{2+} chelating activity of methanol extract from mangosteen shell was estimated by the method as described by Li.[7] Briefly, 200 μL samples (200, 400, 600, 800, 1000 and 1200 μg/mL in methanol) were added to 100 μL $FeCl_2$ aqueous solutions (250 μM). The reaction was initiated by the addition of 150 μL ferrozine aqueous solutions (1 mM) and total volume of the system was adjusted to 1000 μL with methanol. Then, the mixture was shaken vigorously and stood at room temperature for 10 min. Absorbance of the solution was measured spectrophotometrically at 562 nm. The percentage of chelating effect was calculated by the following formula:

$$\text{Chelating effect \%} = (1-A/A_0)\times 100\%$$

Where A_0 is the absorbance without sample, and A is the absorbance with sample.

Cu^{2+}-chelating activity

The Cu^{2+}-chelating activity of methanol extract from mangosteen shell measured by a complexometric method using murexide.[7] Briefly, 60 μL $CuSO_4$ aqueous solution (20 mM) was added to hexamine HCl buffer (pH 5.0, 30 mM) containing 30 mM KCl and 0.20 mM murexide. After incubation for 1 min at room temperature, 20-120 μL sample solutions (2 mg/mL in methanol) were added. The final volume was adjusted to 1500 μL with methanol. Then, the mixture was shaken vigorously and left at room temperature for 10 min. Absorbance of the solution was then measured spectrophotometrically at 485 nm and 520 nm. The absorbance ratio (A485/A520) reflected the free Cu^{2+} content. Therefore, the percentage of cupric chelating effect was calculated by the following formula:

$$\text{Relative chelating effect \%} = [(A_{485}/A_{520})_{max}-(A_{485}/A_{520})]/[(A_{485}/A_{520})_{max}-(A_{485}/A_{520})_{min}]\times 100\%$$

Where (A_{485}/A_{520}) is the absorbance ratio in the presence of the samples, while $(A_{485}/A_{520})_{max}$ is the maximum absorbance ratio and $(A_{485}/A_{520})_{min}$ is the minimum absorbance ratio in the test.

DPPH• radical-scavenging assay

DPPH• radical-scavenging activity was determined as described.[8] Briefly, 1 mL DPPH• ethanolic solutions (0.1 mM) were mixed with 10 mg/mL sample methanolic solutions (2-12 μL). The mixtures were kept at room temperature for 30 min, and then measured with a spectrophotometer (Unico 2100, Shanghai, China) at 519 nm. The DPPH• inhibition percentages were calculated:

$$\text{Inhibition }\% = (1\text{-}A/A_0)\times 100\%$$

Where A is the absorbance with samples, while A_0 is the absorbance without samples. Trolox and BHA were used as the positive controls.

$ABTS^{+}$• radical-scavenging assay

The $ABTS^{+}$• scavenging activity was measured as described,[9] with some modifications. The $ABTS^{+}$• was produced by mixing 0.35 mL ABTS diammonium salt aqueous solution (7.4 mM) with 0.35 mL $K_2S_2O_8$ aqueous solution (2.6 mM). The mixture was kept in the dark at room temperature for 12 h to allow completion of $ABTS^{+}$• generation. Before usage, it was diluted with 95% ethanol (about 1:50) so that its absorbance at 734 nm was 0.70 ± 0.02. Then, 1.2 mL diluted $ABTS^{+}$• reagent was mixed with 0.3 mL sample ethanolic solution. After incubation for 6 min, the absorbance at 734 nm was read on a spectrophotometer (Unico 2100, Shanghai, China). The percentage inhibition was calculated as:

$$\text{Inhibition }\% = (1\text{-}A/A_0)\times 100\%$$

Where A_0 is the absorbance of the mixture without sample, A is the absorbance of the mixture with sample (or positive control).

Reducing power (Fe^{3+}) assay

Ferric (Fe^{3+}) reducing power was determined by the method of Oyaizu.[10] In brief, x μL sample methanolic solution (1 mg/mL) was mixed with (350-x) μL Na_2HPO_4/KH_2PO_4 buffer (0.2 M, pH 6.6) and 250 μL $K_3Fe(CN)_6$ aqueous solution (1 g/100 mL). After the mixture was incubated at 50 °C for 20 min, 250 μL trichloroacetic acid (10 g/100 mL in distilled water) was added. The mixture was then centrifuged at 3500 rpm for 10 min. As soon as 400 μL supernatant was mixed with 400 μL $FeCl_3$ (0.1 g/100 mL in distilled water), the timer was started. At 90 s, absorbance of the mixture was read at 700 nm. Samples were analyzed in groups of three, and when the analysis of one group has finished, the next group of three samples were mixed with $FeCl_3$ to avoid oxidization by air. The relative reducing ability of the sample was calculated by using the formula:

$$\text{Relative reducing power}\% = [(A\text{-}A_{min})/(A_{max}\text{-}A_{min})]\times 100\%$$

Here, A_{max} is the maximum absorbance in the test and A_{min} is the minimum absorbance in the test. A is the absorbance of sample. BHA and Trolox were used as the positive controls.

Reducing power (Cu^{2+}) assay

The cupric ions (Cu^{2+}) reducing power capacity was determined by the method,[11] with a slight modification. Briefly, 125 μL $CuSO_4$ aqueous solution (10 mM), 125 μL neocuproine ethanolic solution (7.5 mM) and 500 μL CH_3COONH_4 buffer solution (100 mM, pH 7.0) were brought to test tubes with different volumes of samples (1 mg/mL, 2-12 μL). Then, the total volume was adjusted to 1000 μL with the buffer and mixed vigorously. Absorbance against a buffer blank was measured at 450 nm after 30 min. The relative reducing power of the sample as compared with the maximum absorbance, was calculated by using the formula:

$$\text{Relative reducing power}\% = [(A\text{-}A_{min})/(A_{max}\text{-}A_{min})]\times 100\%$$

Here, A_{max} is the maximum absorbance in the test and A_{min} is the minimum absorbancein the test. A is the absorbance of sample.

Results and Discussion

It has been demonstrated that there are many xanthones in the mangosteen shell[1,12,13](Figure 1).

As seen in Figure 1, all xanthones bear a phenolic –OH and they can beconsidered as the phenolics. The result in the present study suggested a high level of total phenolics content (317.14±5.16 mg Pyr./g) in mangosteen shell extract. Obviously, these phenolic xanthones can be responsible for the antioxidant ability of mangosteen shell. Here we use a typical xanthone, γ-mangostin, as a reference compound for the following discussion.

As we know, hydroxyl radical (·OH) can be generated via Fenton reaction (Eq. **1**):

$$Fe^{2+} + H_2O_2 \rightarrow HO\cdot + OH^- + Fe^{3+} \qquad \text{Eq. } \mathbf{1}$$

As the most reactive ROS, hydroxyl radical can easily attack DNA to bring about various classes of oxidative lesions from base, nucleoside, nucleotide, oligonucleotide and DNA fragment. In addition, malondialdehyde (MDA) was also yielded. As discussed in our previous report,[5,14] MDA could reflect the protective percentages well. In the study, the protective percentages of mangosteen shell increased in a dose-dependent manner (Figure 2A). As listed in Table 1, the IC_{50} values of mangosteen shell, BHA and Trolox were respectively 727.85±2.21, 979.29±54.05, 285.27±56.33 μg/mL. It means that mangosteen shell can more effectively protect against hydroxyl-induced DNA oxidative damage than a standard antioxidant BHA.

Previous works have demonstrated that there are two approaches for natural phenolic antioxidant to protect DNA oxidative damage: one is to fast repair the deoxynucleotide radical cations damaged by free radicals,[15,16] one is to scavenge ROS (especially ·OH radicals) prior to DNA damage. To explore whether the protective effect of mangosteen shell is associated to ROS scavenging, we further determined its ·OH radical-scavenging ability by deoxyribose degradation assay.

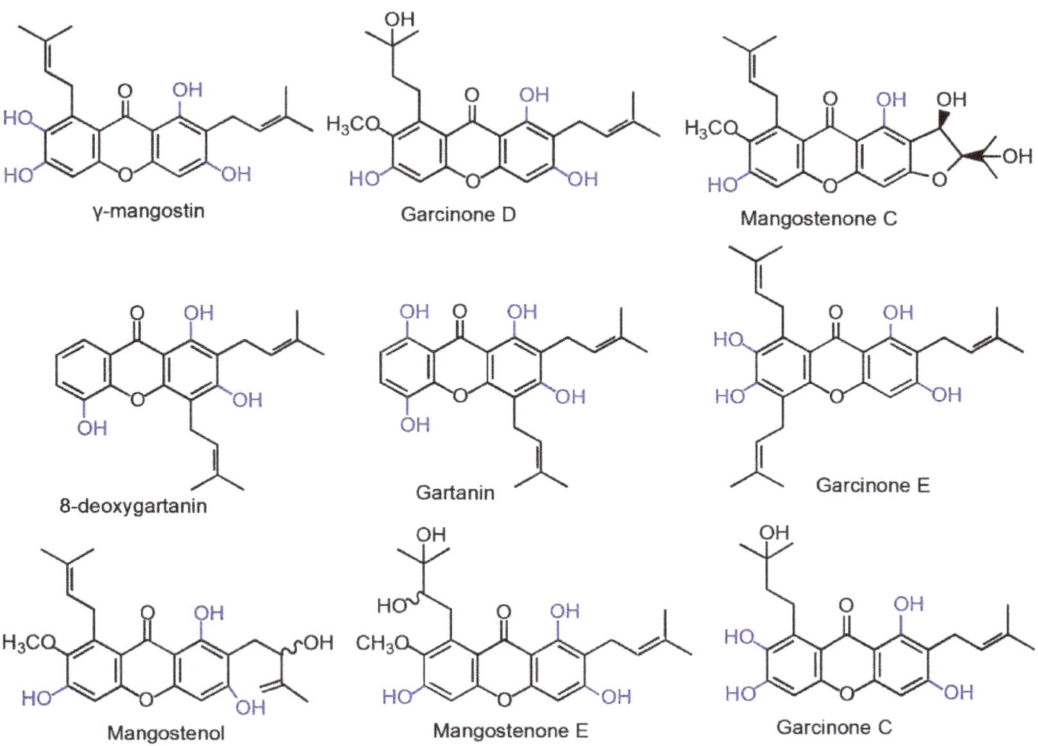

Figure 1. The structures of main xanthones in mangosteen shell.

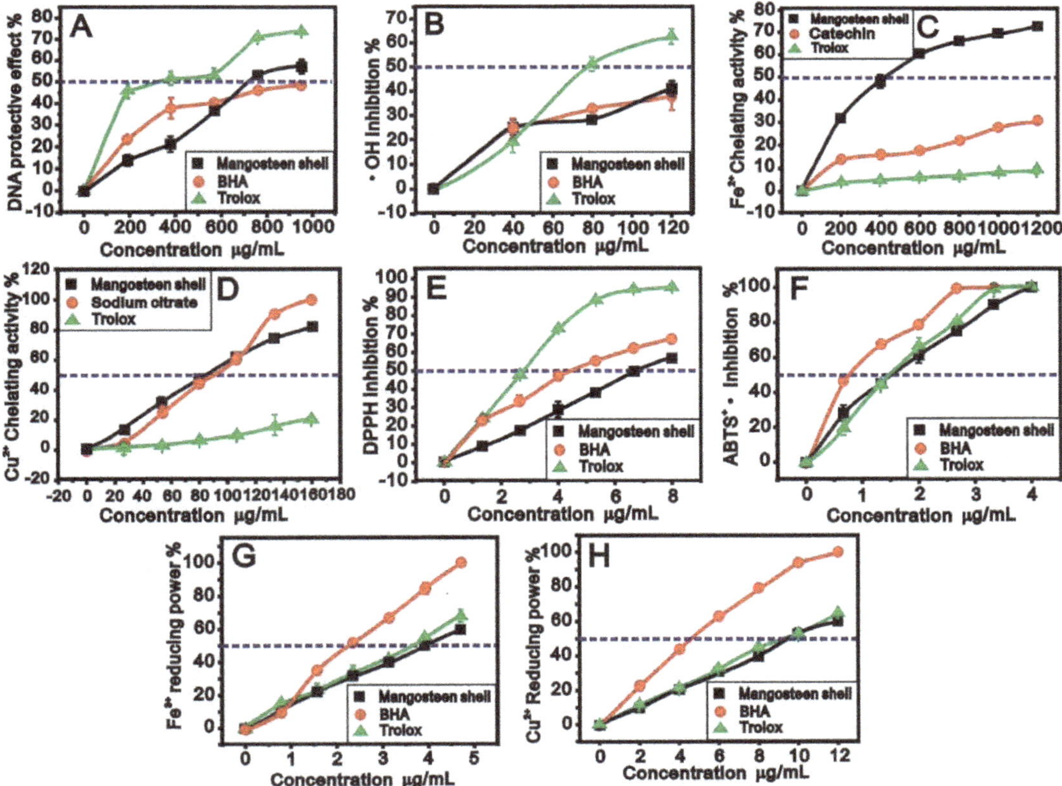

Figure 2. The dose response curves of mangosteen shell in various assays. A: DNA damage assay, B: hydroxyl radical (·OH) scavenging assay, C: Fe^{2+}-chelating assay, D: Cu^{2+}-chelating assay, E: DPPH• scavenging assay, F: $ABTS^{+}$• scavenging assay, G: Fe^{3+} reducing power assay, H: Cu^{2+} reducing power assay. Values are means ± SD (*n* = 3).

Since there is a strong solvent interference in ·OH scavenging assay, we have improved the experimental procedure.[6] Using our method, mangosteen shell was analyzed and the dose response curves are shown in Figure 2B. In terms of IC_{50} values (Table 1), mangosteen shell exhibited a similar ·OH radical-scavenging ability to BHA. It suggests that a possible approach for mangosteen shell to protect against oxidative DNA damage is ROS scavenging.

Table 1. The IC_{50}values of mangosteen shell extract and the positive controls (μg/mL)

Assays	Mangosteen shell	Positive controls	
		BHA	Trolox
DNA damage assay	727.85±2.21 ^{b}	979.29±54.05 ^{c}	285.27±56.33 ^{a}
•OH scavenging	176.94±19.25 ^{b}	172.97±33.04 ^{b}	79.08±3.54 ^{a}
Fe^{2+}-Chelating	453.91±6.47 ^{a}	1878.71±35.83 ^{b} *	5896.73±1574.22 ^{c}
Cu^{2+}-Chelating	84.60±2.47 ^{a}	89.96±0.48 ^{a} **	308.38±10.60 ^{b}
DPPH• scavenging	6.81±0.28 ^{c}	4.39±0.03 ^{b}	2.76±0.03 ^{a}
$ABTS^{+}$•scavenging	1.55±0.10 ^{b}	0.74±0.00 ^{a}	1.51±0.09 ^{b}
Fe^{3+} reducing	3.93±0.17 ^{b}	2.51±0.09 ^{a}	3.58±0.06 ^{b}
Cu^{2+} reducing	9.52±0.53 ^{b}	4.65±0.03 ^{a}	9.23±0.10 ^{b}

IC_{50} value is defined as the concentration of 50% effect percentage and calculated by linear regression analysis and expressed as mean ± SD (n = 3). The linear regression was analyzed by Origin 6.0 professional software. Means values with different superscripts in the same row are significantly different ($p < 0.05$), while with same superscripts are not significantly different ($p < 0.05$). * The positive control was Catechin, instead of BHA. ** The positive control was Sodium citrate, instead of BHA.

As illustrated in Eq. 1, the generation of •OH radical relies on the catalysis of transition metals (especially Fe and Cu). We then explored the metal-chelating ability of mangosteen shell. The dose-response curves in Figure 2C&D indicated an effective metal-chelating ability of mangosteen shell. The IC_{50} values in Table 1 suggest that mangosteen shell had the stronger metal chelating ability than positive controls Trolox and BHA. Now it is clear that metal-chelating may be one approach for mangosteen shell to scavenge ·OH radical. For example, γ-mangostin naturally occurring in mangosteen shell, may bind metal ions via the following proposed mechanism (Figure 3).

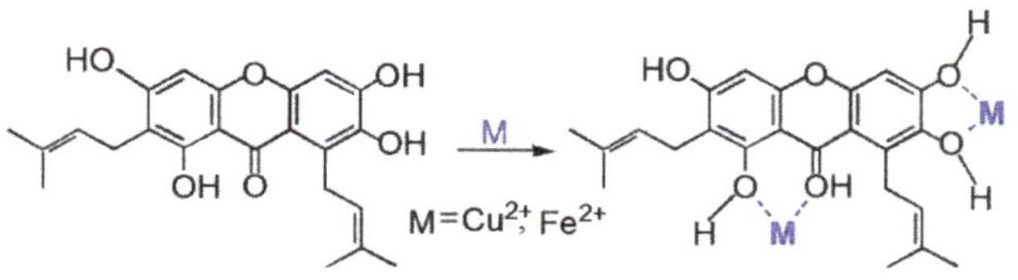

Figure 3. The proposed reaction for γ- mangostin to bind Cu^{2+} and Fe^{2+}.

To verify whether mangosteen shell can directly scavenge free radicals, we further investigated the radical-scavenging effects on DPPH· and $ABTS^{+}$· which don't require metal catalysis.

The DPPH assay confirmed that mangosteen shell could efficiently eliminate DPPH· radical (Figure 2E) and its IC_{50} was 6.81±0.28 μg/mL (Table 1). The previous studies suggested that DPPH· may be scavenged by an antioxidant through donation of hydrogen atom (H·) to form a stable DPPH-H molecule.[17] On the basis of previous reports,[18,19] γ-mangostin, for example, may scavenge DPPH• via the following proposed mechanism (Figure 4).

It has been demonstrated that *ortho*-dihydroxyl groups in benzenze ring play a critical role in the antioxidant ability of phenolic antioxidants.[20] Hence, in γ-mangostin molecule, *ortho*-dihydroxyl groups were thought to homolysis to produce H· and γ-mangostin· radical (I). H· then combined DPPH· to generate DPPH-H molecule and the γ-mangostin· radical might transform into (II), which could be further extracted H· by excess DPPH·to form the stable quinone form (III) (Figure 4).

Figure 2F showed that mangosteen shell could also scavenge $ABTS^{+}$· in a dose-dependent manner and the IC_{50} value was 1.55±0.10μg/mL (Table 1). Hence, mangosteen shell was an effective radical scavenger on $ABTS^{+}$· as well. Unlike DPPH· radical, $ABTS^{+}$· radical cation however needs only an electron (***e***) to neutralize the positive charge. Therefore, $ABTS^{+}$· scavenging is an electron (***e***) transfer process.[21] For example, γ-mangostin scavenged $ABTS^{+}$· possiblyvia the following mechanism. At first, γ-mangostin produced electron (***e***) and H^{+} cation. The electron (***e***) was then donated to $ABTS^{+}$· to form stable ABTS molecule. Meanwhile, γ-mangostin molecule was changed to γ-mangostin· radical (I), which could also be further converted to (II), even (III) in excess $ABTS^{+}$· (Figure 5).

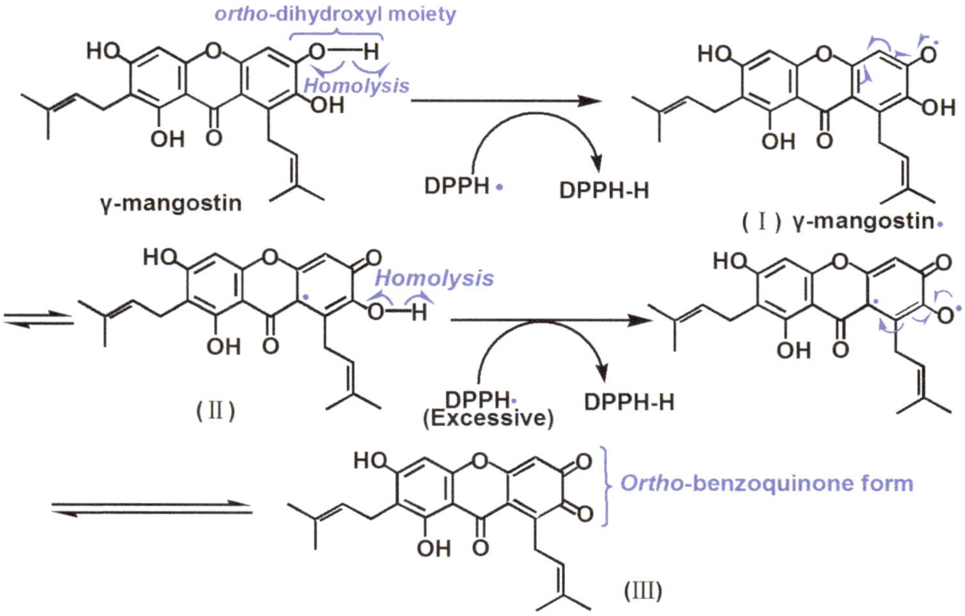

Figure 4. The proposed reaction for γ- mangostin to scavenge DPPH• radical

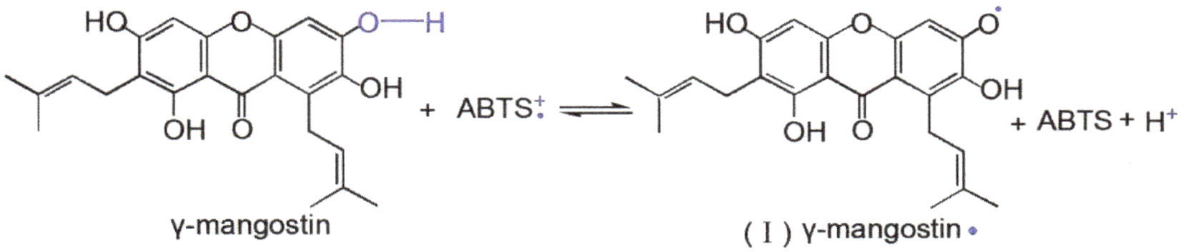

Figure 5. The proposed reaction for γ- mangostin to scavenge ABTS⁺• radical cation.

The electron (*e*) transfer mechanism of ABTS assay was also supported by the Cu & Fe-reducing power assays, in which mangosteen shell exhibited a good dose response. The IC_{50} values (3.93±0.17 and 9.52±0.53 μg/mL, Table 1) suggest that mangosteen shell could successfully reduce Cu^{2+} to Cu^{+}, and Fe^{3+} to Fe^{2+}. As we know, reductive reaction is actually accepting electron (*e*) process, so it agrees with the findings of ABTS assay above.

Conclusion

In conclusion, mangosteen shell can effectively protect against hydroxyl-induced DNA oxidative damage. The protective effect can be attributed to the xanthones. One approach for xanthones to protect against hydroxyl-induced DNA oxidative damage may be ROS scavenging. ROS scavenging may be mediated via metal-chelating, and direct radical-scavenging which is through donating hydrogen atom (H·) and electron (*e*). However, both donating hydrogen atom (H·) and electron (*e*) can result in the oxidation of xanthone to stable quinone form.

Conflict of interest

The authors report no conflicts of interest.

References

1. Yu LM, Zhao M, Yang B, Zhao QZ, Jiang Y. Phenolics from hull of Garcinia mangostana fruit and their antioxidant activities. *Food Chem* 2007;104:176-81.
2. Zheng R, Wang C, Lin C, Shi Y, Li J, Zhao C, et al. The earliest stage of carcinogenesis blocked by the fast repair of DNA transient damage. *Acta Biophys Sinica* 2012;28(3):185-99.
3. Tanaka R. Inhibitory effects of xanthone on paraquat- and NaNO(2)-induced genotoxicity in cultured cells. *J Toxicol Sci* 2007;32(5):571-4.
4. Li X, Wu X, Huang L. Correlation between antioxidant activities and phenolic contents of radix Angelicae Sinensis (Danggui). *Molecules* 2009;14(12):5349-61.

5. Li X, Mai W, Wang L, Han W. A hydroxyl-scavenging assay based on DNA damage in vitro. *Anal Biochem* 2013;438(1):29-31.
6. Li X. Solvent effects and improvements in the deoxyribose degradation assay for hydroxyl radical-scavenging. *Food Chem* 2013;141(3):2083-8.
7. Li X, Lin J, Gao Y, Han W, Chen D. Antioxidant activity and mechanism of Rhizoma Cimicifugae. *Chem Cent J* 2012;6(1):140.
8. Li X, Chen C. Systematic evaluation on antioxidant of magnolol *in vitro*. *Int Res J Pure Appl Chem* 2012;2(1):68-76.
9. Gao Y, Hu Q, Li X. Chemical composition and antioxidant activity of essential oil from *Syzygium samarangense* (BL.) Merr.et Perry flower-bud. *Spatula DD* 2012;2(1):23-33.
10. Oyaizu M. Studies on product of browning reaction prepared from glucoseamine. *Jpn J Nutr* 1986;44(6):307-15.
11. Wang L, Li X. Antioxidant Activity of Durian (Durio zibethinus Murr.) Shell *in vitro*. *Asian J Pharm Biol Res* 2011;1(4):542-51.
12. Chaivisuthangkura A, Malaikaew Y, Chaovanalikit A, Jaratrungtawee A, Panseeta P, Ratananukul P, et al. Prenylated xanthone composition of Garcinia mangostana (Mangosteen) Fruit Hull. *Chromatographia* 2009;69:315-8.
13. Obolskiy D, Pischel I, Siriwatanametanon N, Heinrich M. Garcinia mangostana L.: a phytochemical and pharmacological review. *Phytother Res* 2009;23(8):1047-65.
14. Li X, Chen W, Chen D. Protective effect against hydroxyl-induced DNA damage and antioxidant activity of Radix Glycyrrhizae (Liquorice Root). *Adv Pharm Bull* 2013;3(1):167-73.
15. Zheng R, Huang Z. Free radical biology. Beijing: Higher Education Press; 2007.
16. Cerutti PA. Prooxidant states and tumor promotion. *Science* 1985;227(4685):375-81.
17. Bondet V, Williams W, Berset C. Kinetics and mechanisms of antioxidant activity using the DPPH• free radical method. *LWT-Food Sci Technol* 1997;30(6):609-15.
18. Dimitrios IT, Vassiliki O. The contribution of flavonoid C-ring on the DPPH free radical scavenging efficiency. A kinetic approach for the 3′, 4′-hydroxy substituted members. *Innov Food Sci Emerg Technol* 2006;7(1-2):140-6.
19. Khanduja KL, Bhardwaj A. Stable free radical scavenging and antiperoxidative properties of resveratrol compared in vitro with some other bioflavonoids. *Indian J Biochem Biophys* 2003;40(6):416-22.
20. Zhang D, Liu Y, Chu L, Wei Y, Wang D, Cai S, et al. Relationship Between the Structures of Flavonoids and Oxygen Radical Absorbance Capacity Values: A Quantum Chemical Analysis. *J Phys Chem A* 2013;117(8):1784-94.
21. Aliaga C, Lissi EA. Reaction of 2, 2′-azinobis (3-ethylbenzothiazoline-6-sulfonic acid (ABTS) derived radicals with hydroperoxides.Kinetics and mechanism. *Int J Chem Kine*1998;30(8):565-70.

22

Composition and Antibacterial Activity of *Heracleum Transcaucasicum* and *Heracleum Anisactis* Aerial Parts Essential Oil

Mohammadali Torbati[1], Hossein Nazemiyeh[2], Farzaneh Lotfipour[3], Solmaz Asnaashari[4], Mahboob Nemati[3], Fatemeh Fathiazad[2]*

[1] Students' Research Committee, Faculty of Pharmacy, Tabriz University of Medical Sciences, Iran.

[2] Department of Pharmacognosy, Faculty of Pharmacy, Tabriz University of Medical Sciences, Iran.

[3] Pharmaceutical and Food Control, Faculty of Pharmacy, Tabriz University of Medical Sciences, Iran.

[4] Drug Applied Research Centre, Tabriz University of Medical Sciences, Iran.

ARTICLEINFO

Keywords:
Heracleum transcaucasicum
Heracleum anisactis
Umbelliferae
Essential oil composition
GC/MS Spectrometry
Myristicin

ABSTRACT

Purpose: Two plant essential oils (EOs), including those from *Heracleum transcaucasicum and Heracleum anisactiss* (Umbeliferae) were studied to detect the chemical constituents and evaluated for their antibacterial activities against *Staphylococcus aureus*, *Staphylococcus epidermidis*, *Escherichia coli and Pseudomonas aeruginosa.* ***Methods:*** The EOs of *H. transcaucasicum and H.anisactis* (Apiacae) were obtained by hydrodistillation from aerial parts of the plants. The chemical analyses of the EOs were performed by GC/Mass spectrometry (GC/MS). Myristicin was found to be the principal constituent in both EOs. The susceptibility tests of EOs were performed by agar disc diffusion technique against Gram-positive and Gram-negative bacterial strains. ***Results:*** Eight components comprising 99.97% of the total essential oil of *H. transcaucasicum* and a total of three compounds accounting for 98.5% of the total oil composition of aerial parts of *H. anisactis* were identified, of which myristicin was the main compound in both EOs. The EOs of *H. transcaucasicum and H. anisactis* showed weak antibacterial property against Gram-positive strains of *Staphylococcus aureus* and *Staphylococcus epidermidis* with no measurable effect on *Escherichia coli and Pseudomonas aeruginosa.* ***Conclusion:*** Our GC-MS study revealed myristicin to be the major constituent of *H. transcaucasicum and H.anisactis* aerial parts. In spite of all the information available on the antibacterial properties of plants essential oils, we were not able to find significant antibacterial activity for both EOs.

Introduction

The genus *Heracleum* is one of the largest genera of Umbellifereae (Apiaceae) and there are almost 125 Heracleum species in the world. This genus is widely distributed in Asia[1] and represented by 10 species in the flora of Iran.[2] Umbelliferous plants have been used not only as food-stuff and spice, but also as traditional folk medicine. In Iran *H. persicum* (Golpar) fruits are used commonly as spices, while the fruits and stems are used as a flavoring agent for making pickles. The fruits and leaves of this genus are also used as antiseptic, carminative, digestive and analgesic in Iranian traditional medicine.[3] Consequently, phytochemical analysis in much Heracleum species has been focused on EOs of their various parts[4] and a diversity of compounds have been isolated so far. Aliphatic esters such as hexyl butylate, octyl acetate, hexyl 2-methylbutanoate, hexyl hexanoate, octyl-2-methyl butanoate and monoterpenes including limonene and γ-terpinene have been reported as the major components of *H. persicum* fruits essential oil,[5] while, (E)-anethole, octyl acetate, n- octanol and hexyl butanoate were reported in leaves of *H. persicum.*[6]

As evident from the literature, the essential oils of Heracleum species have been extensively studied for their antibacterial,[7,8] antifungal,[9,10] anti-dermatophytic[11] and insecticidal activity.[12]

It has been found that medicinal plants, spice and EOs bearing plants possess a diversity of pharmacological activities. In particular, for EOs inhibition a wide range of microorganisms have been described.[13]

To the best of our knowledge, according to the literature there is no report on the essential oil composition and antibacterial activity of *Heracleum transcaucasicum* and *Heracleum anisactis* (from Azarbyjan) aerial parts. In this study we report the

***Corresponding author:** Fatemeh Fathiazad, Department of Pharmacognosy, Faculty of Pharmacy, Tabriz University of Medical Sciences, Tabriz, Iran. Email: fathiazad@tbzmed.ac.ir

essential oil constituents and antibacterial activities of the plants.

Materials and Methods

Plant material

Aerial parts of *H. transcaucasicum and H. anisactis* (in full fruiting stage) were collected from Varzeghan in East Azarbaijan province, Iran, in June 2011. A voucher specimen of the plants has been deposited at the Herbarium of the Faculty of Pharmacy, Tabriz University of Medical science, Iran.

Essential oil extraction

Air-dried plants material of aerial parts of *H. transcaucasicum and H. anisactis* were subjected to hydrodistillation using a Clevenger-type apparatus. The obtained essential oils were stored in sealed glass vials at 4-5 °C prior to analysis.

Test organism and Antibacterial assay

Two strains of Gram-negative bacteria [*Escherichia coli* ATCC (8739), *Pseudomonas aeruginosa ATCC* (9027)], and two strains of Gram-positive bacteria [*Staphylococcus epidermidis* ATCC (12228) and *Staphylococcus aureus* (ATCC 6538)] were used. The bacterial strains in lyophilized form were purchased from institute of pasture, Iran. After activating, the cultures of bacteria were maintained in their appropriate agar media at 4 °C throughout the study and used as stock cultures. A single colony from the stock plate was transferred into Mueller Hinton Broth and incubated over night at 37 °C. After incubation time the cells were harvested by centrifugation at 3000 rpm for 15 min and washed twice and re-suspended in Saline solution to provide an optical density equal to 0.5 McFarland or bacterial concentration around 10^8 CFU/ml. Then the final concentration of inocolum was adjusted to approximately 10^6CFU/ml with sterile Saline solution.

Antibacterial activity of essential oils was evaluated by the agar disc diffusion method. One hundred microliters of the suspensions were spread over the plates containing Mueller-Hinton agar using a sterile cotton swab in order to get a uniform microbial growth on both control and test plates. The essential oils were dissolved in 10% aqueous dimethylsulfoxide (DMSO) and sterilized by filtration through a 0.45 µm membrane filter. Sterilized discs (Whatman no.1, 6 mm diameter) were impregnated with 50 µL of different concentrations (1:1, 1:5, 1:10) of the respective essential oils and placed on the agar surface. A paper disc moistened with aqueous DMSO was placed on the seeded plate as a vehicle control. A standard disc containing Amikacin (30mg) was used as reference control. The plates were incubated for 30 min in refrigerator to allow the diffusion of oil, and then they were incubated at 37°C for 18 h. After the incubation period, the zone of inhibition was measured with a calliper. All experiments were performed in triplicate, and mean value was calculated.

Gas Chromatography-Mass Spectrometry (GC-MS)

Essential oils were analysed using GC/MS (Shimadzu capillary GC-quadrupole MS system QP 5050A) with capillary column DB-1 (60 m, 0.25 mm i.d, film thickness 0.25 µm) and a flame ionization detector (FID) which was operated in EI mode at 70 eV. Injector and detector temperatures were set at 210°C and 240°C, respectively. One microliter essential oils were injected and analyzed with the column held initially at 60 °C for 2 min and then increased by 3°C/min up to 240 °C. Helium was employed as carrier gas (1.3 ml/min). The MS operating parameters were as follows: ionization potential, 70 eV; ion source temperature 270 °C; quadrupole 100 °C; Solvent delay 2 min; scan speed 2000 amu/s; scan range 30-600 amu and EV voltage 3000 volts. The relative amount of individual components of the total oil is expressed as percentage peak area relative to total peak area. Qualitative identification of the different constituents was performed by comparison of their relative retention times and mass spectra with those of authentic reference compounds, or by mass spectra.

Identification of the compounds

The identification of compounds was based on direct comparison of the retention times and mass spectral data with those for the standards and by computer matching with the Wiley 229, Nist 107, Nist 21 Library, as well as by comparing the fragmentation patterns of the mass spectra with those reported in the literature.[14] For quantification purpose, relative area percentages were obtained by FID without the use of correction factors.

Results

The Pale yellow EOs were obtained in the yields of 0.2% and 0.3% (V/W) on a dry weight basis respectively. EOs were analyzed by GC-FID and GC-MS and the compositions of both essential oils were identified qualitatively and quantitatively. Analysis of *H. transcaucasicum* aerial parts essential oil revealed seven components accounting for 99.95% of the essential oil (Table 1). The aerial parts of *H. anisactis* were investigated for their essential oil and three ingredients were found representing 99.98% of the essential oil (Table 2). Myristicin, as a major component, was characterized by high amounts in both EOs. It was identified as 70% and 93.5% of the essential oil composition of *H. transcaucasicum* and *H. anisactis* aerial parts, respectively.

The EOs were tested against 4 microorganisms in order to estimate their antimicrobial potentials. Both EOs were almost inactive against the tested microbial strains as compared with Amikacin.

Table 1. Chemical constituent of the essential oil from aerial parts of *H. transcaucasicum*.

No.	Compounds	Rt*	Area (%)
1	n- octanol	19.47	14.285
2	octyl acetate	30.619	7.79
3	isobutyl 2-methylpropanoate	46.23	1.29
4	myristicin	56.04	70.12
5	3,4-dimethyl-1-pentanol	62.45	1.29
6	geranyl nitrile	77.36	3.89
7	alpha.-methylpentenal	82.38	1.29
Total			99.95%

*Rt: Retention time

Table 2. Chemical constituent of the essential oil from aerial parts of *H. anisactis*

No.	Compounds	Rt*	Area (%)
1	3-Methylpentanol	19.24	1.61
2	Myristicin	56.04	93.54
3	5-cyano-2,2,3-rimethyl-2H-pyrrole 1-oxide	77.43	4.83
Total			99.98%

*Rt: Retention time

Discussion

Plant essential oils have been used for many thousands of years. It is necessary to scientifically investigate those plants which have been used in traditional medicine to improve the quality of healthcare. Some biological activities, to mention a few, such as antimicrobial, antioxidant, anti-inflammatory, antispasmodic and relaxing properties have been described for Eos.[14] Since the biological activities of medicinal plants are linked to their complex chemical components, analysis of the EOs begins to be considered an important goal for researchers in order to justify their bioactivities.

The constituents of essential oils of Heracleum species have been isolated by many researchers.[15,6,16] Characteristic constituents Heracleum species have frequently been reported as octyl acetate,n- octanol, myristicin and elemicin. Moreover, myristicin was reported as a major compound (53%) in *H. pastinacifolium*[6] and n- octanol was the main component of *H. Sphondylium.*[17] Octyl acetate was detected as a major compound (29%) followed by elemicin (23%) in *H. Rechingeri.*[18] In the present study, the volatile pattern of *H. transcaucasicum*, was characterized by myristicin (77%), n-octanol (14.2%) and octyl acetate (7.7%) and myristicin were the major components (93%) of *H. anisactis*.

Our results are somewhat similar to those of the previous reports. The presence of myristicin as a predominant compound is in accordance with many other studies but in terms of the number of components both EOs contain a small number of compounds.

Furthermore, in the present study both *H. transcaucasicum* and *H. anisactis* aerial parts EOs exhibited no activity against the selected bacterial strains.

These results are consistent with the previous study that proved myristicin was ineffective against *Staphylococcus aureus*, *Staphylococcus epidermidis*, *Escherichia coli*, and *Pseudomonas aeruginosa.*[19] This report also showed that myristicin induced antiproliferative activity against K-562 (human chronic myelogenous leukemia), NCI-H460 (human lung tumor), and MCF-7 (human breast adenocarcinoma) cell lines.

Conclusion

In conclusion, the high amounts of myristicin in these plants EOs suggest some limitations for using these two Heracleum species as spices in diet. Furthermore, these results suggest more in-depth studies aimed at defining the safety of these oils and elucidating their anti tumor and other biological activities. The results also concluded that the presence of myristicin as a main compound provides the rationale to take into account the key role of myristicin in biological activity of both EOs.

Acknowledgments

The authors would like to thank Drug Applied Research Center of Tabriz University of Medical Sciences for recording the mass spectra. Financial support of this work by the Research Vice-Chancellor of Tabriz University of Medical Sciences is faithfully acknowledged. This article was written based on a data set of Ph.D. thesis, registered in Tabriz University of Medical Sciences (5/52/5691).

Conflict of Interest

The authors report no conflict of interest in this study.

References

1. Pimenov MG, Leonov MV. The Asian Umbelliferae Biodiversity Database (ASIUM) with Particular Reference to South-West Asian Taxa. *Turk J Bot* 2004;28:139-45.
2. Mozaffarian VA. Dictionary of Iranian Plant Names (In Persian). 6th ed. Tehran, Iran: Farhang Moaser Press; 2010.
3. Amin G. Popular medicinal plants of Iran. Tehran: Tehran University of Medical Sciences Press; 2008.
4. Karlson AKB, Valterova I, Nilsson LA. Volatile compounds from flowers of six species in the family Apiaceae: Bouquets for different pollinators? *Phytochemistry* 1994;35(1):111-9.
5. Hajhashemi V, Sajjadi SE, Hashemi M. Anti-inflammatory and analgesic properties of *Heracleum persicum* essential oil and hydroalcoholic extract in animal models. *J Ethnopharmacol* 2009;124(3):475-80.

6. Firuzi O, Asadollahi M, Gholami M, Javidnia K. Composition and biological activities of essential oils from four *Heracleum species*. *Food Chem* 2010;122(1):117-22.
7. Ozkirim A, Keskin N, Kurkcuoglu M, Baser KHC. Evaluation of some essential oils as alternative antibiotics against American foulbrood agent Paenibacillus larvae on honey bees Apis mellifera L. *J Essent Oil Res* 2012;24(5):465-70.
8. Jagannath N, Ramakrishnaiah H, Krishna V, Gowda PJ. Chemical composition and antimicrobial activity of essential oil of Heracleum rigens. *Nat Prod Commun* 2012;7(7):943-6.
9. Ozçakmak S, Dervisoglu M, Akgun A, Akcin A, Akcin TA, Seyis F. The effects of *Heracleum platytaenium* boiss essential oil on the growth of ochratoxigenic penicillium verrucosum (D-99756) isolated from Kashar Cheese. *J Appl Bot Food Qual* 2012;85(1):97-9.
10. Ciesla L, Bogucka-Kocka A, Hajnos M, Petruczynik A, Waksmundzka-Hajnos M. Two-dimensional thin-layer chromatography with adsorbent gradient as a method of chromatographic fingerprinting of furanocoumarins for distinguishing selected varieties and forms of Heracleum spp. *J Chromatogr A* 2008;1207(1-2):160-8.
11. Khosravi RA, Shokri H, Farahnejat Z, Chalangari R, Katalin M. Antimycotic efficacy of Iranian medicinal plants towards dermatophytes obtained from patients with dermatophytosis. *Chin J Nat Med* 2013;11(1):43-8.
12. Chu SS, Cao J, Liu QZ, Du SS, Deng ZW, Liu ZL. Chemical composition and insecticidal activity of *Heracleum moellendorffii* Hance essential oil. *Chemija* 2012;23(2):108-12.
13. Tognolini M, Barocelli E, Ballabeni V, Bruni R, Bianchi A, Chiavarini M, et al. Comparative screening of plant essential oils: phenylpropanoid moiety as basic core for antiplatelet activity. *Life Sci* 2006;78(13):1419-32.
14. Adams RP. Identification of Essential oil Components by Gas Chromatography/ Quadrupole Mass Spectroscopy. USA: Allured Publishing Corporation; 2004.
15. Mojab F, Nikavar B. Composition of the Essential Oil of the Root of Heracleum persicum from Iran. *Iran J Pharm Res* 2003;2(4):245-7.
16. Mirza M, Najafpour NM. Comparative study on chemical composition of fruit essential oil of Heracleum gorganicum Rech. F. in different altitudes. *Iran J Med Aromat Plants* 2012;28(2):324-9.
17. Iscan G, Demirci F, Kurkcuoglu M, Kivanc M, Baser KH. The bioactive essential oil of Heracleum sphondylium L. subsp. ternatum (Velen.) Brummitt. *Z Naturforsch C* 2003;58(3-4):195-200.
18. Habibi Z, Eshaghi R, Mohammadi M, Yousefi M. Chemical composition and antibacterial activity of essential oil of Heracleum rechingeri Manden from Iran. *Nat Prod Res* 2010;24(11):1013-7.
19. Stefano VD, Pitonzo R, Schillaci D. Antimicrobial and antiproliferative activity of Athamanta sicula L. (Apiaceae). *Pharmacogn Mag* 2011;7(25):31-4.

23

HPLC-Analysis of Polyphenolic Compounds in *Gardenia jasminoides* and Determination of Antioxidant Activity by using Free Radical Scavenging Assays

Riaz Uddin[1], Moni Rani Saha[1], Nusrat Subhan[2], Hemayet Hossain[3], Ismet Ara Jahan[3], Raushanara Akter[1], Ashraful Alam[4]*

[1] *Department of Pharmacy, Stamford University Bangladesh, Dhaka-1217, Bangladesh.*

[2] *School of Biomedical Sciences, Charles Sturt University, Wagga Wagga (NSW), Australia.*

[3] *BCSIR Laboratories, Bangladesh Council of Scientific and Industrial Research (BCSIR), Dhaka-1205, Bangladesh.*

[4] *Department of Pharmacy, North-South University, Dhaka-1229, Bangladesh.*

ARTICLEINFO

Keywords:
Gardenia jasminoides
DPPH
Free radical
Reducing power

ABSTRACT

Purpose: *Gardenia jasminoides* is a traditional medicinal plant rich in anti-inflammatory flavonoids and phenolic compounds and used for the treatment of inflammatory diseases and pain. In this present study, antioxidant potential of *Gardenia jasminoides* leaves extract was evaluated by using various antioxidant assays.
Methods: Various antioxidant assays such as 1, 1-diphenyl-2-picrylhydrazyl (DPPH) radical scavenging assay, reducing power and total antioxidant capacity expressed as equivalent to ascorbic acid were employed. Moreover, phenolic compounds were detected by high-performance liquid chromatography (HPLC) coupled with diode-array detection.
Results: The methanol extract showed significant free radical scavenging activities in DPPH radical scavenging antioxidant assays compared to the reference antioxidant ascorbic acid. Total antioxidant activity was increased in a dose dependent manner. The extract also showed strong reducing power. The total phenolic content was determined as 190.97 mg/g of gallic acid equivalent. HPLC coupled with diode-array detection was used to identify and quantify the phenolic compounds in the extracts. Gallic acid, (+)-catechin, rutin hydrate and quercetin have been identified in the plant extracts. Among the phenolic compounds, catechin and rutin hydrate are present predominantly in the extract. The accuracy and precision of the presented method were corroborated by low intra- and inter-day variations in quantitative results in leaves extract.
Conclusion: These results suggest that phenolic compounds and flavonoids might contribute to high antioxidant activities of *Gardenia jasminoides* leaves.

Introduction

The role of oxygen derived free radicals in the pathogenesis of a number of degenerative diseases is well known.[1,2] The oxidation induced by reactive oxygen species can result in cell membrane disintegration, membrane protein damage and DNA mutation, which can further initiate and propagate the development of many diseases, such as cancer, liver injury and cardiovascular disease.[3] Mammalian body possesses antioxidant defense mechanisms such as catalase, superoxide dismutase, glutathione peroxidase enzymes and antioxidant nutrients i.e. vitamin e, ascorbic acid which arrest the damaging properties of reactive oxygen species (ROS).[4,5] Certain chemicals and contaminants exposure may lead to an increase in free radicals generation in the body beyond its capacity to control them, and ultimately cause irreversible damage to tissues and cellular components.[6] Recent investigations have shown that the antioxidant properties of plants could be correlated with oxidative stress defense and different human diseases like aging process etc.[7,8] Currently, the possible toxicity of synthetic antioxidants has been criticized. It is generally assumed that frequent consumption of plant-derived phytochemicals from vegetables, fruit, tea, and herbs may contribute to shift the balance toward an adequate antioxidant status.[9] In this respect, flavonoids and other polyphenolic compounds have received greatest attention. *Gardenia jasminoides* Ellis (family

***Corresponding author:** Ashraful Alam, Department of Pharmacy, North-South University, Bangladesh. E mail- sonaliagun@yahoo.com

Rubiaceae) is an evergreen shrub grows all over Bangladesh. They are used as contraceptive, febrifuge, analgesic, diuretic, larvicide, antihypertensive, antibacterial, anxiolytic, antiplasmodial and for the treatment of headaches.[10] It has also been used for the cure of febrile diseases, jaundice, acute conjunctivitis, epistaxis, haematemesis, pyogenic infections and ulcers of the skin.[11] The fruits of *Gardenia jasminoides* are included in oriental herbal medicines and in traditional formulations. It is used for the treatment of inflammation, jaundice, headache, edema, fever and hepatic disorders.[12] In addition, its pigments are used as food colorants in oriental countries.[13] The pharmacological actions of *Gardenia jasminoides,* such as protection against oxidative damage, cytotoxic effects, anti-inflammatory activity, and fibrolytic activity have been described previously.[14,15] The fruits extracts of *Gardenia jasminoides* showed potent antioxidant activities by using *in vitro* antioxidant assay systems.[16,17] The bioactive compound isolated from *Gardenia jasminoides* is crocin and the relationship between total crocin contents and antioxidant activity of ethanol extracts were investigated which showed a positive correlation with the crocin content.[17] However, very few reports have been found in literature which showed the analysis of phenolic compounds present in *Gardenia jasminoides.*[18]

As a part of our ongoing investigations about natural antioxidants from local medicinal plants of Bangladesh,[19-21] in this paper, we analyzed the phenolic compounds present in *Gardenia jasminoides* leaves extracts by using HPLC-diode-array detection system and evaluated antioxidant activities *in vitro* by using DPPH radical scavenging assay, reducing power and total antioxidant capacity assays.

Materials and Methods

Chemicals

DPPH (1, 1-diphenyl, 2-picrylhydrazyl), TCA (trichloroacetic acid) and ferric chloride were obtained from Sigma Chemical Co. USA. Ascorbic acid was obtained from SD Fine Chem. Ltd., Biosar, India. Ammonium molybdate was purchased from Merck, Germany. Gallic acid (GA), (+)-catechin hydrate (CH), vanillic acid (VA), caffeic acid (CA), (-)-epicatechin (EC), *p*-coumaric acid (PCA), rutin hydrate (RH), ellagic acid (EA), and quercetin (QU) were purchased from Sigma–Aldrich (St. Louis, MO, USA). Acetonitrile (HPLC), methanol (HPLC), acetic acid (HPLC), and ethanol was obtained from Merck (Darmstadt, Germany).

Plant material

Leaves of *Gardenia jasminoides* were collected from Dhaka, Bangladesh in May, 2013, and identified by the expert of the National Herbarium of Bangladesh. The accession number of the plant is 32545; a voucher specimen (GR-SK-05.12.12) for this collection has been retained in the National Herbarium, Dhaka, Bangladesh.

Extraction

The shade-dried leaves were coarsely powdered and extracted with 95% methanol by a Soxhlet apparatus at 45°C. The solvent was completely removed by rotary evaporator and obtained greenish gummy exudates (percentage recovery approximately 12%). This crude extract was used for further investigation for potential antioxidant properties.

Phytochemical screening

The freshly prepared extract of *Gardenia jasminoides* was qualitatively tested for the presence of chemical constituents. Phytochemical screening of the extract was performed using the following reagents and chemicals: alkaloids with Dragendorffs reagent, Mayer's reagent and Fehling's Solutions, flavonoids with the use of Mg and HCl; tannins with ferric chloride and potassium dichromate solutions, steroids with sulfuric acid and saponins with ability to produce suds. Gum was tested using Molish reagents and concentrated sulfuric acid. These were identified by characteristic color changes using standard procedures.[19]

Determination of total phenolic content

The total phenolic content of the extract was determined by the modified Folin-Ciocaltu method.[22] Briefly, 1.0 ml of each extract (1 mg/ml) was mixed with 5 ml Folin-Ciocaltu reagent (1:10 v/v distilled water) and 4 ml (75g/l) of sodium carbonate. The mixture was vortexed for 15 second and allowed to stand for 30 min at 40°C for color development. The absorbance was read at 765 nm with a spectrophotometer. Total phenolic content was determined as mg of gallic acid equivalent per gram using the equation obtained from a standard gallic acid calibration curve $y = 6.2548x - 0.0925$, $R^2=0.9962$.

High Performance Liquid Chromatography (HPLC) Analysis of the Extract

High performance liquid chromatography (HPLC) system

Chromatographic analyses were carried out on a Thermo Scientific Dionex UltiMate 3000 Rapid Separation LC (RSLC) systems (Thermo Fisher Scientific Inc., MA, USA), coupled to a quaternary rapid separation pump (LPG-3400RS), Ultimate 3000RS auto sampler (WPS-3000) and rapid separation diode array detector (DAD-3000RS). Phenolic compounds were separated on an Acclaim® C18 (4.6 x 250 mm; 5μm) column (Dionix, USA) which was controlled at 30°C using a temperature controlled column compartment (TCC-3000). Data acquisition, peak integration, and calibrations were performed with Dionix Chromeleon software (Version 6.80 RS 10).

Chromatographic conditions

The phenolic composition of the methanol extract of *Gardenia* was determined by HPLC, as described previously with some modifications.[23] The mobile phase consisted of acetonitrile (solvent A), acetic acid solution at pH 3.0 (solvent B), and methanol (solvent C). The system was run with the following gradient elution program: 0 min, 5%A/95%B; 10 min, 10%A /80%B /10%C; 20 min, 20%A /60%B /20%C and 30min, 100%A. There was a 5 min post run at initial conditions for equilibration of the column. The flow rate was kept constant throughout the analysis at 1 ml/min and the injection volume was 20 µl. For UV detection, the wavelength program was optimized to monitor phenolic compounds at their respective maximum absorbance wavelengths as follows: λ 280 nm held for 18.0 min, changed to λ 320 nm and held for 6 min, and finally changed to λ 380 nm and held for the rest of the analysis and the diode array detector was set at an acquisition range from 200 nm to 700 nm. The detection and quantification of GA, CH, VA, CA, and EC was done at 280 nm, of PCA, RH, and EA at 320 nm, and of QU at 380 nm, respectively.

Standard and sample preparation

A stock standard solution (100µg/ml) of each phenolic compound was prepared in methanol by weighing out approximately 0.0050 g of the analyte into 50 ml volumetric flask. The mixed standard solution was prepared by dilution the mixed stock standard solutions in methanol to give a concentration of 20 µg/ml for each polyphenols except caffeic acid (8 µg/ml) and quercetin (6 µg/ml). All standard solutions were stored in the dark at 5°C and were stable for at least three months.

The calibration curves of the standards were made by serial dilution of the stock standards (five set of standard dilutions) with methanol to yield 1.25 - 20 µg/ml for GA, CH, VA, EC, PCA, RH, EA; 0.5 - 8.0 µg/ml for CA, and 0.375 - 6.0 µg/ml for QU. The calibration curves were constructed from chromatograms as peak area vs. concentration of standard.

A solution of methanolic extract of *Gardenia jasminoides* at a concentration of 5 mg/ml was prepared in ethanol by vortex mixing (Branson, USA) for 30 min. The samples were stored in the dark at low temperature (5°C). Spiking the sample solution with phenolic standards was done for additional identification of individual polyphenols.

Prior to HPLC analysis, all solutions (mixed standards, sample, and spiked solutions were filtered through 0.20 µm nylon syringe filter (Sartorius, Germany) and then degassed in an ultrasonic bath (Hwashin, Korea) for 15 min.

Peak characterization and quantification

The compounds were identified by comparing with standards of each identified compound using the retention time, the absorbance spectrum profile and also by running the samples after the addition of pure standards. Quantification was performed by establishing calibration curves for each compound determined, using the standards. Linear calibration curves for standards (peak area vs concentration) were constructed with R^2 exceeding 0.995. Data are reported as means ± standard deviations of triplicate independent analyses.

Antioxidant Activity Test

DPPH radical scavenging activity

Qualitative analysis DPPH radical scavenging activity: The methanol extract was applied on a TLC plate as a spot (100 µg/ml) for chromatographic separation of the extract using the mobile phase methanol:chloroform (95:5, v/v). It was allowed to develop the chromatogram for 30 minutes. After completion of the chromatogram the whole plate was sprayed with DPPH (0.15 % w/v) solution using an atomizer. The color changes (yellowish color development on pinkish background on the TLC plate) were noted as an indicator of the presence of antioxidant substances.

Quantitative analysis for DPPH radical scavenging activity: The free radical scavenging capacity of the extracts was determined using DPPH.[19] DPPH solution (0.004% w/v) was prepared in 95% methanol. Metahnol extract of *Gardenia jasminoides was* mixed with 95 % methanol to prepare the stock solution (5 mg/ml). Freshly prepared DPPH solution (0.004% w/v) was taken in test tubes and *Gardenia jasminoides* extracts was added followed by serial dilutions (1 µg to 500 µg) to every test tube so that the final volume was 3 mL and after 10 min, the absorbance was read at 515 nm using a spectrophotometer (HACH 4000 DU UV – visible spectrophotometer). Ascorbic acid was used as a reference standard and dissolved in distilled water to make the stock solution with the same concentration (5 mg/ml). Control sample was prepared containing the same volume without any extract and reference ascorbic acid. 95 % methanol was served as blank. % scavenging of the DPPH free radical was measured by using the following equation:

% Scavenging Activity= [(Absorbance of the control – Absorbance of the test sample)/ Absorbance of the control] X 100.

The inhibition curve was plotted for duplicate experiments and represented as % of mean inhibition ± standard deviation.

Determination of total antioxidant capacity: The antioxidant activity of the extract was evaluated by the phosphomolybdenum method according to the procedure describe by Prieto and his colleagues.[24] The assay is based on the reduction of Mo (VI)–Mo (V) by the extract and subsequent formation of a green phosphate/Mo (V) complex at acid pH. 0.3 ml extract was combined with 3 ml of reagent solution (0.6 M sulfuric acid, 28 mM sodium phosphate and 4 mM ammonium molybdate). The tubes containing the reaction solution were incubated at 95°C for 90 min. Then the absorbance of the solution was measured at 695 nm using a spectrophotometer (HACH 4000 DU UV – visible spectrophotometer) against blank after cooling to room temperature. Methanol (0.3 ml) in the place of extract was used as the blank. The antioxidant activity is expressed as the number of equivalents of ascorbic acid.

Reducing power: The reducing power of *Gardenia jasminoides* was determined according to the method described by Oyaizu.[25] Different concentrations of crude extract (100 µg – 1000 µg) in 1 ml of distilled water were mixed with phosphate buffer (2.5 ml, 0.2 M, pH 6.6) and potassium ferricyanide [$K_3Fe(CN)_6$] (2.5 ml, 1%). The mixture was incubated at 50°C for 20 min. A portion (2.5 ml) of trichloroacetic acid (10%) was added to the mixture, which was then centrifuged at 3000 rpm for 10 min. The upper layer of the solution (2.5 ml) was mixed with distilled water (2.5 ml) and $FeCl_3$ (0.5 ml. 0.1%) and the absorbance was measured at 700 nm. Increased absorbance of the reaction mixture indicated increased reducing power. Ascorbic acid was used as the standard. Phosphate buffer (pH 6.6) was used as blank solution. The absorbance of the final reaction mixture of three parallel experiments was taken and is expressed as mean ± standard deviation.

Results and Discussion

In the past few years, there has been growing interest in the involvement of reactive oxygen species (ROS) in several pathological situations. ROS produced *in vivo* include superoxide radical ($O_2^{\bullet-}$), hydrogen peroxide (H_2O_2) and hypochlorous acid (HOCl). H_2O_2 and $O_2^{\bullet-}$ can interact in the presence of certain transition metal ions to yield a highly-reactive oxidizing species, the hydroxyl radical ($^{\bullet}OH$).[26] In this respect, polyphenolic compounds like flavonoids and phenolic acids are getting much interest because of their potent antioxidant activity.[27] Phenolic compounds and flavonoids have been reported to show antioxidant activity in biological systems, acting as scavengers of singlet oxygen and free radicals.[28,29] Many plants contain substantial amounts of antioxidants including Vitamin C and E, carotenoids, flavonoids, tannins and thus can be utilized to scavenge the excess free radicals from the human body.[30-32] Preliminary phytochemical screening of the *Gardenia jasminoides* showed the presence of flavonoids and tannins (Table 1).

Gardenia jasminoides leaves extract was also evaluated for their antioxidant activity by using various *in vitro* assays. DPPH is relatively stable nitrogen centered free radical that can easily accept an electron or hydrogen radical to form a more stable diamagnetic molecule.[32] The DPPH radical scavenging activity of *Gardenia jasminoides* extracts are given in Figure 1. This activity was increased by increasing the concentration of the sample extract. DPPH antioxidant assay is developed based on the ability of 1, 1-diphenyl-2-picryl-hydrazyl (DPPH), a stable free radical, to decolorize in the presence of antioxidants. The DPPH radical contains an odd electron, which is responsible for a visible deep purple color of DPPH in alcoholic solution and the color intensity can be measured at absorbance 515 nm.[32,33] When DPPH accepts an electron donated by an antioxidant compound, the DPPH is decolorized, which can be quantitatively measured from the changes in absorbance. Moreover, the DPPH radical scavenging activity has been shown to be directly related with the total phenolic content present in the extracts as suggested by many previous reports.[34,35]

Table 1. Phytochemical Screening of *Gardenia jasminoides.*

Groups	Status*
Glycosides	+
Alkaloid	+
Flavonoids	+
Tannins	++
Gums	+
Saponin	-
Steroid	++

* (+) means presence in a single method test, (++) means presence experimented in two methods and (-) = absence.

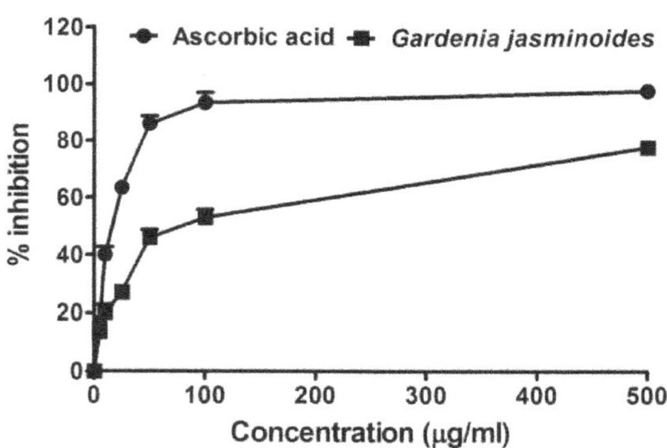

Figure 1. DPPH radical scavenging activity of the methanol extracts *Gardenia jasminoides.* DPPH radical scavenging activity was increased by increasing the concentration of the sample extract. Data was represented as Mean ± SD of duplicate experiments.

Total antioxidant capacity of the *Gardenia jasminoides* extract, expressed as the number of equivalents of ascorbic acid was shown in Table 2. The phosphomolybdenum method was developed based on the reduction of Mo (VI) to Mo (V) by the antioxidant compound which may produce a green phosphate/Mo (V) complex. The color intensity of the phosphate/Mo (V) complex can then be measured with a maximal absorption at 695 nm.

Reducing power of the extracts has been investigated based on the conversion of Fe^{3+} to Fe^{2+} transformation in the presence of extract samples using the method previously described by Oyaizu.[25] The reducing properties are generally associated with the presence of reductones,[36] which have been shown to exert antioxidant action by breaking the free radical chain by donating a hydrogen atom. Reductones are also reported to react with certain precursors of peroxide, thus preventing peroxide formation. Figure 2 shows the reducing capabilities of the plant extract where reducing power of *Gardenia jasminoides* extract was increased in a concentration dependent manner compared to ascorbic acid. Increased absorbance in samples in the reducing power assay implies that extracts are capable of donating hydrogen atoms in a dose dependent manner.[33,37] The reducing power of extract of *Gardenia jasminoides* was found remarkable and the reducing power of the extract was observed to rise as the concentration of the extract gradually increased. Moreover, the amount of total phenolic compound was found quite high in the methanol extract of *Gardenia jasminoides* (190.97 ± 10.37 mg of gallic acid equivalent). Thus higher inhibition values and reducing ability of the methanol extract might be due to the high concentration of phenolic compounds present.[37]

Table 2. Contents of polyphenolic compounds in the methanol extract of ***Gardenia jasminoides***.

Polyphenolic compound	*Gardenia jasminoides*	
	Content	**% RSD**
GA	9.06(mg/100 g of dry extract)	0.96
CH	141.02(mg/100 g of dry extract)	3.05
RH	72.06(mg/100 g of dry extract)	1.25
QU	19.06(mg/100 g of dry extract)	0.97
Total phenolic content (mg of gallic acid equivalent per g of dry extract)	190.97 ± 10.37	-
Average absorbance at 765 nm	141.02(mg/100 g of dry extract)	3.05

GA, gallic acid; CH, (+)-catechin; RH, rutin hydrate; QU, quercetin.

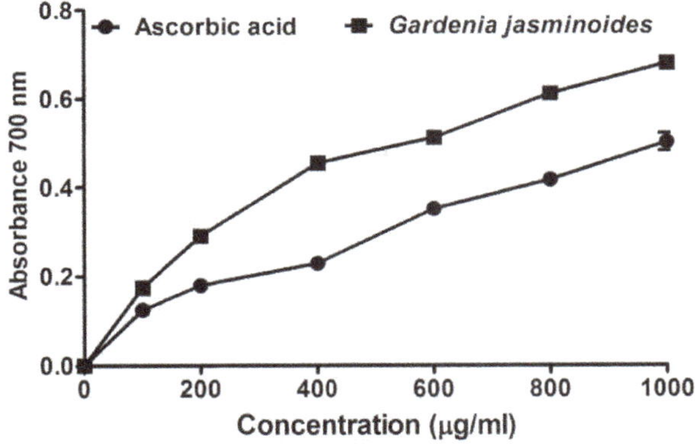

Figure 2. Reducing power of the crude plant extract *of Gardenia jasminoides.* An increase in absorbance in the reducing power method implies that extracts are capable of donating hydrogen atoms in a dose dependent manner. Data was represented as Mean ± SD of duplicate experiments.

Among the many separation systems, the HPLC analysis includes the use of a binary solvent system containing acidified water and a polar organic solvent to specifically measure polyphenolic concentrations.[38,39] For method development, we had followed the previously reported method[23] with some modifications. In this study we used C18 column with 250 mm length, and rapid separation LC (RSLC) systems while other authors used C18 column with 150mm length, and HP 1090, series II, liquid chromatography systems to determine the polyphenolic contents. In this study we also used nine different phenolic standards to compare with the chromatograms produced by the unknown *Gardenia jasminoides* extracts while earlier investigators[23] used six standards for identifying phenolic compounds. From Figure 3, it can be observed that a good separation can be achieved within 30 min using the above condition described. Symmetrical, sharp and well-resolved peaks were observed for the nine polyphenolic standards. The elution order and the retention times for GA, CH, VA, CA, EC, PCA, RH, EA, and QU were 6.16, 13.54, 15.90, 16.16, 16.60, 19.85, 21.01, 21.65, and 26.10 min respectively.

Phenolic compounds are very important plant constituents because of their scavenging ability due to their hydroxyl groups. In HPLC analysis, the presence of gallic acid, (+)-catechin, rutin hydrate and quercetin were confirmed in *Gardenia jasminoides* extracts. Figure 3 and 4 show the HPLC chromatograms obtained from standards and *Gardenia jasminoides* extracts respectively. Out of the four phenolic compounds catechin was found in the highest concentration compared to others amounting 141.02 mg/g in *Gardenia jasminoides* extracts whereas rutin hydrate was found 72.06 mg/g (Table 3). Catechin and rutin both showed beneficial effects such as antioxidant, anti-ageing and may prevent cardiovascular complecations.[40-42] Their beneficial effects are attributed to their ability to reduce oxidative stress, lipid peroxidation, free radical generation and low density lipoprotein (LDL) cholesterol-oxidation.[40,42] Moreover, other phenolic compounds found in the extracts such as gallic acid and quercetin also possess beneficial effects on human health and eases oxidative stresses.[27] Literature reviews suggests that the chemical constituents present in *Gardenia* plants are triterpenes,[43] carotenoids, *e.g.* crocins,[17] iridoid glycosides, quinic acid derivatives, amides and fatty acids.[10] However, very few reports suggest the presence of polyphonic compounds in *Gardenia jasminoides*. Our results confirmed the presence of catechin and rutin hydrate (Figure 5) present in abundant in the extract of *Gardenia jasminoides*. Radical scavenging activity can thus be explained by the presence of flavonoids, catechin and rutin hydrate in this plant.

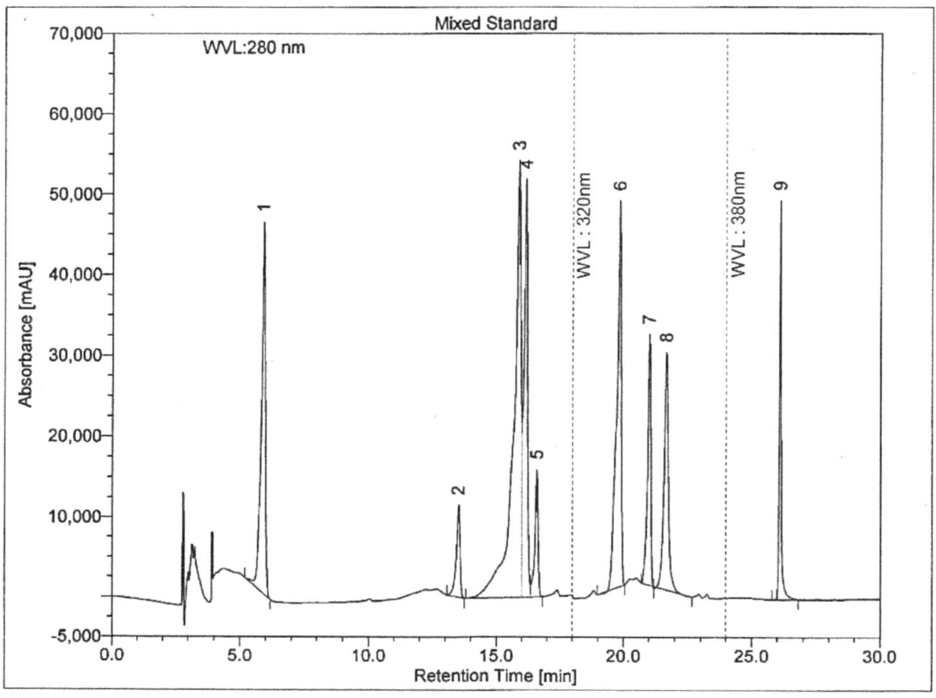

Figure 3. HPLC chromatogram of a standard mixture of polyphenolic compounds. Peaks: 1, gallic acid; 2, (+)-catechin; 3, vanillic acid; 4, caffeic acid; 5, (–)-epicatechin; 6, *p*-coumaric acid; 7, rutin hydrate; 8, ellagic acid; 9, quercetin.

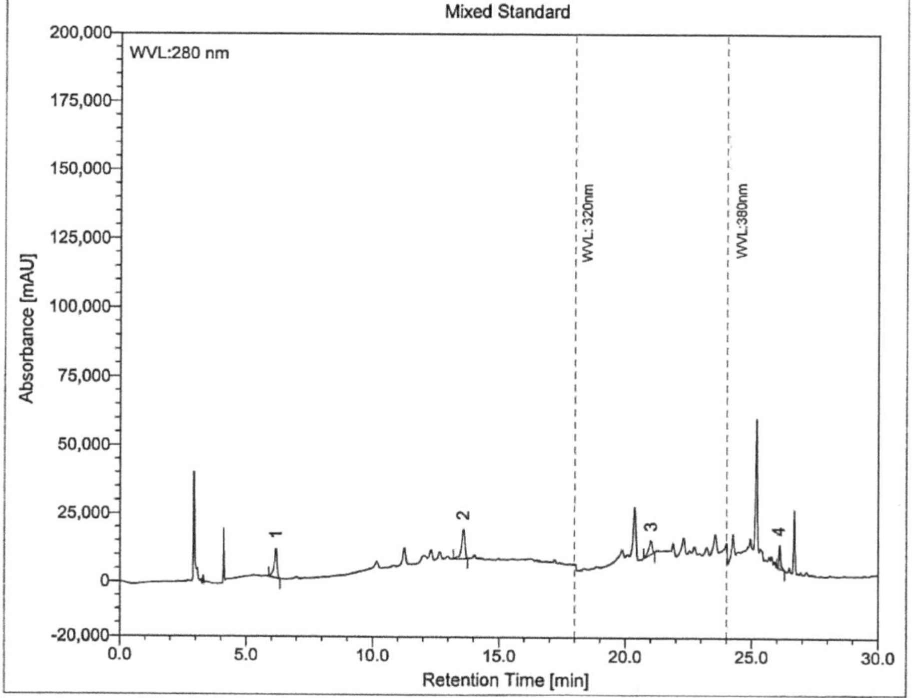

Figure 4. HPLC chromatogram of *Gardenia jasminoides* leaves extract. Peaks: 1, gallic acid; 2, (+)-catechin; 3, rutin hydrate; 4, quercetin.

Table 3. Total antioxidant capacity of methanol leaf extract of *Gardenia jasminoides Ells.*[a]

Materials	Concentration (μg/ml)	Equivalent to ascorbic acid (μg/mg)
Methanol extract of *Gardenia jasminoides*	100	1.00 ± 0.15
	200	1.99 ± 0.07
	400	2.80 ± 0.15
	600	3.41± 0.14
	800	5.37 ± 0.14

[a]Total antioxidant capacity of the *Gardenia jasminoides* extract, expressed as the number of equivalents of ascorbic acid. Values are the average of triplicates experiments and represented as mean± standard deviation.

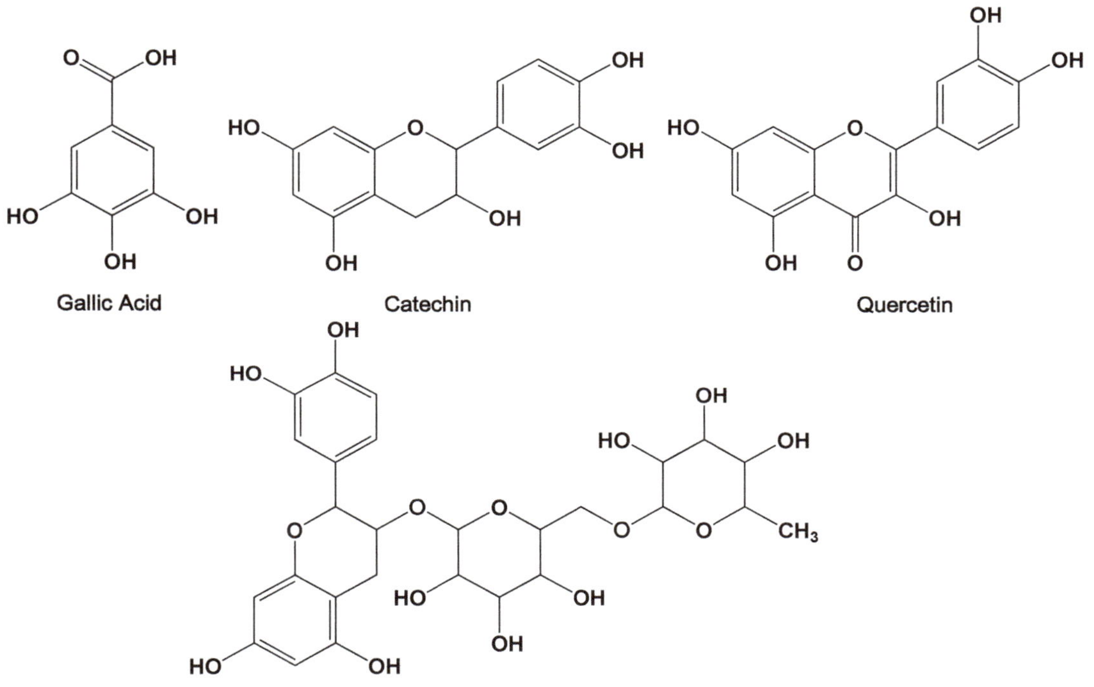

Gallic Acid

Catechin

Quercetin

Rutin

Figure 5. HPLC separated phenolic compounds from *Gardenia jasminoides* leaves extract. 1, gallic acid; 2, (+)-catechin; 3, quercetin and 4, rutin hydrate.

Conclusion

This is the first report on the phytochemical and antioxidant potentials of *Gardenia jasminoides* leaves extract. Our results clearly indicate that *Gardenia jasminoides* leaves extract possess antioxidant activities which are comparable to the standard antioxidant vitamin C. This study showed that the phenolic compounds and flavonoid contents are responsible for its free radical scavenging activity. These antioxidant substances may be responsible for anti-inflammatory and chemoprotective properties of *Gardenia jasminoides* leaves extract as well as justify the use of this plant's extract in folkloric remedies.

Acknowledgements

This project was supported by the Department of Pharmacy, Stamford University Bangladesh.

Conflict of Interest

The authors report no conflict of interest.

References

1. Cross CE, Halliwell B, Borish ET, Pryor WA, Ames BN, Saul RL, et al. Oxygen radicals and human disease. *Ann Intern Med* 1987;107(4):526-45.
2. Khatoon M, Islam E, Islam R, Rahman AA, Alam AK, Khondkar P, et al. Estimation of total phenol and in vitro antioxidant activity of *Albizia procera* leaves. *BMC Res Notes* 2013;6(1):121.
3. Liao K, Yin M. Individual and combined antioxidant effects of seven phenolic agents in human erythrocyte membrane ghosts and phosphatidylcholine liposome systems: importance of the partition coefficient. *J Agric Food Chem* 2000;48(6):2266-70.

4. Halliwell B, Aeschbach R, Loliger J, Aruoma OI. The characterization of antioxidants. *Food Chem Toxicol* 1995;33(7):601-17.
5. Sies H. Strategies of antioxidant defense. *Eur J Biochem* 1993;215(2):213-9.
6. Flora SJS Structural, chemical and biological aspects of antioxidants for strategies against metal and metalloid exposure. *Oxid Med Cell Longev* 2009;2(4):191-206.
7. Lobo V, Patil A, Phatak A, Chandra N. Free radicals, antioxidants and functional foods: Impact on human health. *Pharmacogn Rev* 2010;4:118-26.
8. Rahman K. Studies on free radicals, antioxidants, and co-factors. *Clin Interv Aging* 2007;2(2):219-36.
9. Halliwell B. Oxidative stress, nutrition and health. Experimental strategies for optimization of nutritional antioxidant intake in humans. *Free Radic Res* 1996;25(1):57-74.
10. Fu X-M, Chou G-X, Wang Z-T. Iridoid glycosides from *Gardenia jasminoides* Ellis. *Helv Chim Acta* 2008;91(4):646-53.
11. Lee SJ, Oh PS, Lim KT. Hepatoprotective and hypolipidaemic effects of glycoprotein isolated from Gardenia jasminoides ellis in mice. *Clin Exp Pharmacol Physiol* 2006;33(10):925-33.
12. Koo HJ, Lim KH, Jung HJ, Park EH. Anti-inflammatory evaluation of gardenia extract, geniposide and genipin. *J Ethnopharmacol* 2006;103(3):496-500.
13. Spears K. Developments in food colourings: the natural alternatives. *Trends Biotechnol* 1988;6(11):283-8.
14. Jagadeeswaran R, Thirunavukkarasu C, Gunasekaran P, Ramamurty N, Sakthisekaran D. *In vitro* studies on the selective cytotoxic effect of crocetin and quercetin. *Fitoterapia* 2000;71(4):395-9.
15. Tseng TH, Chu CY, Huang JM, Shiow SJ, Wang CJ. Crocetin protects against oxidative damage in rat primary hepatocytes. *Cancer Lett* 1995;97(1):61-7.
16. Debnath T, Park PJ, Deb Nath NC, Samad NB, Park HW, Lim BO. Antioxidant activity of *Gardenia jasminoides* Ellis fruit extracts. *Food Chem* 2011;128(3):697-703.
17. Chen Y, Zhang H, Tian X, Zhao C, Cai L, Liu Y, et al. Antioxidant potential of crocins and ethanol extracts of *Gardenia jasminoides* ELLIS and *Crocus sativus* L.: A relationship investigation between antioxidant activity and crocin contents. *Food Chem* 2008;109(3):484-92.
18. He W, Liu X, Xu H, Gong Y, Yuan F, Gao Y. On-line HPLC-ABTS screening and HPLC-DAD-MS/MS identification of free radical scavengers in Gardenia (*Gardenia jasminoides* Ellis) fruit extracts. *Food Chem* 2010;123(2):521-8.
19. Alam M, Ghani A, Subhan N, Rahman M, Haque M, Majumder M, et al. Antioxidant and membrane stabilizing properties of the flowering tops of *Anthocephalus cadamba. Nat Prod Commun* 2008;3:65-7.
20. Alam M, Nyeem M, Awal M, Mostofa M, Alam M, Subhan N, et al. Antioxidant and hepatoprotective action of the crude methanolic extract of the flowering top of *Rosa damascena. Oriental Pharm Exp Med* 2008;8:164-70.
21. Talukder FZ, Khan KA, Uddin R, Jahan N, Alam MA. In vitro free radical scavenging and anti-hyperglycemic activities of Achyranthes aspera extract in alloxan-induced diabetic mice. *Drug Discov Ther* 2012;6(6):298-305.
22. Wolfe K, Wu X, Liu RH. Antioxidant activity of apple peels. *J Agric Food Chem* 2003;51(3):609-14.
23. Chuanphongpanich S, Phanichphant S. Method development and determination of phenolic compounds in broccoli seeds samples. *Chiang Mai J Sci* 2006;33:103-7.
24. Prieto P, Pineda M, Aguilar M. Spectrophotometric quantitation of antioxidant capacity through the formation of a phosphomolybdenum complex: specific application to the determination of vitamin E. *Anal Biochem* 1999;269(2):337-41.
25. Oyaizu M. Studies on product of browning reaction prepared from glucose amine. *Jap J Nutr* 1986;44:307-15.
26. Aruoma OI, Halliwell B, Hoey BM, Butler J. The antioxidant action of N-acetylcysteine: its reaction with hydrogen peroxide, hydroxyl radical, superoxide, and hypochlorous acid. *Free Radical Biol Med* 1989;6(6):593-7.
27. Pandey KB, Rizvi SI. Plant polyphenols as dietary antioxidants in human health and disease. *Oxid Med Cell Longev* 2009;2(5):270-8.
28. Blokhina O, Virolainen E, Fagerstedt KV. Antioxidants, oxidative damage and oxygen deprivation stress: a review. *Ann Bot* 2003;91 Spec No:179-94.
29. Wilmsen PK, Spada DS, Salvador M. Antioxidant activity of the flavonoid hesperidin in chemical and biological systems. *J Agric Food Chem* 2005;53(12):4757-61.
30. Carocho M, Ferreira IC. A review on antioxidants, prooxidants and related controversy: natural and synthetic compounds, screening and analysis methodologies and future perspectives. *Food Chem Toxicol* 2013;51:15-25.
31. Andre C, Larondelle Y, Evers D. Dietary antioxidants and oxidative stress from a human and plant perspective: A review. *Curr Nutr Food Sci* 2010;6:2-12.
32. Mai W, Chen D, Li X. Antioxidant activity of Rhizoma cibotii *in vitro*. *Adv Pharm Bull* 2012;2(1):107-14.
33. Asirvatham R, Christina AJ, Murali A. *In Vitro* Antioxidant and Anticancer Activity Studies on *Drosera Indica* L. (Droseraceae). *Adv Pharm Bull* 2013;3(1):115-20.

34. Saeed N, Khan MR, Shabbir M. Antioxidant activity, total phenolic and total flavonoid contents of whole plant extracts Torilis leptophylla L. *BMC Complement Altern Med* 2012;12:221.
35. Middha SK, Usha T, Pande V. HPLC evaluation of phenolic profile, nutritive content, and antioxidant capacity of extracts obtained from punica granatum fruit peel. *Adv Pharmacol Sci* 2013;2013:296236.
36. Duh PD, Tu YY, Yen GC. Antioxidant activity of water extract of Harng Jyur (*Chrysanthemum morifolium* Ramat). *LWT - Food Sci Technol* 1999;32(5):269-77.
37. Ganjewala D, Gupta AK. Study on Phytochemical composition, antibacterial and antioxidant properties of different parts of *Alstonia scholaris* Linn. *Adv Pharm Bull* 2013;3(2):379-84.
38. Sakakibara H, Honda Y, Nakagawa S, Ashida H, Kanazawa K. Simultaneous determination of all polyphenols in vegetables, fruits, and teas. *J Agric Food Chem* 2003;51(3):571-81.
39. Tsao R, Yang R. Optimization of a new mobile phase to know the complex and real polyphenolic composition: towards a total phenolic index using high-performance liquid chromatography. *J Chromatogr A* 2003;1018(1):29-40.
40. Thielecke F, Boschmann M. The potential role of green tea catechins in the prevention of the metabolic syndrome - a review. *Phytochemistry* 2009;70(1):11-24.
41. Mandel S, Youdim MB. Catechin polyphenols: neurodegeneration and neuroprotection in neurodegenerative diseases. *Free Radic Biol Med* 2004;37(3):304-17.
42. Augustyniak A, Bartosz G, Cipak A, Duburs G, Horakova L, Luczaj W, et al. Natural and synthetic antioxidants: an updated overview. *Free Radic Res* 2010;44(10):1216-62.
43. Suksamrarn A, Tanachatchairatana T, Kanokmedhakul S. Antiplasmodial triterpenes from twigs of *Gardenia saxatilis*. *J Ethnopharmacol* 2003;88(2-3):275-7.

Development and Evaluation of a Solid Self-Nanoemulsifying Drug Delivery System for Loratadin by Extrusion-Spheronization

Mohammadreza Abbaspour*, Negar Jalayer, Behzad Sharif Makhmalzadeh

Nanotechnology Research Center and school of Pharmacy, Ahvaz Jundishapur University of Medical Sciences, Ahvaz, Iran.

ARTICLEINFO

Keywords:
Solid self-emulsifying drug delivery system
Extrusion-spheronisation
Pellets
Loratadin

ABSTRACT

Purpose: Recently the liquid nanoemulsifying drug delivery systems (SNEDDS) have shown dramatic effects on improving oral bioavailability of poorly soluble drugs. The main purpose of this study was to prepare a solid form of self-nanoemulsifying drug delivery system of loratadin by extrusion-spheronization. The liquid SNEDDS are generally prepared in a soft or hard gelatin capsules which suffers from several disadvantages. Therefore incorporation of SNEDDS into solid dosage form is desirable to get together the advantages of SNEDDS and solid multiparticualte systems.
Methods: The SNEDDS was consisted of liquid paraffin, capriole, span 20, transcutol and loratadin as a poorly soluble drug. A multilevel factorial design was used to formulation of SNEDDS pellets, liquid SNEDDS (20 and 30%) was mixed with lactose, microcrystallin cellulose (40%) and silicon dioxide (0, 5 and 10%), and Na-crosscarmelose (0, 5 and 10%). The resulting wet mass transformed into pellets by extrusion-spheronization. The pellets were dried and characterized for size (sieve analysis), shape (image analysis), mechanical strength (friability test), droplet size (laser light scattering) and drug release rate (dissolution test). Selected SNEDDS pellets were also compared with conventional loratadin pellet or tablet formulation.
Results: The resulting SNE pellets exhibited uniform size and shape. Total friability of pellets did not affected by formulation variables. The in vitro release of SNE pellets was higher than the liquid SNE and powder tablets.
Conclusion: Our studies demonstrated that extrusion-spheronization is a viable technology to produce self-emulsifying pellets in large scale which can improve in vitro dissolution with better solubility.

Introduction

In the drug discovery, a large proportion of new chemical entities and many existing drug molecules exhibit poor water solubility and hence poor oral absorption.[1] An innovation strategy which would overcome this barrier is self-emulsifying drug delivery system (SEDDS) that so results in improving the oral bioavailability of poorly water soluble and lipophilic drugs.[2] Self-emulsifying systems have shown lots of unique and reasonable properties compared to other formulation strategies such as application of cyclodextrins, nanoparticles, solid dispersions, permeation enhancers, micronization, co-solubilization, inclusion complexation, nano suspensions and lipid-based formulations.[1-6] Self-emulsifying (SE) systems are able to emulsify rapidly and spontaneously in the gastrointestinal fluids and create fine oil/water emulsions under the gentle agitation provided by gastro-intestinal motion.[7] Small droplets of oil created by SEDDS increase drug diffusion into intestinal fluids (because of large surface area). Moreover, the emulsion droplets lead to a faster and more uniform distribution of drug in the GI tract. They also minimize the mucosal irritation due to the contact between the drug and the gut wall.[7-9]

SEDDS are normally prepared as liquid dosage forms or encapsulated in soft gelatin capsules[10] which have some limitations such as: high production cost, incompatibility problems with capsule shell[6,10-13], low drug portability and stability, drug leakage and precipitation,[1] low drug loading, few choices of dosage forms and irreversible drugs/excipients precipitation. More importantly the large quantity of surfactants in the formulations can induce GI irritations.[13,14] Incorporating liquid SEDDS into pharmaceutical excipients to create solid dosage forms (SE pellets[15] or SE granules[16]) have recently developed by researchers. To some extent, this combination offers the sum of the benefits of both SEDDS and solid dosage forms. From the perspective of the dosage form, pellets have some desired advantages making them of great attraction to

***Corresponding author:** Mohammadreza Abbaspour, Nanotechnology Research Center and School of pharmacy, Ahvaz Jundishapur University of Medical Sciences, Golestan Blv., Ahvaz, Iran. Email: abbaspourmr@ajums.ac.ir

the pharmaceutical industry. The pellets have improved appearance with fine pharmaceutical elegance, they can decrease the risk of dose dumping and local mucosal irritation, avoid powder dusting in the pharmaceutical industries, also their larger surface area enables better distribution in case of immediate release products.[17] Furthermore, pellets disperse freely in the gastrointestinal tract and invariably maximize drug absorption with a subsequent reduction in peak plasma flactuations, as a result they minimize potential side effects without lowering drug bioavailability. Moreover reduction of intra-and inter patient variability of plasma profiles is achieved by reducing overall transit time.[6]

The method of choice in preparing the pellet dosage forms is extrusion-spheronization since it provides much more benefits than other methods, including large-scale producibility, spherical shape, narrow modal size distribution, good flow, ease of coating,[6] compact packaging, higher density and surface area.[17]

In this study, we intended to prepare and characterize solid self-nanoemulsifying drug delivery system for oral delivery of loratadin as the model insoluble drug. We firstly prepared a liquid SNEDDS formulation containing loratadin.Then solidified it with incorporating liquid SNEDDS into spherical pellets produced by the extrusion-spheronization technique. The developed formulations were characterized by determination of their morphology, size, friability, in-vitro drug release, disintegrating properties, and emulsion droplet size analysis. Optimum SNE pellet formulations were then selected and their in-vitro drug release was evaluated in comparison with liquid SEDDS, conventional loratadin tablets and pellets.

Materials and Methods

Chemicals

Loratadin was kindly donated by Abidi Pharmaceutical Co. (Tehran, Iran). Capriol® and transcutol® were gift from Gattefosse (France). Span® 20, liquid paraffin and hydrochloric acid were provided by Merk (Germany). Aerosil® (silicon dioxide) was purchased from Exir Pharmaceutical Company. Avicel® (MCC, microcrystalin cellulose) from FMC, Biopolymer (USA) was used as a pellet forming material. Sodium crosscarmelose was provided by Fluka, Germany and lactose was purchased from Akbarieh pharmaceutical Co (Iran).

Preparation of the liquid self-nanoemulsifying drug delivery system (SNEDDS)

Based on previous studies,[18] a self-emulsifying system was prepared containing a fixed proportion of loratadin (0.1%), 73.8% of liquid paraffin, 24.55% span 20, and 6.15% capriole as surfactant and co-surfactant, respectively. 0.5% transcutol was added as permeation enhancer. This procedure involved admixing defined amount of the components (oil, surfactant, co-surfactant and transcutol), then adding loratadin 0.1% (w/w) to the mixture. The mixture was stirred at 40 °C for a time period necessary to solve the drug until a solution was obtained. To evaluate self-emulsification properties of the liquid SNEDDS formulation, 1 ml of liquid SNEDDS was added to 0.1 N HCl (100 ml) under continuous stirring (60 rpm) at 37 °C. The formulation was characterized as transparent to milky dispersion.

Experimental design

The solid self-nanoemulsifying drug delivery system (SNE pellets) was prepared using a multi-level full factorial design. Three independent variables, including the percentage of Aerosil (three levels), the Crosscarmellose (three levels), and the amount of liquid SNEDDS (two levels) were used (Table 1). The dependent variables or responses were pellet's disintegration time, friability, MDT and sphericity. The SPSS 16 software was employed for the experimental design and regression analysis of the data to evaluate the effect of the variables on the responses.

Table 1. Independent variables (factors and levels) for factorial design.

Factors	levels		
	-1	0	+1
Aerosil%	0	5	10
Crosscarmelose%	0	5	10
SNEDDS%	20	-	30

Preparation of the SNE pellets

The composition of SNE pellets is shown in Table 2. The pellets were produced by the following processes: initially the resulted liquid SNEDDS was added into Aerosil (or mixture of Avicel and lactose for formulations that had 0% Aerosil), and mixed in a kneader until the liquid SNEDDS were completely adsorbed to form a fine mixture. Then, the adsorbed mixture was blended with other components (MCC, lactose and crosscarmelose) for 5 minutes. After that, drops of distilled water were added until a mass with suitable consistency was obtained for extrusion. The wet mass was extruded at 100 rpm in a screw extruder (Dorsa, Iran) with a die of 1mm thickness and 1mm diameter holes. The extrudates were spheronized for 2 minutes, at 1000 rpm on a spheronizer (Dorsa, Iran). The produced pellets were then dried for 15 h at 40 °C in an oven drier. The pellets were stored in sealed bags.

Size distribution of SNE pellets

25 mg of SNE pellet formulations were vibrated by a set of standard sieves (0.35, 0.5, 0.71, 1.18, 1.4, and 1.7 mm) for determination of size distribution. The subsequent tests were carried out on the modal size fraction (1180-1400 µm).

Table 2. Compositions of the SNE pellets

-	Aerosil %	crosscarmelose %	lactose%	avicel%	SNEDDS%	Water (mL) (mL)
F1	10	10	10	40	30	9
F2	10	5	15	40	30	8
F3	10	0	20	40	30	5
F4	5	10	15	40	30	7
F5	5	5	20	40	30	9
F6	5	0	25	40	30	3
F7	0	10	20	40	30	9
F8	0	5	25	40	30	7
F9	0	0	30	40	30	5
F10	10	10	20	40	20	10
F11	10	5	25	40	20	11
F12	10	0	30	40	20	8
F13	5	10	25	40	20	12
F14	5	5	30	40	20	9
F15	5	0	35	40	20	3
F16	0	10	30	40	20	9
F17	0	5	35	40	20	7
F18	0	0	40	40	20	3

Image analysis of SNE pellets

Shape analysis was performed using a stereo microscope (ZSM-1001-3E, Iran) and a digital camera connected to a personal computer with SCION image analysis software. This test was performed on 50 pellets within the 1180-1400 (µm) fraction and two shape factors were determined using projected two-dimensional images of pellets:[19]

$$Aspect\ ratio = d_{max}/\ d_{min} \quad (1)$$

$$Sphericity\ (circularity) = 4\pi\ A/P_m{}^2 \quad (2)$$

Where d_{max} and d_{min} are maximum and minimum ferret diameters of pellets, Ferret diameter is the distance between two tangents on opposite sides of the particle parallel to some fixed direction; so, based on direction several Ferret diameters can be determined for the particle. A is the pellet's projected area and P_m is the pellet's perimeter.

Friability test of SNE pellets

5 mg SNE pellets (d ≥1mm) were placed in the friabilator (ERWEKA, Germany) together with 5 (g) of glass spheres, and rotated for 15 minutes at 25 rpm. Then the rotated SE pellets were sieved by mesh 60 sieve and weighed in order to determine friability.[6]

$$\%\,F = \frac{Mb-Ma}{Mb} \times 100 \quad (3)$$

Where M_b is the weight of pellets before friability test, and M_a is the weight of pellets after friability test.

Disintegration of SNE pellets

Using a disintegration apparatus (ERWEKA, Germany) 50 mg pellet samples from each formulation were tested (n=3) in 700 ml distilled water at 37 °C, and the end point was taken as the time at which no obvious particles were remained on the sieve in each disintegration baskets.[1]

Dissolution test

The dissolution tests were carried out on, liquid SNEDDS, SE pellets, conventional pellets and tablets formed by drug powder in order to compare drug release profiles. The dissolution medium was 900 ml of HCl 0.1N solution at 37± 0.5 °C. Each formulation weighed to be equivalent to 3 mg loratadin. The USP dissolution apparatus (basket method) was used for pellets and tablets and paddle method was used for liquid SNEDDS, at 50 rpm. 2 ml of dissolution medium was sampled at predetermined intervals and fresh dissolution medium was replaced in flasks to achieve sink condition.[20] The samples were assayed by a UV spectrophotometer at 276 nm to determine the dissolved drug concentration[18] (it was found that SEDDS or pellet compositions had no considerable absorbance in this wavelength), the dissolution data were then converted to mean dissolution time (MDT) by following equation:[21]

$$MDT = \frac{\sum \bar{t}_i . \Delta Mi}{\sum \Delta M_i} \quad (4)$$

$$\bar{t}_i = (t_i + t_{i+1})/2 \quad (5)$$

$$\Delta M_i = (M_{i+1} - M_i) \quad (6)$$

Where t_i is the midpoint of the time period during which the fraction ΔM_i of the drug has been released from the dosage form. A high MDT value for a drug delivery system means that it has a slow in vitro drug release.

Emulsion droplet size determination

To determine the size of the droplets formed by liquid SNEDDS and SNE pellets 1 ml of liquid SNEDDS and 1 g of selected pellet formulations were gently agitated in 50 ml distilled water with a magnetic stirrer. After 30 minutes, samples were filtered through 0.45 µm micropore filters.[1] Then the resulted size of the emulsion droplet was determined by laser diffraction (Scatteroscope Qudix I, Korea). The experiments were carried out in triplicates and reported as mean droplet size and poly dispersity index (PDI).

Statistical analysis

The effects of independent variables on the experimental response were modeled using a second order polynomial equation with a backward, stepwise linear regression technique. Only significant terms ($p<0.05$) were chosen for the final model. ANOVA and modeling process were performed using SPSS for Windows®, Version 16.0 (SPSS Inc., USA). The related surface plots were obtained by Statgraphics for Windows®, Version 5.1 plus (Statistical Graphics Corp., USA).

Results and Discussion

Preparation and characterization of SNE pellets

Size distribution

Acceptable loratadin SNE pellets were successfully prepared by extrusion-spheronization technique, using different factors and levels applied in this study. The calculated pelletization yield for most of the formulation was over 80% (Table 3).

Quality assessment of the produced pellets was made by evaluating their size and shape,[22] and percentages of the SE pellets in the sieve fraction are shown in Table 3. The size of modal fraction was 1 – 1.7 mm which more than 60% of pellets were in this range.

Table 3. Results of sieve analysis and experimental responses of different SE pellets.

Formulation	Sieve Analysis							Friability (%)	MDT (min)	Sphericity	Aspect ratio	Disintegration Time (min)
	Total weight(g)	0.5-0.71 (mm)	0.71-1 (mm)	1-1.18 (mm)	1.18-1.4 (mm)	1.4-1.7 (mm)	Formulation yield (%)					
1	14.5	6.6	10.3	23.9	44.6	7.4	86.1	0.2±0.3	9.7±0.30	0.53±0.11	1.24±0.13	4.66±2.08
2	21.5	1.9	5.9	21.8	34.3	35.8	97.8	0±0	23.0±2.68	0.56±0.09	1.17±0.09	38±2.64
3	21.42	0.3	3.3	10.4	21.2	55.6	90.4	0.6±0.04	24.7±5.41	0.57±0.07	1.23±0.22	158.67±5.50
4	11.07	11.2	18.3	21.4	42.5	1.5	83.7	3.8±0.05	12.0±1	0.58±0.08	1.16±0.1	0.97±0.05
5	22.47	0.1	1.2	5.1	12.2	72.5	91.1	0.2±0.09	14.9±2.07	0.59±0.10	1.13±0.09	13.33±3.21
6	15.6	4.2	8.4	17.2	31.7	38.3	95.6	0.4±0.1	15.1±1.46	0.57±0.08	1.17±0.13	34.67±5.50
7	17.54	1.8	5.4	10.1	37	46.6	99	1.2±0.04	7.4±0.2	0.63±0.08	1.18±0.11	0.51±0
8	20.5	0.1	0.9	6.1	16.3	59.9	83.2	4.6±0.8	8.6±0.11	0.63±0.12	1.21±0.09	1.5±0
9	19.7	0.1	0.3	4.1	11.9	51.2	67.5	0.6±0.54	9.8±1.17	0.63±0.07	1.19±0.07	27.33±3
10	18.53	2.7	3.9	10.1	14.1	68.2	96.3	0.4±0.62	19.0±0.85	0.63±0.09	1.15±0.1	107±45
11	19.5	1	2.6	7.1	20	27.3	57	0.6±0.09	25.8±2.56	0.58±0.11	1.17±0.14	95.33±35
12	20.4	1.7	5.4	17.6	40.2	34.3	97.6	0.1±0.78	26.6±0.37	0.59±0.06	1.20±0.14	100.67±5.03
13	10.08	1.8	4.4	12.9	52.4	10.1	79.8	0±0.54	15.1±3.71	0.64±0.07	1.21±0.10	41±17
14	22	0.6	2	6.1	15.2	73.9	97.2	0.4±0.4	22.8±3.84	0.64±0.09	1.16±0.10	95.67±2.08
15	20.04	0.5	1.5	5	13.3	76.4	96.3	0.1±0.71	18.5±2.47	0.64±0.06	1.16±0.09	108.33±10.7
16	11.25	9.9	11.3	13.7	54	7.6	86.6	1±0.67	7.1±0.33	0.65±0.09	1.14±0.07	2.5±1
17	14.6	8.2	11.5	18.8	44	12	86.3	0±0.025	7.8±0.92	0.62±0.08	1.18±0.09	4±1
18	21.54	0	0.3	2.8	9.5	66.5	79.1	0.3±0.6	10.8±2.69	0.64±0.09	1.17±0.09	13.33±6.1

Image analysis

The image analysis was based on the consideration that for a perfect spherical particle the aspect ratio shows the value of unity and values deviating from unity (greater than 1) indicate the degree of spheroid elongation. For the sphericity a value of unity considers a perfect spheroid and smaller values show the deviation from spherical form.

Details of shape analysis results are brought in Table 3. The regression analysis did not show any significant relevancy between aspect ratio and studied formulation factors; while it is indicated that the sphericity could be affected by the factors. As shown in the surface plot (Figure 1) increasing the amount of Aerosil as an absorbent and pelletization aid lead to improve pellets sphericity. Although the amount of crosscarmelose as disintegrating agent and the percent of SNEDDS had no significant effect on sphericity, in formulations containing higher levels of Aerosil, increasing the amount of crosscarmelose showed a negative impact on pellets' sphericity.

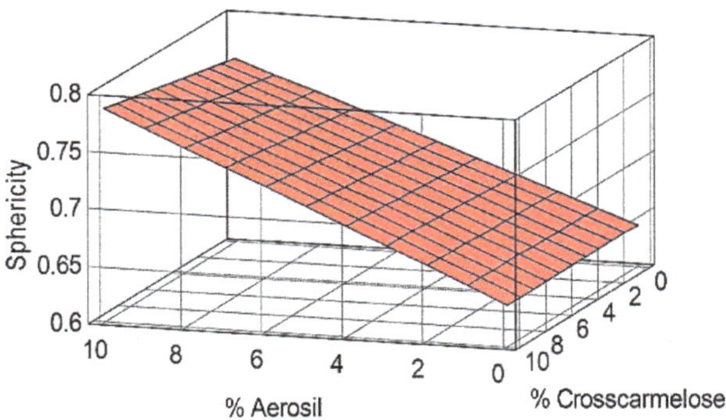

Figure 1. Effect of %Aerosil and %Crosscarmelose on pellets sphericity.

Friability test

The summary of friability test results is shown in Table 3. In this study the mechanical strength of pellets was not significantly affected by studied factors. However it is reported that increasing the amount of SEDDS of the pellets or granules would weaken the interaction within the pellets due to incomplete adsorption on pellets components and decrease their hardness.[1,22] This could be attributed to utilization of different amounts of granulating water in different formulations to achieve suitable consistency which can affects the pellets mechanical strength.

Disintegration of SNEDDS pellets

The effect of both Aerosil and crosscarmelose on disintegration time is shown as a surface plot (Figure 2). The plot demonstrates that increasing the amount of crosscarmelose lead to faster pellet disintegration. It is well known that crosscarmelose possesses wicking and swelling abilities and hence favors the water ingress inside the pellets and improve disintegration of pellets.[23] Moreover, increasing the quantity of Aerosil as a pelletization aid would be useful to improve pellets integrity and the disintegration time. As we found out in this test and according to a previous study, adding the lactose had less effect on disintegration time, but would be useful to improve appearance of the pellets.[1] However, the amount of liquid SNEDDS, had no significant effect on disintegration time.

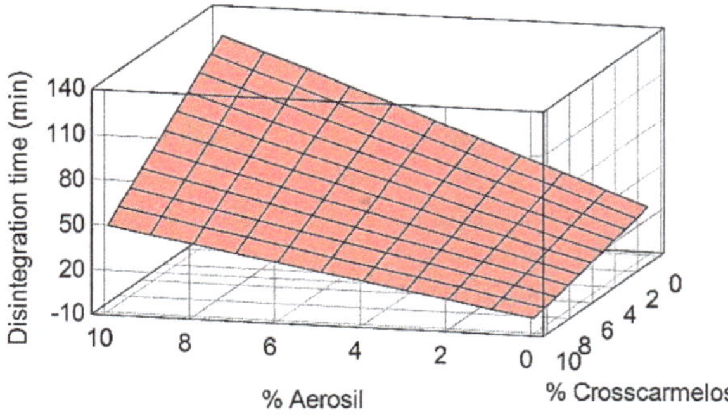

Figure 2. Effect of %Aerosil and %Crosscarmelose on pellets disintegration time.

In vitro dissolution test

In vitro dissolution profile of different pellets formulations are shown in Figure 3. The mean dissolution time (MDT) was used to compare the release profiles easily, (Table 3). The results are shown in Figure 4 as a surface plot. According to the plot increasing amount of Aerosil, increasing the (MDT), is in accordance with the disintegration time of the pellets, while increasing crosscarmelose cause to decrease MDT.

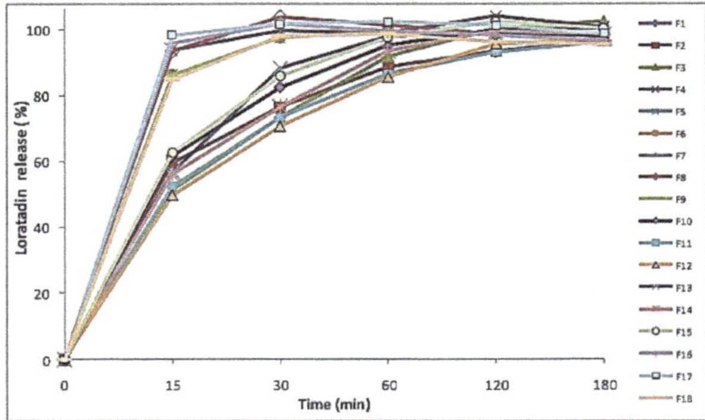

Figure 3. In vitro dissolution profile of different pellets formulation.(n=3)

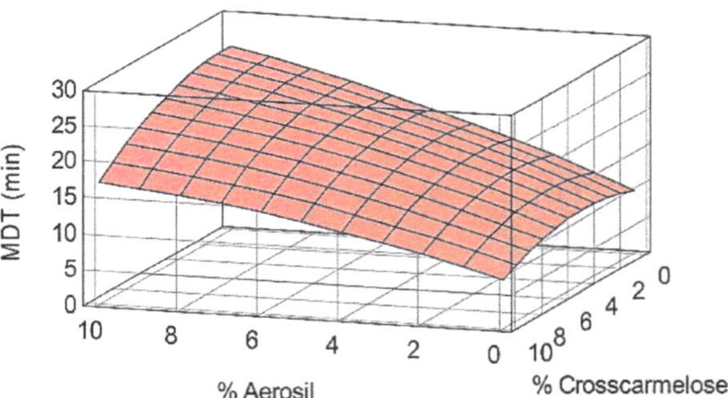

Figure 4. Effect of %Aerosil and %Crosscarmelose on pellets MDT

Formulations F_7 (30% SNEDDS) and F_{16} (20% SENDDS) which had lowest MDT and highest drug release rate, were selected as optimal formulations; moreover, their release profiles were compared with liquid SNEDDS, pellets and tablets, which were prepared in our lab based on powder drug with the same fraction of components as selected formulations (Figure 5).

As shown in Figure 5 and using MDT results, the selected SSNEDDS had a faster drug release than liquid SNEDDS and powder drug pellets ($p<0.01$). This finding could be primarily attributed to the effects of pellet components particularly crosscarmelose on enhancing water absorption into the pellets and improve interfacial surface between liquid SNEDDS and dissolution medium. Secondly the result could be related to the role of fine solid components of pellet formulations as an auxiliary emulsifying agent. It has been shown that finely divided solid particles can be used as emulsifying agents and emulsion stabilizer.[24]

As shown in Table 4, pelletization process did not affect the emulsifying efficiency of the SNEDDS. However, the F_{16} pellets resulted in smaller droplet size compare to the liquid SNEDDS ($p<0.05$). This may explained by emulsifying effect of solid components in the formulation. The efficiency of self-emulsification could be estimated by determining the rate of emulsification and droplet size distribution.[20] The droplet size of the emulsion is a crucial factor in self-emulsification performance because it determines the extent of drug release as well as absorption.[25] Furthermore, F_{16} have a slightly faster drug release than F_7 (Table 4). This result could be related to the smaller droplet size of F_{16}.[26]

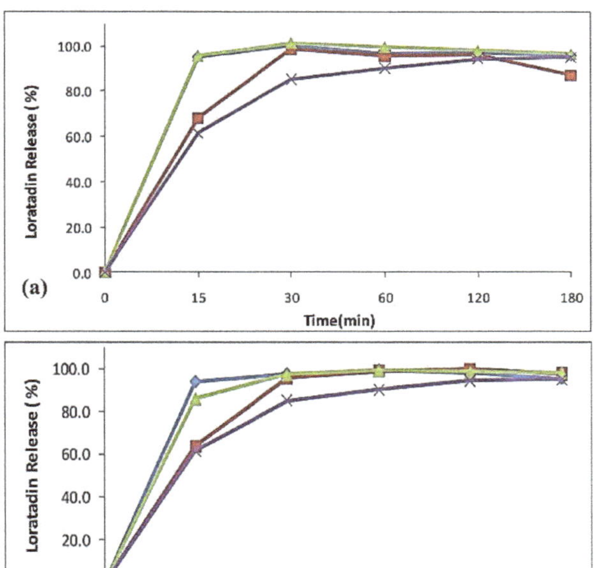

Figure 5. In vitro dissolution profile of the selected SNE pellets (▲), liquid SEDDS(×), tablets(■) and pellets formed by powder drug (♦) ; a: F_7 , b: F_{16} (n=3)

Table 4. Droplet size, PDI and MDT results of liquid SNEDDS and two selected pellet formulations.

Formulation	Mean Droplet size (nm)	PDI	MDT (min)
Liquid SNEDDS	190±42	0.39	17.6±5.9
SSNEDDS (F_7)	213.3±46	0.34	7.4±0.2
SSNEDDS (F_{16})	87.0±27	0.34	7.1±0.33

Conclusion

The overall results of this study indicated that an improved formulation of loratadin SNEDDS pellets was successfully developed using the extrusion-spheronization technique. The resulting SE pellets exhibit uniform size and spherical shape and suitable hardness. The results of in vitro dissolution revealed that the pelletization process of loratadin SNEDDS not only had no inappropriate effect on its self-emulsification properties, but also improve the drug release rate from resulted nano-emulsions.

Acknowledgments

This study was a Pharm. D thesis of Ms. N. Jalayer and was supported by a grant from Ahvaz Jundishapur University of Medical Sciences.

Conflict of Interest

The authors report no conflicts of interest.

References

1. Wang Z, Sun J, Wang Y, Liu X, Liu Y, Fu Q, et al. Solid self-emulsifying nitrendipine pellets: preparation and in vitro/in vivo evaluation. *Int J Pharm* 2010;383(1-2):1-6.
2. Iosio T, Voinovich D, Perissutti B, Serdoz F, Hasa D, Grabnar I, et al. Oral bioavailability of silymarin phytocomplex formulated as self-emulsifying pellets. *Phytomedicine* 2011;18(6):505-12.
3. Aungst BJ. Novel formulation strategies for improving oral bioavailability of drugs with poor membrane permeation or presystemic metabolism. *J Pharm Sci* 1993;82(10):979-87.
4. Wong JW, Yuen KH. Improved oral bioavailability of artemisinin through inclusion complexation with beta- and gamma-cyclodextrins. *Int J Pharm* 2001;227(1-2):177-85.
5. Patravale VB, Date AA, Kulkarni RM. Nanosuspensions: a promising drug delivery strategy. *J Pharm Pharmacol* 2004;56(7):827-40.
6. Abdalla A, Mader K. Preparation and characterization of a self-emulsifying pellet formulation. *Eur J Pharm Biopharm* 2007;66(2):220-6.
7. Iosio T, Voinovich D, Grassi M, Pinto JF, Perissutti B, Zacchigna M, et al. Bi-layered self-emulsifying pellets prepared by co-extrusion and spheronization: influence of formulation variables and preliminary study on the in vivo absorption. *Eur J Pharm Biopharm* 2008;69(2):686-97.
8. Charman SA, Charman WN, Rogge MC, Wilson TD, Dutko FJ, Pouton CW. Self-emulsifying drug delivery systems: formulation and biopharmaceutic evaluation of an investigational lipophilic compound. *Pharm Res* 1992;9(1):87-93.
9. Pouton CW. Formulation of self-emulsifying drug delivery systems. *Adv Drug Deliver Rev* 1997;25(1):47-58.
10. Yi T, Wan J, Xu H, Yang X. A new solid self-microemulsifying formulation prepared by spray-drying to improve the oral bioavailability of poorly water soluble drugs. *Eur J Pharm Biopharm* 2008;70(2):439-44.
11. Franceschinis E, Voinovich D, Grassi M, Perissutti B, Filipovic-Grcic J, Martinac A, et al. Self-emulsifying pellets prepared by wet granulation in high-shear mixer: influence of formulation variables

and preliminary study on the in vitro absorption. *Int J Pharm* 2005;291(1-2):87-97.
12. Tuleu C, Newton M, Rose J, Euler D, Saklatvala R, Clarke A, et al. Comparative bioavailability study in dogs of a self-emulsifying formulation of progesterone presented in a pellet and liquid form compared with an aqueous suspension of progesterone. *J Pharm Sci* 2004;93(6):1495-502.
13. Tang B, Cheng G, Gu JC, Xu CH. Development of solid self-emulsifying drug delivery systems: preparation techniques and dosage forms. *Drug Discov Today* 2008;13(13-14):606-12.
14. Chen Y, Li G, Wu X, Chen Z, Hang J, Qin B, et al. Self-microemulsifying drug delivery system (SMEDDS) of vinpocetine: formulation development and in vivo assessment. *Biol Pharm Bull* 2008;31(1):118-25.
15. Hu X, Lin C, Chen D, Zhang J, Liu Z, Wu W, et al. Sirolimus solid self-microemulsifying pellets: formulation development, characterization and bioavailability evaluation. *Int J Pharm* 2012;438(1-2):123-33.
16. Beg S, Jena SS, Patra Ch N, Rizwan M, Swain S, Sruti J, et al. Development of solid self-nanoemulsifying granules (SSNEGs) of ondansetron hydrochloride with enhanced bioavailability potential. *Colloids Surf B Biointerfaces* 2013;101:414-23.
17. Setthacheewakul S, Mahattanadul S, Phadoongsombut N, Pichayakorn W, Wiwattanapatapee R. Development and evaluation of self-microemulsifying liquid and pellet formulations of curcumin, and absorption studies in rats. *Eur J Pharm Biopharm* 2010;76(3):475-85.
18. Lavanya K, Senthil V, Rathi V. Pelletization technology: a quick review. *Int J Pharm Sci Res* 2011;2(6):1337-55.
19. Zadeh BSM, Dahanzadeh S, Rahim F. Preparation and evaluation of the self-emulsifying drug delivery system containing loratadine. *Int J Adv Pharm Sci* 2010;1(3);239-48.
20. Kleinebudde P. Application of low substituted hydroxypropylcellulose (L-HPC) in the production of pellets using extrusion/spheronization. *Int J Pharm* 1993;96(1-3):119-28.
21. Balakrishnan P, Lee BJ, Oh DH, Kim JO, Hong MJ, Jee JP, et al. Enhanced oral bioavailability of dexibuprofen by a novel solid self-emulsifying drug delivery system (SEDDS). *Eur J Pharm Biopharm* 2009;72(3):539-45.
22. Costa FO, Sousa JJ, Pais AA, Formosinho SJ. Comparison of dissolution profiles of Ibuprofen pellets. *J Control Release* 2003;89(2):199-212.
23. Abdalla A, Klein S, Mader K. A new self-emulsifying drug delivery system (SEDDS) for poorly soluble drugs: characterization, dissolution, in vitro digestion and incorporation into solid pellets. *Eur J Pharm Sci* 2008;35(5):457-64.
24. Rowe RC, Sheskey PJ, Owen SC. *Handbook of pharmaceutical excipients*. 2nd ed. London: Pharmaceutical Press; 2006.
25. Levine S, Sanford E. Stabilisation of emulsion droplets by fine powders. *Can J Chem Eng* 1985;63(2):258-68.
26. Kohli K, Chopra S, Dhar D, Arora S, Khar RK. Self-emulsifying drug delivery systems: an approach to enhance oral bioavailability. *Drug Discov Today* 2010;15(21-22):958-65.

Formulation and Physicochemical Characterization of Buccoadhesive Microspheres Containing Diclofenac Sodium

Mitra Jelvehgari[1], Hadi Valizadeh[2], Ramin Jalali Motlagh[3], Hassan Montazam[4]

[1] *Drug Applied Research Center and Faculty of Pharmacy, Tabriz University of Medical Sciences, Tabriz, Iran.*

[2] *Biotechnology Research Center and Faculty of Pharmacy, Tabriz University of Medical Sciences, Tabriz, Iran.*

[3] *Student Research Committee, Tabriz University of Medical Sciences, Tabriz, Iran.*

[4] *Islamic Azad University of Bonab Unit, Bonab, Iran.*

ARTICLEINFO

Keywords:
Buccal-mucoadhesive
Microparticle
Diclofenac
Emulsion dehydration
Carboxymethylcellulose sodium

ABSTRACT

Purpose: The present study involves preparation and evaluation of diclofenac buccal-mucoadhesive microparticles for prolongation of buccal residence time.
Methods: The microparticles were prepared by modified double-emulsion dehydration method ($O_{1}/W/O_2$) using sodium carboxymethylcellulose (CMC-Na) as mucoadhesive polymer. Calcium chloride was used as a cross-linking agent. Buccal-mucoadhesive microparticles with different drug to polymers ratios were prepared and characterized by encapsulation efficiency, particle size, DSC (Differential Scanning Calormetric), flowability, degree of swelling, surface pH, mucoadhesive property and drug release studies.
Results: The best drug to polymer ratio in microparticles was 1:5 (F_3) with CMC-Na. F_1 microparticles showed loading efficiency 51.43% and mean particle size 1013.92 µm. The DSC showed stable character of drug in microparticles and revealed amorphous form. Microparticles had slower release than the commercial tablet (p<o.o5). The results of mucoadhesion study showed better retention of diclofenac microparticles in mucosa (>50 min). Histopathological studies revealed no buccal mucosal damage.
Conclusion: It may be concluded that drug loaded buccal-mucoadhesive microparticles are a suitable delivery system for DS.

Introduction

Drugs supplied through the buccal route induce a quick onset of effect and enhanced bioavailability. The buccal mucosa offers several advantages for controlled drug delivery for extended periods of time. The mucosa is well supplied with both vascular and lymphatic drainage. Besides, first-pass metabolism and pre-systemic elimination in the gastrointestinal tract are avoided. Furthermore, there is a good potential for prolonged delivery through the mucosal membrane within the oral mucosal cavity.[1] Delivery of drugs is grouped into three various classes of drug delivery within the oral cavity (i.e., sublingual, buccal, and local drug delivery). Choosing one over another is principally established on anatomical and permeability differences that is between the different oral mucosal areas. The permeability of the buccal mucosa is 4-4000 times larger than that of the skin.[2] The buccal mucosa is thicker and significantly less permeable than the sublingual area. It is usually not able to supply the quick absorption and good bioavailability seen with sublingual administration. The buccal mucosa has an extent of smooth muscle (non-keratinized) and relatively immobile mucosa which makes it a more desirable region for oral transmucosal drug delivery. Thus the buccal mucosa is further suited for sustained delivery applications, delivery of less permeable molecules, and possibly peptide drugs. Similar to any other mucosal membrane, the buccal mucosa as a site for drug delivery has limitations as well. One of the major disadvantages associated with buccal drug delivery is the low flux which results in low drug bioavailability. Hydrogels are hydrophilic bioadhesive matrices that are able of swelling when put in aqueous medium. Usually, hydrogels are cross-linked so that they would not dissolve in the medium and would only absorb water. As water is absorbed into the matrix, chain relaxation happens and drug molecules are released through the spaces or channels within the hydrogel network.

Samaligy *et al*, formulated diclofenac sodium (DS) buccoadhesive discs containing CP 974, polycarbophil, PEO, SCMC-medium viscosity (SCMCMV), SCMC-

***Corresponding author:** Hadi Valizadeh, Department of Pharmaceutics, Faculty of Pharmacy, Tabriz University of Medical Sciences, Tabriz, Iran.
Email: valizadeh@tbzmed.ac.ir

ultrahigh viscosity (SCMC-UHV) or their combinations. Discs were prepared by directly compressing the polymer powder or polymer powder mixture with DS using a hydraulic press.[3] Dhanaraju *et al.* prepared sustained release particulate beads of CMC-Na and Na alginate with DS by the ionotropic gelation method using calcium chloride as a cross-linking agent. Beads of DS were produced with different concentrations of polymers.[4] Abha *et al.* formulated the buccal films of DS using PVA and HPMC.[5]

DS is a non-steroidal anti-inflammatory drug (NSAID) which may cause gastro-intestinal inflammation and ulceration in long term therapy. The buccal delivery of DS prevents direct exposure to mucosa therefore decreases the probability of gastrointestinal ulceration.[6] Buccal drug delivery has become important route of administration; thus when it is joined with mucoadhesive drug delivery, it can be called as transbuccal mucoadhesive drug delivery system.[6] The aim of this research was to formulate the buccal disc of DS using mucoadhesive polymers like carboxymethylcellulose sodium.

Materials and Methods

Diclofenac sodium (DS), carboxymethylcellulose sodium (CMC-Na), acetone, almond oil, chloride calcium, isopropyl alcohol, buffer phosphate and buffer phosphate saline (pH 6.8) were obtained from Merck (Darmstadt, Germany). All solvents and reagents were of analytical grade.

Experimental Methods

Method of preparation of CMC-Na microspheres

Double-emulsification method was utilized for the preparation of microspheres followed by cross-linking with calcium chloride according to published method with some modifications.[7] Briefly, 1 ml of almond oil (O_1, containing 50, 66.7and 100 mg DS) was emulsified for 1-2 min in 10 ml of aqueous phase (containing 500 mg CMC-Na) by stirring at 500 rpm with magnetic stirrer. The primary emulsion (O_1/W) was poured into 50 ml light liquid paraffin oil (O_2) containing span 80 (1 %w/w) at 70°C to form $O_1/W/O_2$ double emulsion. Different ratios of drug to polymer (1:5, 1:7.5 and 1:10) were prepared. After formation of emulsion 2 ml of $CaCl_2$ (2M) was added dropwise under stirring at 1000 rpm for 10 min at 70°C. The mixture was rapidly cooled to 15°C and then, 50 ml of acetone was added in order to dehydrate the droplets. The particles were isolated by filtration and washing the microspheres with 3 X 30 ml aliquots of isopropyl alcohol. Microspheres were allowed to dry at room temperature.

Determination of Loading Efficiency and production yield

Loading efficiency (%) = (actual drug content in microparticles/theoretical drug content) × 100

The production yield of the microparticles was determined by calculating the initial weight of the raw materials and the last weight of the polymeric particles obtained to the initial weight of the raw materials. Each determination was performed in triplicate manner (Table 1).

Table 1. Effect of drug to polymer ratio on the loading efficiency, production yield and particle size of diclofenac sodium microparticles

Formulation	Drug : Polymer ratio	Production yield (%±SD)	Theoretical drug Content (%)	Mean drug Entrapped (%±SD)	Drug loading Efficiency (%±SD)	Mean particle size (µm±SD)
F_1	1:10	99.99 ± 3.54	9.09	4.67 ± 1.78	51.43 ± 4.19	13.92 ± 0.47
F_2	1:7.5	94.99 ± 6.07	11.77	5.04 ± 2.49	42.830 ± 7.98	14.01 ± 0.49
F_3	1:5	91.67 ± 2.48	16.67	5.15 ± 2.37	30.907 ± 4.73	8.34 ± 0.60

Physicochemical properties of discs

Each disc contained 200 mg of DS microspheres (with different drug to polymer ratios of 1:10, 1:7.5 and 1:5). The discs were round and flat with an average diameter of 7 ± 0.1 mm compressed with a constant compression force (2 tones). Hardness of the discs was determined for six discs using Erweka hardness tester (Erweka, Germany). Friability of the prepared discs was assessed using friability tester (Erweka, Germany).

Differential Scanning Colorimetry (DSC)

The physical state of drug in the microspheres was analyzed by Differential Scanning Calorimeter (Shimadzu, Japan). The thermograms were obtained at a scanning rate of 10 °C/min conducted over a temperature range of 25-300 °C.

Flowability characterization of microparticles

Angle of repose of different formulations was measured according to fixed funnel standing method.

$$\theta = \tan^{-1} h / r$$

Where θ is the angle of repose, r is the radius, and h is the height.

Bulk and tapped densities were measured by using 10 ml of graduated cylinder. The sample poured in cylinder was tapped mechanically for 200 times, then tapped volume was noted down and bulk density and tapped density were calculated. Each experiment was performed in triplicate. Compressibility index (Ci) or Carr's index value of microparticles was computed according to the following equation:

$$\text{Carr's index (\%)} = (\text{Tapped density} - \text{bulk density}) \times 100 / \text{Tapped density}$$

Hausner's ratio of microparticles was determined by comparing the tapped density to the bulk density using the equation:

Hausner's ratio = Tapped density / Bulk density

Surface pH

The surface pH of the formulation was determined in order to investigate their possible side effects *in vivo.* An acidic or alkaline formulation will cause irritation of the mucosal membrane and hence this is an important parameter in developing a mucoadhesive dosage form. A combined glass electrode was used for determination of surface pH. pH was measured at time intervals of 15, 30, 60, 90 and 120 min. The discs were first allowed to swell by keeping them in contact with 5 ml phosphate buffer pH 6.8 for two hours in 50 ml beakers. pH was then noted by bringing the electrode near the surface of the formulation and allowing equilibrating for 1 min. The experiments were carried out in triplicate.

Swelling Studies

Upon application of the bioadhesive material to a tissue a process of swelling may occur. The swelling rate of buccoadhesive discs was evaluated by placing the discs after weighting (W_1) in phosphate buffer solution pH 6.8 at 37°c. Swelling was measured at time intervals of 15, 30, 60, 90 and 120 min. The disc was removed from the beaker and excess surface water was removed carefully using the filter paper. The swollen disc was then weighed again (W_2) and the swelling index was calculated.

$$\text{Swelling index} = (W_2 - W_1)/ W_1 \times 100$$

Ex vivo mucoadhesion time

Male Wistar rats (260±30 g) were used in this study. The animals were given food and water ad libitum. They were housed in the Animal House of Tabriz University of Medical Sciences at a controlled ambient temperature of 25±2 °C with 50±10% relative humidity and a 12-h light/ 12-h dark cycle. The present study was performed in accordance with Guide for the Care and Use of Laboratory Animals of Tabriz University of Medical Sciences, Tabriz-Iran (National Institutes of Health Publication No 85-23, revised 1985). The selected batch was subjected to ex vivo mucoadhesion test. The disintegration medium was composed of 900 ml phosphate buffer pH 7.4 maintained at 37°C. An abdominal segment of rat, 3 cm long, was glued to the surface of a glass slab, vertically attached to the disintegration apparatus (Erweka, Germany).[8] The mucoadhesive discs were hydrated from one surface and then were brought into contact with the mucosal membrane. The glass slab was vertically fixed to the apparatus and allowed to move up and down so that the disc was completely immersed in the buffer solution at the lowest point and was out of solution at the highest point. The time necessary for complete erosion or detachment of the discs from the mucosal surface was recorded. The experiment was carried out in triplicate.

Permeation studies

The *in vitro* study of DS permeation through the mucosal area of rat abdominal was performed using a Franz diffusion cell at 37 ± 0.2°C. Mucosa was obtained from mucosal area of rat in animal center. Freshly obtained rat mucosa was mounted between the donor and receptor compartments so that the smooth surface of the mucosa faced the donor compartment. The discs were placed on the mucosa and the compartments clamped together. The donor compartment was filled with 3 ml simulated saliva, pH 6.8 (sodium chloride 4.50 g, potassium chloride 0.30 g, sodium sulfate 0.30 g, ammonium acetate 0.40 g, urea 0.20 g, lactic acid 3 g, and distilled water up to 1,000 mL, adjusting pH of the solution to 6.8 by 1 M NaOH solution). The receptor compartment was filled with 22-25 ml phosphate buffer pH 7.4 and by stirring with a magnetic bead at 700 RPM. 3ml sample was withdrawn at predetermined time intervals and analyzed for drug content at 224 nm.

Bioadhesion strength

The tensile strength required to detach the bioadhesive discs from the mucosal surface was applied as a measure of the bioadhesive performance. The apparatus was locally assembled. The device was mainly composed of a two-arm balance. The mucoadhesive forces of discs were determined by means of the mucoadhesive force-measuring device,[8] using tissue cut from mucosal area abdominal of rat. The pieces of mucosa were stored frozen in phosphate buffer pH 7.4, thawed to room temperature before use.[9] At the time of testing, a section of mucosa was secured to the upper glass vial (C) using a cyanoacrylate adhesive (E). The diameter of each exposed mucosal membrane was 1.5 cm. The vials were equilibrated and maintained at 37°C for 10 min. Next, one vial with a section of tissue (E) was connected to the balance (A) and the other vial was fixed on a height-adjustable pan (F). To exposed tissue on this vial, a constant amount of discs (D) was applied. The height of the vial was adjusted so that the discs could adhere to the mucosal tissues of both vials. Immediately, a constant force of 0.5 N was applied for 2 minutes to ensure intimate contact between the tissues and the samples. The vial was then moved upwards at constant speed, it was connected to the balance. Weights were added at a constant rate to the pan on the other side of the modified balance of the used device until the two vials were separated. During measurement, 150 µl of phosphate buffer, (pH 6.8) was evenly spread onto the surface of the test membrane. The bioadhesive force, expressed as the detachment stress in g/cm^2, was determined from the minimal weights that detached the tissues from the surface of each formulation using the following equation.[1]

$$\text{Detachment Stress } (g/cm^2) = \frac{m}{A}$$

Where m is the weight added to the balance in grams and A is the area of tissue exposed. Measurements were repeated thrice for each of the discs. All the above three experiments were conducted in triplicates.

Histopathological Evaluation of mucosa

Histopathological effects of mucoadhesive discs were evaluated. The tissue was fixed with 10% formalin, routinely processed, and embedded in paraffin. Paraffin sections were cut on glass slides and stained with hematoxylin and eosin. Any damage to tissue was recorded by a light microscope.[9]

In vitro release Studies

In order to carry out *In-vitro* release studies dissolution test apparatus type II (USP) rotating paddle method was used. The studies were carried out for all formulation combination in triplicate, using 900 ml (37°C, 100 rpm) of isotonic phosphate buffer (pH 6.8) as the dissolution medium. An aliquot of 5ml sample was withdrawn at 0.25, 0.5, 1, 2, 3, 4 hours intervals and similar volume was replaced with fresh phosphate buffer (pH 6.8) maintained at same temperature. Samples were then analyzed at 224 nm with UV spectrophotometer.

Results

Physicochemical Properties of microparticles/discs

Mucoadhesive buccal discs of DS were prepared using CMC-Na as a matrix. The discs were characterized for their physical characteristics (Table 1). The production yield of the beads was increases with the increase in the concentration of drug. A lower drug entrapment was observed with increasing concentration of CMC-Na. This is in accordance with the results previously reported on DS beads.[10] This phenomenon could be due to the difficulty of formation of microspheres due to the high concentration of hydrophilic polymer (F_1, 1:10 drug to polymer ratio).[11] Particle analysis of microspheres prepared is shown in Table 1. An increase in polymers ratio from 1:5 to 1:10 results in a significant effect on the mean particle size of microparticles. The analysis of data showed that all obtained microparticles followed a log-probability distribution.

Angle of repose of microspheres was between 29.745° to 33.693°, indicating poor flow property for microspheres (Table 2). DS showed an amorphous state (Figure 1). Pure DS exhibits a melting exotherm around 281°C (Figure 1). CMC-Na showed wide endotherm peak in rang of 50-120°C and calcium chloride demonstrated abrupt or drastic change in the thermal behavior at 47.48 °C. It is obvious from thermograms that the DSC curves of physical mixtures of drug with polymer and the microparticle formulations are almost the same.

Table 2. Flowability Characteristics of microparticle formulations, physicochemical characteristics of disc formulations

Variables	Formulation code			
	F_1	F_2	F_3	Untreaed diclofenac
Drug : Polymer ratio	1:10	1:7.5	1:5	-
Bulk density (g/cm^3± SD)	0.187 ± 0.01	0.232 ± 0.00	0.191 ± 0.00	0.455±0.00
Tapped density (g/cm^3± SD)	0.287 ± 0.02	0.408 ± 0.00	0.283 ± 0.01	0.625±0.01
Carr's index (%±SD)	34.78 ± 0.00	43.18 ± 0.01	32.57 ± 0.00	27.20±0.00
Hausner ratio (±SD)	1.53 ± 0.00	1.76 ± 0.01	1.48 ± 0.00	1.48 ± 0.00
Angle of repose (°θ ±SD)	29.745 ± 0.22	31.820 ± 1.14	33.690 ± 0.56	21.413±0.85
Weight variation (mg ± SD)	194 ± 3.63	193 ± 4.13	190 ± 6.25	-
Hardness (N ± SD)	14.99 ± 0.72	19.28 ± 2.14	16.19 ± 0.83	-
Friability (%±SD)	6.15±0.43	5.01±1.63	6.42±0.85	-
Content uniformity (%±SD)	97.19 ± 0.47	94.00± 0.47	91.29 ± 0.85	-
***pH surface** (±SD)	5.95 ± 0.01	5.13 ± 0.01	5.96 ± 0.01	-
***Swelling** (%±SD)	76.47 ± 3.55	94.74 ± 2.24	111.11 ± 4.43	-
Mucoadhesive strength (g/cm^2±SD)	8.95±0.53	7.89±0.69	5.88±0.15	-
Residence time (min±SD)	53.43 ± 0.93	51.51 ± 0.19	50.69 ± 5.67	-

* Results of pH and swelling index was determined after 2h in phosphate buffer (pH=6.8).

All formulations consisted of 91.29-97.19% drug content, 14.99-19.28 N hardness, and 5.01-6.42% friability (Table 2).

The results revealed that all microsphere formulations swelled rapidly when immersed in 0.2 M phosphate buffer (pH 6.8). The swelling percent of different microparticle formulations was found to follow the rank order of 31.58±1.61% (F_2), 33.33±2.013% (F_3) and 41.18±1.72% (F_1). After 2 h of incubation swelling percent was observed to be 76.47±3.55% (F_1), 94.74±2.24% (F_2) and 111.11±4.43% (F_3), respectively (Table 2).

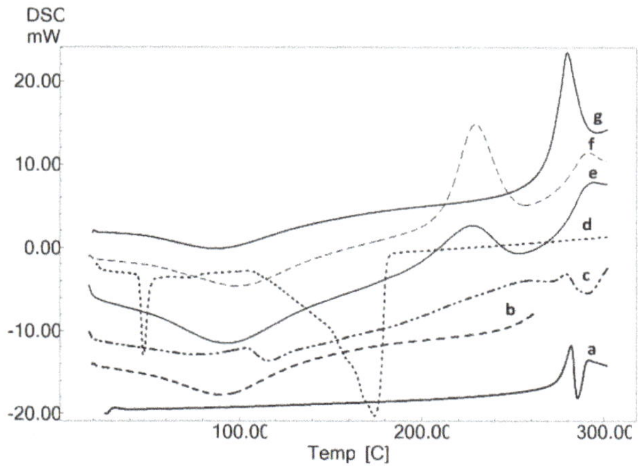

Figure 1. DSC thermogram of; diclofenac sodium (a); CMC-Na (b); microspheres of F_1 (c); Cacl2 (d); , F_5 (e); F_3 (f) and physical mixture of F_5 (g).

The surface pH of all the discs was within the range of salivary pH (5.13-5.96). No significant difference was found in surface pH of different discs (Table 2).

The *in vitro* mucosal residence time in phosphate buffer (pH 6.8) varied for microparticles from 0 to 120 min (Table 2). Microparticles showed high mucoadesion and did not dissolve in 0.2 M phosphate buffer (pH 6.8) for about 2 h.

The results of *in vitro* bioadhesive strength study are shown in the Table 2. The bioadhesion characteristics were affected by the concentration of the bioadhesive polymers. F_3 Formulation containing 1:10 ratio (drug: polymer) showed the highest mucoadhesive property (8.95±0.53 g/cm^2).

Figure 2 gives comparison of permeation of DS through rat abdominal mucosa for formulations containing different drug to polymer ratio. Slopes of the linear portion of the release profiles were calculated. These slopes represented the rate of penetration per unite area or flux of DS from different formulations (Table 3). The fluxes for formulations F_1, F_2 and F_3 were 0.0004, 0.0016 and 0.0015 mg/cm^2.h, respectively.

The microscopic observations indicated that the microparticles had no significant effect on the microscopic structure of mucosa. As shown in Figure 3, no cell necrosis was observed.

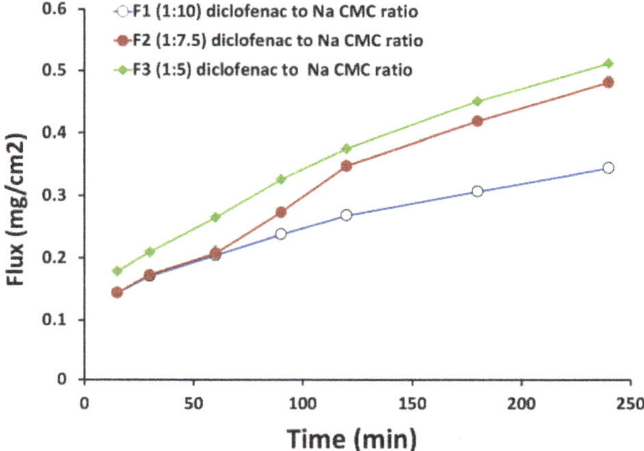

Figure 2. Cumulative amount of drug penetration per unit area (Flux) through abdominal mucosal of rat

Table 3. Flux or amount of drug release per unit surface area after 4 h, intercept and regression coefficient for different formulation and comparison of various release characteristics of diclofenac from different formulations and commercial® tablet

Formulation	^{a}Rel$_{0.5}$ (%)	^{b}Rel$_2$ (%)	^{c}DE	^{d}t$_{50\%}$ (min)	^{e}f$_1$	^{f}Flux (mg/cm^2/min)	Intercept (mg/cm^2)	r^2
F_1	6.98±1.47	44.56±13.90	27.79	90.34	62.55	0.0004	0.0763	0.9686
F_2	6.64±0.23	56.57±2.35	29.70	113.99	54.34	0.0016	0.1291	0.9811
F_3	6.81±2.13	66.67±7.52	32.07	124.41	59.15	0.0015	0.1741	0.9815
Commercial Tablet®	0	73.62±0.59	49.41	78.93	0	-	-	-

^{a}Rel$_{0.5}$ = amount of drug release after 0.5 h; ^{b}Rel$_2$ = amount of drug release after 2 h; ^{c}DE = dissolution efficiency; ^{d}t$_{50\%}$ = dissolution time for 50% fractions; ^{e}f$_1$ = Differential factor, ^{f}Flux was obtained from regression analysis between the amount of drug release per unit surface area and time.

In vitro release

The release profiles for all microparticles are illustrated in Figure 4. In order to have better comparison between the dissolution profiles, dissolution efficiency, $t_{50\%}$, $Q_{0.5}$ and Q_2 were calculated. Microparticles with high loading efficiency or high drug entrapment showed faster dissolution rate. This could be due to lower level of polymers corresponding to higher level of the drug in the formulation (F_3, 1:5 drug to polymer ratio) which resulted in a decrease in the drug release rate $p<0.05$. As more drugs are released from the microparticles, more channels and pores are probably produced, contributing to faster drug release rates. Figure 4 and Table 3 show that the initial drug releases for the microparticle formulations are high. The release of drug from microparticles ($t_{50\%}$ =90.34-124.41 min) was slower than the release of drug from commercial tablet ($t_{50\%}$ =78.93 min) ($p > 0.05$). However, a significant difference was observed between the percentages of drug released at 2 hours (Rel$_2$) between discs and commercial tablet ($p > 0.05$). There was a significant difference between dissolution profiles of commercial tablets and microparticles. During dissolution, CMC-Na containing microparticles swelled forming a gel layer on the exposed beads surfaces.

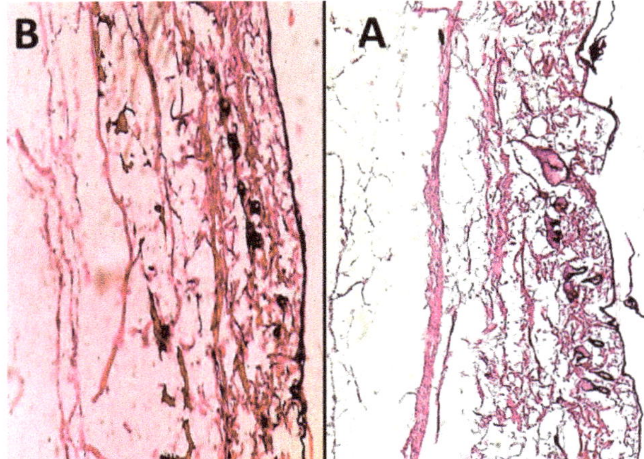

Figure 3. Histopathological evaluation of sections of mucosal area abdominal of rat (A) un-treated (B) treated with microparticles discs containing DS (magnitude X).

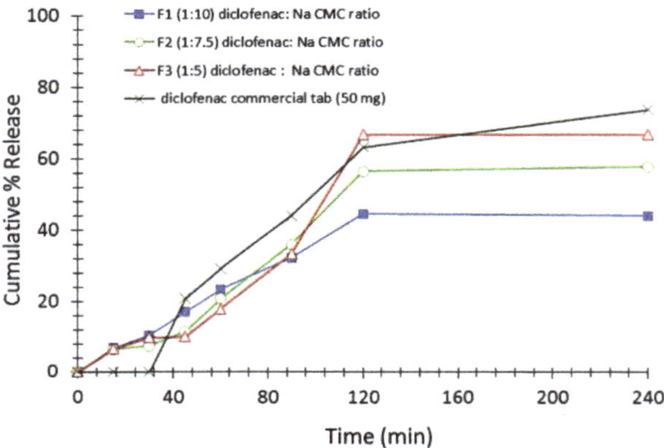

Figure 4. Cumulative percent release of DS from discs prepared with different drug to polymer ratios.

Discussion

Hydrogels are three dimensionally cross-linked polymer chains with capacity to hold water within its porous structure. The water holding capacity of the hydrogels is mainly due to the presence of hydrophilic functional groups like hydroxyl, amino and carboxyl groups.[12] As water is absorbed into the matrix, chain relaxation occurs and drug molecules inside matrix are released through the spaces or channels within the hydrogel network through the dissolution and/or the disintegration of the matrix.[13]

The influence of drug on the swelling properties of polymer is primarily dependent on the substituted groups of the polymer. The hydroxyl group in the molecules plays an important role in the matrix integrity of the swollen hydrophilic cellulose matrices. The amount and properties of the incorporated drug determine matrix integrity. Hydration is required for a mucoadhesive polymer to expand and create a proper macromolecular mesh of sufficient size, and also to induce mobility in the polymer chains in order to enhance the interpenetration process between polymer and mucin. Polymer swelling permits a mechanical entanglement by exposing the bioadhesive sites for hydrogen bonding and/or electrostatic interaction between the polymer and the mucous network.[14] However, a critical degree of hydration of the mucoadhesive polymer exists where optimum swelling and bioadhesion occurs.[15]

The effect of DS on the swelling behaviour and the residence time of various mucoadhesive polymer was also observed (Table2).

The comparative percentage swelling for various formulations was in order of $F_3 > F_2 > F_1$. CMC-Na containing beads showed high percent swelling due to presence of more hydroxyl group in the CMC-Na molecules. The weight of these formulations was increased to the extent of 30 to 110% from the initial value within 2 h (Table 2). Although the marked increase in surface area during swelling can promote drug release but the increase in diffusion path length of the drug may paradoxically delay the release.

Considering the fact that acidic or alkaline pH may cause irritation to the buccal mucosa and influence the degree of hydration of polymers, the surface pH of the buccal discs was determined to optimize both safety as well as drug permeation and mucoadhesion. Attempts were made to keep the surface pH as close to buccal/salivary pH as possible.

Increase in the ratio of polymer increased bio-adhesive strength of formulation. The incorporation of the drug induced significant reduction of the residence time of various formulations. As the particle swells, the matrix experiences intra-matrix swelling force which promotes disintegration and leaching of the drug leaving behind a highly porous matrix. Water influx weakens the network integrity of the polymer, thus influencing structural resistance of the swollen matrices, which in turn results in pronounced erosion of the lose gel layer.[4] DS, with logP value of 1.13, exhibits low permeability through buccal mucosa. Similar to the other studies the obtained results showed that generally an increase in the ratio of drug to polymer ratio resulted in a reduction in release of DS from discs (Table 3 and Figure 2).[16]

Cellular membrane was intact and no damage was observed to the treated rat mucosa (was used in the disintegration test). Thus, formulation containing microparticles appeared to be safe with respect to buccal administration (Figure 3).

The ionic interactions between calcium ion and negatively charged polymer (CMC-Na) might have been reduced at pH 6.8, forming a loose network with induced porous surface. In pH 6.8 phosphate buffer, slow dissociation of the CMC membrane may occur leading to drug release with a burst effect.

The release of DS from CMC-Na beads was slow (Figure 4), because of the formation of a loose network of CMC which dissociates and disintegrates slowly in phosphate buffer. With an increase in DS concentration, the interaction between the polymer and drug increased with the formation of a closer network, which showed a decrease in the diffusion of drug from the beads. The reason for the burst release ($Rel_{0.5}$)

could be due to the presence of some DS particles close to the surface of the microspheres. When water-soluble drugs don't have a tendency to migrate to the non-polar medium (liquid paraffin), thereby drug did not concentrate at the surface of the microspheres and did not induce the burst effect.[17]

The pores present in CMC-Na polymer act as a channels for the entrance of the liquid medium through the microparticles wall, causing it to swell. Hydrogen bonding between the hydroxyl groups of the carboxylic moiety and the carbonyl oxygen of ester group increases the degree of solidity of the polymer and decreases its porosity and permeability. Thus, by varying the ratio of drug to polymer the release rate of DS can be controlled.

According to the obtained results, Carr's (compressibility) index was greater than 25, indicating poor flow characterizes. The DSC themograms showed amorphous character of drug in the drug loaded microparticles.

Conclusion

Sustained release diclofenac loaded buccal-mucoadhesive microparticles with prolonged buccal residence time was designed. From the obtained results it may be concluded that the proposed drug loaded CMC-Na buccoadhesive microparticles could be suitable for diclofenac delivery.

Acknowledgments

The financial support from the Drug Applied Research Center and Research Council of Tabriz University of Medical Sciences is greatly acknowledged.

Conflict of Interest

The authors declare that they have no conflict of interest.

References

1. Macfarlane GT, Hay S, Macfarlane S, Gibson GR. Effect of different carbohydrates on growth, polysaccharidase and glycosidase production by Bacteroides ovatus, in batch and continuous culture. *J Appl Bacteriol* 1990;68(2):179-87.
2. Alagusundaram M, Chetty CM, Dhachinamoorthi D. Development and evaluation of novel-trans-buccoadhesive films of famotidine. *J Adv Pharm Technol Res* 2011;2(1):17-23.
3. El-Samaligy MS, Yahia SA, Basalious EB. Formulation and evaluation of diclofenac sodium buccoadhesive discs. *Int J Pharm* 2004;286(1-2):27-39.
4. Dhanaraju MD, Sundar VD, NandhaKumar S, Bhaskar K. Development and evaluation of sustained delivery of diclofenac sodium from hydrophilic polymeric beads. *J Young Pharm* 2009;1(4):301-4.
5. Doshi A, Koliyote S, Joshi B. Design and evaluation of buccal film of diclofenac sodium. *Int J Pharm Biol sci* 2011;1(1):17-30.
6. Shojaei AH. Buccal mucosa as a route for systemic drug delivery: a review. *J Pharm Pharm Sci* 1998;1(1):15-30.
7. Arica B, Caliş S, Kaş H, Sargon M, Hincal A. 5-Fluorouracil encapsulated alginate beads for the treatment of breast cancer. *Int J Pharm* 2002;242(1-2):267-9.
8. Wong CF, Yuen KH, Peh KK. An in-vitro method for buccal adhesion studies: importance of instrument variables. *Int J Pharm* 1999;180(1):47-57.
9. Shidhaye SS, Thakkar PV, Dand NM, Kadam VJ. Buccal drug delivery of pravastatin sodium. *AAPS PharmSciTech* 2010;11(1):416-24.
10. Manjunatha KM, Ramana MV, Satyanarayana D. Design and evaluation of diclofenac sodium controlled drug delivery systems. *Ind J Pharm Sci* 2007;69(3):384-9.
11. Fernandez-Hervas MJ, Holgado MA, Fini A, Fell JT. *In vitro* evaluation of alginate beads of a diclofenac salt. *Int J Pharm* 1998;163(1-2):23-34.
12. Cerezo A, Godfrey TJ, Sijbrandij SJ, Smith GDW, Warren PJ. Performance of an energy-compensated three-dimensional atom probe. *Rev Sci Instrum* 1998;69(1):49-58.
13. Gonzalez-Rodriguez ML, Holgado MA, Sanchez-Lafuente C, Rabasco AM, Fini A. Alginate/chitosan particulate systems for sodium diclofenac release. *Int J Pharm* 2002;232(1-2):225-34.
14. Shojaei AH, Chang RK, Guo X, Burnside BA, Couch RA. Systemic drug delivery via the buccal mucosal route. *Pharm Technol* 2001;25(6):70-81.
15. Shukla S, Jain D, Verma K, Verma S. Formulation and *in vitro* characterization of alginate microspheres loaded with diloxanide furoate for colon-specific drug delivery. *Asian J Pharm* 2010;4(4):199-204.
16. Pasparakis G, Bouropoulos N. Swelling studies and *in vitro* release of verapamil from calcium alginate and calcium alginate-chitosan beads. *Int J Pharm* 2006;323(1-2):34-42.
17. Lu W, Park TG. Protein release from poly(lactic-co-glycolic acid) microspheres: protein stability problems. *PDA J Pharm Sci Technol* 1995;49(1):13-9.

Anxiogenic Effects of Acute Injection of Sesame oil May be Mediated by β-1 Adrenoceptors in the Basolateral Amygdala

Mahnaz Kesmati, Maysam Mard-Soltani*, Lotfolah Khajehpour

Department of Biology, Faculty of Science, Shahid Chamran University, Ahvaz, Iran.

ARTICLEINFO

Keywords:
Sesame oil
Anxiety
β-1 Adrenoceptors
Basolateral Amygdala
Elevated Plus-Maze

ABSTRACT

Purpose: A few studies have indicates that the sesame oil influences anxiety, but many reports show that β-1 adrenoceptors (ARs) of the basolateral amygdala (BLA) plays a pivotal role in this regard. Therefore, in this study the effect of acute injection of sesame oil on anxiety-like behavior in the presence and absence of the BLA β-1 ARs in the male Wistar rats were investigated.

Methods: Guide cannulas, for seven groups of rats, were implanted bilaterally into the BLA. Two weeks after the stereotaxic surgery, anxiety-like behaviors (the OAT%, OAE % and locomotor activity) were evaluated by Elevated Plus-Maze (EPM) for all groups. 3 groups received different volumes of sesame oil (i.p.) and they were compared with control group (received saline via i.p.), and the anxiogenic volume of sesame oil (1.5ml/kg) was determined. Then, 3 other groups received constant effective volume of sesame oil (1.5ml/kg) along with 3 different doses of betaxolol, selective β-1 ARs antagonist, intra BLA microinjection in order to be compared with sesame oil group (1.5 ml/kg).

Results: The acute injection of sesame oil with the volume dependent manner showed an anxiogenic effect with reduction of the OAT% and OAE% which the maximum effect of sesame oil was observed in the dose of 1.5mg/kg. Also, betaxolol with dose dependent manner attenuated the anxiogenic effects of sesame oil (1.5mg/kg), but this reduction could not remove the anxiety effects completely.

Conclusion: It seems that the sesame oil acute (i.p.) injection induces anxiety, and this effect is attenuated by inhibition of β-*1ARs in the BLA.*

Introduction

Anxiety is known as a complex and compatible behavior in human and animals.[1] If it exists in the right level, it has appropriate effects on the learning and human's routine activities.[2] Nowadays, it is revealed that the anxiety-like behaviors are affected by the central/peripheral nervous systems (CNS/PNS) and different mediators such as hormones and neurotransmitters.[3-6] For example, high level of norepinephrine in limbic region has anxiety effects on human and animals.[7-10] In this regard, many studies show that the adrenergic/noradrenergic system plays a critical role in anxiety-like behaviors and these effects are mediated by two groups of α and β adrenoceptors (ARs) in different regions of the brain.[11-14] Among the different types of ARs, the regulatory role of β ARs, especially β-1 ARs, is confirmed on the anxiety-like behaviors in many studies.[12,14] For instance, betaxolol, as a selective β-1 ARs antagonist, has been used for treating anxiety disorders.[14] Furthermore it is revealed that the β-1 ARs, in the CNS, have effects on the anxiety-like behaviors.[12,14] Also, many studies show that the selective β-2 ARs antagonists are effective in treating acute anxiety, but they don't have any effects on treating chronic anxiety.[12,14,15] In addition, it is confirmed that the β-1 gene expression in amygdala obviously increases the cocaine-induced anxiogenesis.[14] In the different parts of limbic system such as amygdala and hippocampus, there is a powerful noradrenergic system which imposes effects on anxiety-like behaviors.[12,14] Also, β-1 and β-2 ARs elevation in amygdala, hippocampus and other parts of limbic system has been confirmed in anxiety complications.[16] Mammalians studies revealed that the amygdala complex, especially basolateral amygdala (BLA), has regulatory role via β ARs on anxiety-like behaviors.[12,17] Fu and et al. (2008) confirmed that intra BLA injection of metaproponolol, as a selective β-1 ARs antagonist, attenuates the anxiety.[12] Also, their western blot analyses confirmed that after anxiety condition, the β-1 ARs gene expression significantly increases in the BLA.[12]

***Corresponding author:** Maysam Mard-Soltani, Department of Biology, Faculty of Science, Shahid Chamran University, Ahvaz, Iran.
Email: maysam.mardsoltani@modares.ac.ir

On the other hand, the sesame seed and its products such as sesame oil are used in large quantities in medicine and food industries.[18] The sesame oil is mainly composed of stearic and poly unsaturated fatty acids (PUFAs) such as linolenic acid and it has antioxidant effects through containing high levels of vitamin E.[18-21] Also, different studies confirmed that the sesame oil contain metallic ions such as magnesium, copper, calcium, iron, zinc and also vitamin B.[21] Traditional medicine reports explained that sesame oil is a good medicine for treating arthritis romatoid, lung complication, colon cancer, osteoporosis, blood pressure, and migraine.[18] On the other investigations, the effect of sesame oil has been proved on memory and learning.[22] The PUFAs in the sesame oil increases the dendrite branches, number of neural synapses, and synapses efficiency.[23,24] It is believed that neurophysiological effects of sesame oil on the learning process and emotional behavior may be performed through its antioxidant effects on cholesterol and modulation of neurotransmitter systems.[25,26] Also, sesame oil anti-depression characteristics have been confirmed through its effects on plasma cholesterol.[25] The results of many studies show that sesame oil produces low serum cholesterol which changes the plasma cholesterol level in the neurons membrane in certain areas of CNS. It will change production of some neurotransmitter receptors, especially serotonergic receptors, in these areas and which finally changes emotional and anxiety-like behaviors.[27-30] Based on our collected data about sesame oil effects on anxiety and its correlation with β-1 ARs of amygdala, there are very little evidence related to this issue. So, due to the widespread uses of the sesame oil, as a vehicle oil in the many steroid drugs and food industry, our team research conducted this study for discovering the effects of acute i.p. injection of sesame oil on the anxiety-like behaviors and its interaction with BLA β-1 ARs.

Materials and Methods

Animal

This study was conducted using the adult intact male Wistar rats with weight range of 180±20gr and age range of 13±2 weeks in the surgery time. The rats were divided into seven groups. Each group contains 8 animals. The rats were housed four per cage in the colony room with a 12-hour reverse- light/dark cycle (7:00AM-19:00PM light off) at 22±1 °C and relative humidity of 30% to 50%. All the animals one week before the surgery were compatible with conditions and handling was taken 5min daily for all animals. In the study, all of the behavioral sessions were taken in the light period from 9:00 to 14:00 when rats usually have the most activities. Each animal was used once and had stereotaxic surgery.

Surgery

Two week before behavioral testing, rats were implanted with stainless-steel guide cannulas aimed at the BLA. Rats were anesthetized with interperitoneal injection (i.p.) of ketamine hydrochloride (50mg/kg) and xylazine (4mg/kg), and mounted in a stereotaxic instrument (Stalling Co, Illinois, and USA). The scalp was incised and retracted, and the head was positioned to place bregma and lambda in the same horizontal plane. Two small holes were drilled through the skull for bilateral placement of stainless-steel guide cannulas (21gauge; 14mmin length; Samen Mashhad, Iran) into the BLA (2.8mm from Bregma, 5mm lateral, and 6.8mm through the skull surface) along with three jeweler's screws.[31] Cannulas were affixed to the skull, and the scalp incision was closed with dental cement. After surgery, stainless-steel obturators (27gauge; 15mm in length; Samen Mashhad, Iran) were placed in the guide cannulas. The obturators were replaced every other day throughout the experiment.

Drug and injections

The sesame oil approved by Berovich Company (Berovich, Tehran, Iran) with different volume of 0.5, 1, and 1.5 ml/kg per rats were injected interperitoneally (i.p.). Betexolol hydrochloride (Tocris Bioscience, IO Center Moorend Farm Avenue, Bristol BS 11,OL, UK), as a selective β-1 ARs antagonist, was diluted in the normal saline (Samen Mahhad, Iran) to provide appropriate doses of betaxolol (0, 0.025, 0.1 and 0.4 μg/rat) and microinjected intra BLA.[32] For Betaxolol or its vehicle intra BLA microinjection in 60 seconds, a stainless steel needle (15mm stainless steel 27gauge tubing) connected to the Hamilton syringe of 2 μl by a polyethylene tube were placed into guiding cannulas. The volume of all the intra BLA injections into each cannula was 0.5 μl and for complete betaxolol and vehicles diffusion, top of the needle was kept in the cannula for 90 additional seconds. 15min after intra BLA injections saline or different volume of sesame oil: 0.5, 1, and 1.5 ml/kg per rat were injected to animals.

Behavioral testing

The Elevated Plus-Maze (EPM) test was applied to investigate the anxiety-like behavior. The EPM is an unconditional anxiety model which is used for measuring the anxiety like parameters.[33,34] The EPM is consisted of two open arms (50×10 cm, surrounded by a 0.5-cm-high border) and two closed arms (50×10 cm, surrounded by 30-cm-high walls). The apparatus was elevated 50cm above the floor. A 40W red light was placed at the upper part of EPM center in the height of one meter in order to shed light on the arms equally. The test session was initiated by placing the rat on the central platform of the EPM, facing one of the open arms, and letting it move freely. Each session lasted 5min, being recorded by a high quality Sony handycam (Sony Handycam HDR-CX 110 Camcorder-1080i). All test sessions were carried out under lighting phase between the 9:00 to 14:00. The criterion to determine the rat's entrance to each arm was entering of two rat's hind legs on the arm. The number of entries and the time spend on the open and close arms were recorded and after each test, the EPM was thoroughly cleaned by sterilized cotton and 70% ethyl alcohol. Using the collected data, the percentage of open arms entries to total arms entries (%OAE), the percentage of time spend on the open arm to total spending time on the all arms (%OAT), and the number of total arms entries (Locomotor activity), were evaluated.

Ethics of Animal Care and Use

In the present study, all experiments and methods were carried out in accordance with the Institutional Guidelines for Animal Care and Use of Laboratory Animals, and approved by the Biology Department of Shahid Chamran University (Ahvaz, Khuzestan Province, Iran).

Experiment I: Effects of sesame oil acute injection alone on the anxiety-like behaviors

Four rat groups received saline (1ml/kg rat), as betaxolol vehicles, intra BLA (1 µl/rat). After 15min, each group received saline or different volume of sesame oil: 0.5 ml/kg, 1 ml/kg and 1.5 ml/kg via i.p. respectively, and constitutes Control, Sesame 0.5, Sesame1, and Sesame 1.5 groups. The behavioral test session was performed 45min after the i.p. injection and the percentage of open arm time (%OAT), the percentage of open arm entries (%OAE) and locomotors activity were assessed (Figure 1).

Experiment II: Effects of betaxolol against anxiogenesis effects of sesame oil acute injection in the Experiment I

Three groups of rats received different doses of betaxolol: 0.025, 0.1, and 0.4 µg/rat intra-BLA, After 15min, the effective volume of sesame oil on the anxiety in the experiment 1, 1.5 ml/kg, i.p., was applied and injected into the all groups and constitute: bet. 0.025, bet.1 and bet.4 groups, respectively, and it was compared with control and Sesame 1.5 groups, as mentioned earlier. The behavioral test session was performed, using the EPM, 45min after the i.p. injection and the percentage of open arm time (%OAT), the percentage of open arm entries (%OAE) and locomotor activity were assessed (Figure 2)

Cannula verification

The animals were immediately killed with chloroform after the completion of the two experiments. Subsequently, 0.5µl per cannula of ink (0.1% aquatic methylene blue) was injected intra-BLA by a 15mm stainless steel 27gauge. Following that the animals' brain was removed and fixed in 10% formalin two weeks before sectioning. All sections were examined to determine the location of the cannula aimed for the BLA. The cannula placement was verified using the Atlas of Paxinos and Watson (1998).[31] The data from rats with cannula placement outside the BLA were excluded from the analyses.

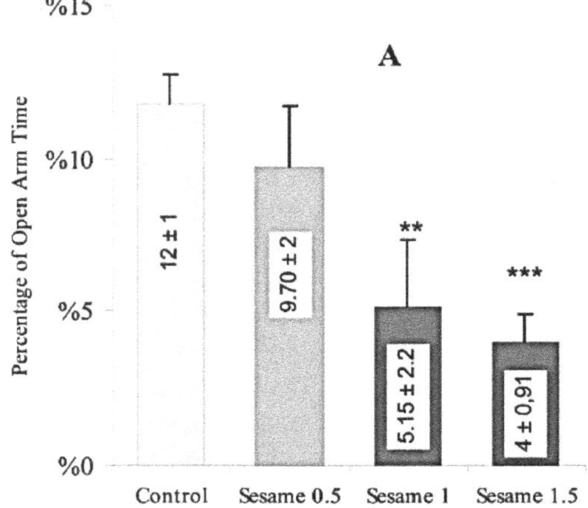

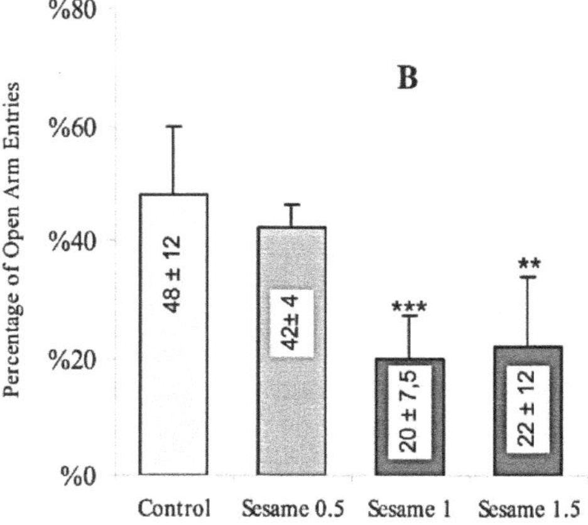

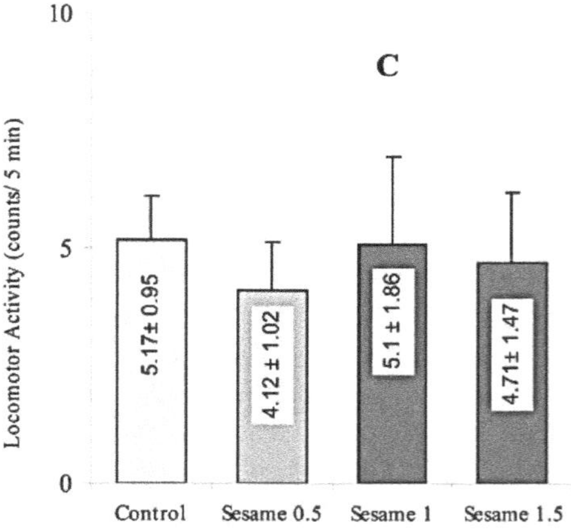

Figure 1. The effects of different volume of sesame oil on the anxiety like behaviors in the EPM: (A) OAT%, (B) OAE% and (C) locomotor activity. $^{**}p<0.01$ $^{***}p<0.001$

Statistical analyses

Statistical analyses were performed using SPSS software (SPSS-PC, version 15. SPSS, Inc., Chicago, IL). Graphical data are expressed as means±SEM. The data analysis for the experiments 1 and 2 was performed by one-way analysis of variance (ANOVA) followed by Tukey test for assessing specific group comparisons. The differences between the experimental groups at each point were considered as statistically significant ($P < 0.05$).

Results

Effects of sesame oil acute injection alone on the anxiety-like behaviors in the EPM

Figure 1, shows the comparison between measurement anxiety behaviors in four groups: control (saline), Sesame 0.5, Sesame 1, and Sesame 1.5. As it can be seen in Figure 1A regarding OAT%, there was a significant difference with $p<0.01$, and $p<0.001$ between control group and two groups of sesame 1 and sesame 1.5. Also, regarding the number of rats` entering into open arms (%OAE), there was a significant difference, $p<0.001$, $p<0.01$, between control group and sesame 1, and sesame 1.5 (Figure 1B). But, as Figure 1C shows, there was not any significant difference among four groups in regard to locomotor activity. So, the sesame oil with volume dependent manner increases anxiety in the adult male rats.

Effects of betaxolol (B) on anxiogenesis effects of sesame oil acute injection in the EPM

Figure 2, Part A, B and C, shows the anxiety assessment behaviors in each group of: sesame 1.5, B 0.025, B 0.1, B 0.4 and control. As mentioned earlier regarding the control and sesame 1.5, the sesame oil in the maximum volume, regarding the Experiment I, was injected to the three groups of: B 0.025, B 0.1, and B 0.4, but they had received different doses of betaxolol intra-BLA. As the Figure 2A, there was a significant difference with $p<0.01$, $p<0.001$, and $p<0.001$ between OAT%, of sesame 1.5 with OAT% of: B 0.1, B 0.4 and control group, respectively. Also, a significant difference, $p<0.01$, $p<0.001$, was observed in regard to %OAE among sesame 1.5 group with control and B 0.4 groups, respectively (Figure 2B). In the Figure 2C, there was not seen any significant difference between sesame 1.5 with control group and any other groups. Figure 2 contains the analyses of control group in the first step of the study to assure the effect of sesame oil on anxiety. It should be noted that, although rats had received different doses of betaxolol, but the anxiogenesis effect of sesame oil was not completely removed even in maximum dose of betaxolol.

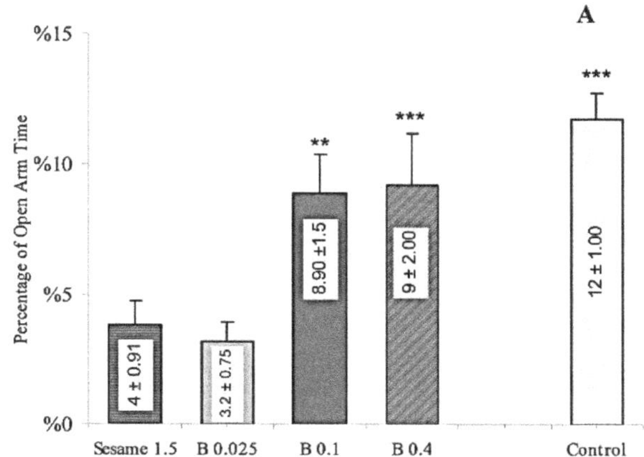

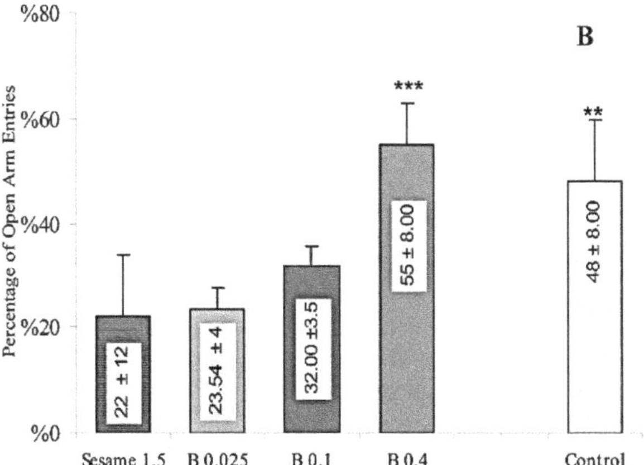

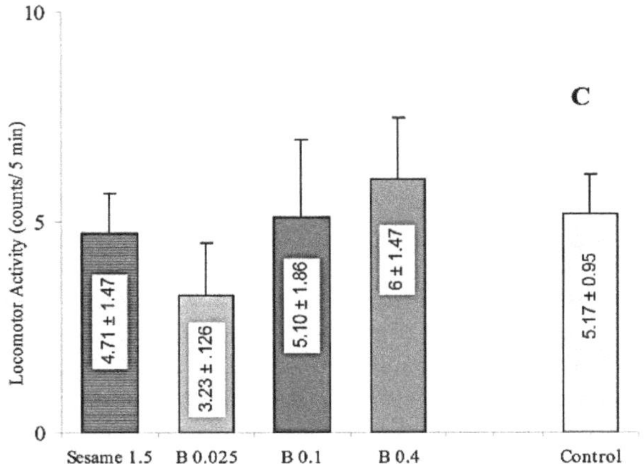

Figure 2. The comparison between anxiogenesis effect of sesame oil (1.5 ml/kg) in the presence and absence of different doses of betaxolol (0.025, 0/1, 0.4 µl/rat) on the anxiety like behaviors in the EPM: (A) OAT%, (B) OAE% and (C) locomotor activity. The significant value is showed comparing the Sesame 1.5 group. **$p<0.01$ ***$p<0.001$

Discussion

In the present work, our data revealed the anxiogenic effects of acute injection of sesame oil using the EPM. Our findings clarified reduction of the OAT% and OAE% by sesame oil volume dependent manner and showed it has significant anxiogenic effects. Also, these acute injections didn't impose meaningful effect on the rats' locomotor activity. So, this note show that the sesame oil anxiogenesis effects was not due to reduction of the rats' locomotor activity.

The results of other studies support the neurophysiologic and antioxidant effects of sesame oil.[18] These activities could be the result of sesame oils' poly unsaturated fatty acids (PUFAs).[18-20] The previous studies confirmed that the sesame oil is enrichment of PUFAs such as linoleic acid. PUFAs can be effective on the neurophysiological processes e.g. learning and memory processes.[18,19,22] Also, other studies show that the unsaturated fatty acids such as oleic acid, other chemical compound in sesame oil, can change in membrane fluidity by reduction in dendrites' plasma membrane cholesterol level.[25] They showed that there is a negative correlation between cholesterol level with emotional disorders such as anxiety and depression.[35-38] Therefore, the evidences have supported significant relationship between anxiety/stress with lipids reduction e.g. cholesterol reduction.[35-38] Herstin and et al. found that females who have total cholesterol lower than 4.7mM/L shows the depression symptoms 2-fold more than others.[39] Also, there are some hypothesis to support the effect of cholesterol level in plasma and neural membrane on anxiety-like behavior.[30,40] The first hypothesis suggests that anxiety can leads to decrease in appetite, and this will cause losing weight and decrease in level of cholesterol, therefore, the anxious individuals have hypocholestermia.[30] But, other studies rejected this possibility.[40] The second hypothesis is about the cholesterol impact on the anxiety and stress and its role in changing serotonergic receptors activities and their down regulation, and finally decreasing in serotonergic system in CNS.[35] According to this theory, serotonin system down regulation leads to the decrease of neurons` activities in this area.[35] In this regard, many studies confirmed the hyperserotonemia in anxious individuals.[41-44] So, these studies revealed that the hypocholestermia may be mediated by down-regulation of serotonin receptors.[40,44] Perhaps, these anxiogenic effects of sesame oil in our experiment caused by reduction of the lipids content of the neurons and then serotonergic system down regulation in CNS. Also, another study confirmed that monkeys which received foods with lower level of cholesterol showed more invasive behaviors where similar cases have been observed in human studies.[28] Further, it is proved that patients whom received anti-cholesterol drugs, revealed much anxiety and depression.[45] In the present study, also, it seems that sesame oil can lead to cholesterol reduction by affecting the blood cholesterol and following that, it will affect some tissues such as CNS and BLA cholesterol contain. Considering the relationship between serotonin and level of cholesterol, it seems that part of its effect is because of the increase of the blood serotonin which finally leads to the increase of anxiety.

It should be noted that there are contradictory studies regarding the effects of serotonergic system on anxiety.[35,41,42,43,46] De-Almeida and et al (1998) suggested that the low serotonin level would cause to the increase of anxiety.[46] But, many studies approved anxiogenic effects role of high level of serotonin in CNS.[35,41,42,43]

Basically, due to the increase of β-1 and β-2 ARs in amygdala, hippocampus and other parts of the limbic system during anxiety conditions,[47,48] and the controlling role of β-1 receptors in the BLA on decreasing the anxiety behaviors,[12,14] our team research, as other alternative procedure, applied the EPM and then injecting the sesame oil in presence and absence of β-1 ARs into BLA to find another possible interaction between the sesame oil with β-1 ARs in this area.

The results showed that β-1 ARs in the BLA would cause to the attenuation of sesame oil anxiety effects, with different doses of betaxolol, in maximum volume of sesame oil. In this study, interaction between anxiogenic effects of sesame oil and β-1 ARs in the BLA can be seen. Besides, the findings show that microinjection of betaxolol in the maximum dose can't remove the anxiogenic effect of sesame oil completely (Figure 2).

The studies somewhat reconfirmed that the BLA noradrenergic system is mostly innervated from other brain nucleus, especially locus coeruleus,[49,50] and when these postsynaptic neurons discharge in the BLA, they can leads to anxiety-like behavior.[51] Although there are a powerful evidences related to the neurons discharge of locus coeruleus and anxiety in the BLA, but the results state that noradrenergic has a controlling role on BLA.[12,14] Fu and et al. (2008) and other researcher confirmed the anxiolytic effects of β-1 ARs antagonist administration in the BLA.[12,14] Also, their study showed that the β-1 ARs in BLA in anxiety conditions were elevated, and the inhibition of β-1 ARs, by selective β-1 ARs antagonist, metoprolol, would relieve anxiety in anxiety conditions.[12] In their study the up regulation of β-1 ARs in the BLA after the anxiety condition was confirmed by Western Blot analysis.[12] The inhibition of β-1 ARs in the BLA by another selective β-1 antagonist, betaxolol, was also confirmed in other studies.[14] Our result showed that in the absence of β-1 ARs, the sesame oil could not impose anxiety-like effects, in other words, for execution of these effects, β-1 ARs in the BLA is needed.

As we discussed the probability of anxiogenic effects of sesame oil by hypocholestermia earlier, it didn't seem that the sesame oil impose its effects directly via β-1 ARs in the BLA, because the previous studies confirmed that hypercholesterolemia leads to up-regulation of β-1 ARs in the other organs and therefore hypocholestermia, by this mechanism, must be leads to down-regulation of the β-1 ARs.[52] Furthermore, the studies on marmosets maintained on a high cholesterol diet showed 3-fold increase in the β-1 ARs mRNA in endothelial cells, but hypocholestermia made contradiction results.[52] On the other hands, the higher

membrane cholesterol levels led to a decrease in Na/K-ATPase activity and other membrane bounded enzymes,[53] therefore, perhaps down regulation of plasma membrane cholesterol level with sesame oil effects, in the BLAs' neurons, causes anxiogenic effects, as a mentioned earlier.
However, due to the dyssynchrony between intra BLA injection of betaxolol and i.p. injection of sesame oil and then test session in the present study, it is impossible that the sesame oil hasn't enough time to change the level of plasma cholesterol to affect the target β-1 ARs in the BLAs' neurons and other receptor systems such as serotonin or GABA and etc in this area. So, more studies should be done to confirm the precise anxiogenic mechanism of acute injection of sesame oil, but our study revealed the anxiogensis effects of acute injection sesame oil and the existence of unknown interaction between sesame oil and BLA β-1 ARs. In the future studies, research teams can change the administering procedure of sesame oil in order to consider its effect by inhibiting β-1 ARs and serotonin receptors in the appropriate methods.

Conclusion

The present study suggests that the sesame oil i.p. acute injection induces anxiety, and this anxiogenic effect of sesame oil is attenuated by inhibition of β-1 ARs in the BLA, but this reduction could not remove the anxiety effects completely. Therefore, sesame oil and β-1 ARs have an unknown precise interaction in the BLA.

Acknowledgments

This study was supported by Shahid Chamran University of Ahvaz, Iran, grant number 90/302/18672. Hereby, researchers of this study would like to express their sincere gratitude to the Esteemed Vice-presidency for Research of Shahid Chamran University for their financial and moral supports.

Conflict of Interest

The authors report no conflicts of interest.

References

1. Zhou W, Hou P, Zhou Y, Chen D. Reduced recruitment of orbitofrontal cortex to human social chemosensory cues in social anxiety. *Neuroimage* 2011;55(3):1401-6.
2. Mathews A, Mackintosh B. A cognitive model of selective processing in anxiety. *Cognit Ther Res* 1998;22(6):539-60.
3. Fernandez-Guasti A, Martinez-Mota L. Anxiolytic-like actions of testosterone in the burying behavior test: role of androgen and GABA-benzodiazepine receptors. *Psychoneuroendocrinology* 2005;30(8):762-70.
4. Zuloaga DG, Jordan CL, Breedlove SM. The organizational role of testicular hormones and the androgen receptor in anxiety-related behaviors and sensorimotor gating in rats. *Endocrinology* 2011;152(4):1572-81.
5. Gilhotra N, Dhingra D. Thymoquinone produced antianxiety-like effects in mice through modulation of GABA and NO levels. *Pharmacol Rep* 2011;63(3):660-9.
6. Karg K, Burmeister M, Shedden K, Sen S. The serotonin transporter promoter variant (5-HTTLPR), stress, and depression meta-analysis revisited: evidence of genetic moderation. *Arch Gen Psychiatry* 2011;68(5):444-54.
7. Galvez R, Mesches MH, Mcgaugh JL. Norepinephrine release in the amygdala in response to footshock stimulation. *Neurobiol Learn Mem* 1996;66(3):253-7.
8. Hatfield T, Spanis C, Mcgaugh JL. Response of amygdalar norepinephrine to footshock and GABAergic drugs using in vivo microdialysis and HPLC. *Brain Res* 1999;835(2):340-5.
9. Crippen D. Agitation in the ICU: part one Anatomical and physiologic basis for the agitated state. *Crit Care* 1999;3(3):R35-R46.
10. Wang DV, Wang F, Liu J, Zhang L, Wang Z, Lin L. Neurons in the amygdala with response-selectivity for anxiety in two ethologically based tests. *PLoS One* 2011;6(4):e18739.
11. Roozendaal B, Hui GK, Hui IR, Berlau DJ, Mcgaugh JL, Weinberger NM. Basolateral amygdala noradrenergic activity mediates corticosterone-induced enhancement of auditory fear conditioning. *Neurobiol Learn Mem* 2006;86(3):249-55.
12. Fu A, Li X, Zhao B. Role of beta1-adrenoceptor in the basolateral amygdala of rats with anxiety-like behavior. *Brain Res* 2008;1211:85-92.
13. Bremner JD, Krystal JH, Southwick SM, Charney DS. Noradrenergic mechanisms in stress and anxiety: II. Clinical studies. *Synapse* 1996;23(1):28-51.
14. Mard-Soltani M, Kesmati M, Khajehpour L, Rasekh A, Shamshirgar-Zadeh A. Interaction between Anxiolytic Effects of Testosterone and β-1 Adrenoceptors of Basolateral Amygdala. *Int J Pharmacol* 2012;8(5):344-54.
15. Rudoy CA, Van Bockstaele EJ. Betaxolol, a selective beta(1)-adrenergic receptor antagonist, diminishes anxiety-like behavior during early withdrawal from chronic cocaine administration in rats. *Prog Neuropsychopharmacol Biol Psychiatry* 2007;31(5):1119-29.
16. Buffalari DM, Grace AA. Noradrenergic modulation of basolateral amygdala neuronal activity: opposing influences of alpha-2 and beta receptor activation. *J Neurosci* 2007;27(45):12358-66.
17. Kryger R, Wilce PA. The effects of alcoholism on the human basolateral amygdala. *Neuroscience* 2010;167(2):361-71.

18. Morris JB. Food, industrial, nutraceutical, and pharmaceutical uses of sesame genetic resources. In: Janick J, Whipkey A, editors. Trends in new crops and new uses. Alexandria, VA: ASHS Press; 2002:153-6.
19. Annussek G. Sesame oil. In: Gale encyclopedia of alternative medicine. Gale Group and Looksmart; 2001.
20. Cooney RV, Custer LJ, Okinaka L, Franke AA. Effects of dietary sesame seeds on plasma tocopherol levels. *Nutr Cancer* 2001;39(1):66-71.
21. Steve Dounis S. Nuts and Seeds Provide Health Benefits. USA: HealthyNutrition.me; [cited 8 July 2009]; Available from: http://healthynutrition.me/?p=977.
22. Zare K, Fatemi Tabatabaei SR, Shahriari A, Jafari RA. Effect of Butter and Sesame Oils on Avoidance Memory of Diabetic Rats. *Iran J Diabetes Obesity* 2011;3(2):65-71.
23. Fernandez ML, West KL. Mechanisms by which Dietary Fatty Acids Modulate Plasma Lipids. *J Nutr* 2005;135(9):2075-8.
24. Bendich A, Brock PE. Rational for introduction of long chain polyunsa turated fatty acid for concomitant in infant formulas. *Int J Vitam Nutr Res* 1997;67(4):213-31.
25. Bourre JM, Dumont OL, Clement ME, Durand GA. Endogenous synthesis cannot compensate for absence of dietary oleic acid in rats. *J Nutr* 1997;127(3):488-93.
26. Um MY, Ahn JY, Kim S, Kim MK, Ha TY. Sesaminol glucosides protect beta-amyloid peptide-induced cognitive deficits in mice. *Biol Pharm Bull* 2009;32(9):1516-20.
27. Engelberg H. Low serum cholesterol and suicide. *Lancet* 1992;339(8795):727-9.
28. Kaplan JR, Manuck SB, Fontenot MB, Muldoon MF, Shively CA, Mann JJ. The cholesterol-serotonin hypothesis: interrelationships among dietary lipids, central serotonergic activity and social behavior in monkeys. In: Hillbrand M, Spitz RT, editors. Lipids, Health and Behavior. Washington, DC: American Psychological Association; 1997:139-65.
29. Steegmans PH, Hoes AW, Bak AA, Van Der Does E, Grobbee DE. Higher prevalence of depressive symptoms in middle-aged men with low serum cholesterol levels. *Psychosom Med* 2000;62(2):205-11.
30. Wardle J. Cholesterol and psychological well-being. *J Psychosom Res* 1995;39(5):549-62.
31. Paxinos G, Watson C. The rat brain in stereotaxic coordinates, CD-ROM. 4th ed. San Diego: Academic Press;1998.
32. Cecchi M, Capriles N, Watson SJ, Akil H. Beta-1 adrenergic receptors in the bed nucleus of stria terminalis mediate differential responses to opiate withdrawal. *Neuropsychopharmacol* 2007;32(3):589-99.
33. Walf AA, Frye CA. The use of the elevated plus maze as an assay of anxiety-related behavior in rodents. *Nat Protoc* 2007;2:322-8.
34. Matuszewich L, Karney JJ, Carter SR, Janasik SP, O'brien JL, Friedman RD. The delayed effects of chronic unpredictable stress on anxiety measures. *Physiol Behav* 2007;90(4):674-81.
35. Morgan RE, Palinkas LA, Barrett-Connor EL, Wingard DL. Plasma cholesterol and depressive symptoms in older men. *Lancet* 1993;341(8837):75-9.
36. Brown SL, Salive ME, Harris TB, Simonsick EM, Guralnik JM, Kohout FJ. Low cholesterol concentrations and severe depressive symptoms in elderly people. *BMJ* 1994;308(6940):1328-32.
37. Lindberg G, Larsson G, Setterlind S, Rastam L. Serum lipids and mood in working men and women in Sweden. *J Epidemiol Community Health* 1994;48(4):360-3.
38. Neaton JD, Blackburn H, Jacobs D, Kuller L, Lee DJ, Sherwin R, et al. Serum cholesterol level and mortality findings for men screened in the Multiple Risk Factor Intervention Trial. Multiple Risk Factor Intervention Trial Research Group. *Arch Intern Med* 1992;152(7):1490-500.
39. Horsten M, Wamala SP, Vingerhoets A, Orth-Gomer K. Depressive symptoms, social support, and lipid profile in healthy middle-aged women. *Psychosom Med* 1997;59(5):521-8.
40. Suarez EC. Relations of trait depression and anxiety to low lipid and lipoprotein concentrations in healthy young adult women. *Psychosom Med* 1999;61(3):273-9.
41. Coccaro EF, Siever LJ, Klar HM, Maurer G, Cochrane K, Cooper TB, et al. Serotonergic studies in patients with affective and personality disorders. Correlates with suicidal and impulsive aggressive behavior. *Arch Gen Psychiatry* 1989;46(7):587-99.
42. Delgado PL, Charney DS, Price LH, Aghajanian GK, Landis H, Heninger GR. Serotonin function and the mechanism of antidepressant action. Reversal of antidepressant-induced remission by rapid depletion of plasma tryptophan. *Arch Gen Psychiatry* 1990;47(5):411-8.
43. Kahn RS, Van Praag HM, Wetzler S, Asnis GM, Barr G. Serotonin and anxiety revisited. *Biol Psychiatry* 1988;23(2):189-208.
44. Steegmans PH, Fekkes D, Hoes AW, Bak AA, van der Does E, Grobbee DE. Low serum cholesterol concentrations and serotonin metabolism in men. *Br Med J* 1996;312(7025):221.
45. Ketterer MW, Brymer J, Rhoads K, Kraft P, Goldberg AD, Lavallo WA. Lipid lowering therapy and violent death: is depression a culprit? *Stress Med* 2006;10(4):233-7.
46. De Almeida RM, Giovenardi M, Charchat H, Lucion AB. 8-OH-DPAT in the median raphe nucleus decreases while in the medial septal area it may increase anxiety in female rats. *Neurosci Biobehav Rev* 1998;23(2):259-64.

47. Rainbow TC, Parsons B, Wolfe BB. Quantitative autoradiography of beta 1- and beta 2-adrenergic receptors in rat brain. *Proc Natl Acad Sci U S A* 1984;81(5):1585-9.
48. Ordway GA, Gambarana C, Tejani-Butt SM, Areso P, Hauptmann M, Frazer A. Preferential reduction of binding of 125I-iodopindolol to beta-1 adrenoceptors in the amygdala of rat after antidepressant treatments. *J Pharmacol Exp Ther* 1991;257(2):681-90.
49. Fallon JH, Koziell DA, Moore RY. Catecholamine innervation of the basal forebrain. II. Amygdala, suprarhinal cortex and entorhinal cortex. *J Comp Neurol* 1978;180(3):509-32.
50. Clayton EC, Williams CL. Adrenergic activation of the nucleus tractus solitarius potentiates amygdala norepinephrine release and enhances retention performance in emotionally arousing and spatial memory tasks. *Behav Brain Res* 2000;112(1-2):151-8.
51. Bracha HS, Garcia-Rill E, Mrak RE, Skinner R. Postmortem locus coeruleus neuron count in three American veterans with probable or possible war-related PTSD. *J Neuropsychiatry Clin Neurosci* 2005;17(4):503-9.
52. Elshourbagy NA, Korman DR, Wu HL, Sylvester DR, Lee JA, Nuthalaganti P, et al. Molecular characterization and regulation of the human endothelin receptors. *J Biol Chem* 1993;268(6):3873-9.
53. McMurchie EJ. Dietary lipids and the regulation of membrane fluidity and function. In: Liss AL, editor. Physiologic regulation of membrane fluidity. Philadelphia: Saunders; 1988.

Cytotoxic Effects of Alcoholic Extract of Dorema Glabrum Seed on Cancerous Cells Viability

Maryam Bannazadeh Amirkhiz[1,2], Nadereh Rashtchizadeh[1]*, Hosein Nazemieh[3], Jalal Abdolalizadeh[1], Leila Mohammadnejad[4], Behzad Baradaran[4]*

[1] *Drug Applied Research Center, Tabriz University of Medical Sciences, Tabriz, Iran.*

[2] *student of Tabriz International University of Medical Sciences (Aras), Tabriz University of Medical Sciences, Tabriz, Iran.*

[3] *Research Center for Pharmaceutical Nanotechnology, Tabriz University of Medical Sciences, Tabriz, Iran.*

[4] *Immonuology Research Center, Tabriz University of Medical Sciences, Tabriz, Iran.*

ARTICLEINFO

Keywords:
Cancer
Apoptosis
Dorema Glabrum
WEHI-164 cell
Plant extract
Cytotoxicity

ABSTRACT

Purpose: In the present study cytotoxic effects of the alcoholic extract of Dorema Glabrum seed on viability of WEHI-164 cells, mouse Fibrosarcoma cell line and L929 normal cells were compared with the cytotoxic effects of Taxol (anticancer and apoptosis inducer drug). ***Methods:*** To find out the plant extract cytotoxic effects, MTT test and DNA fragmentation assay, the biochemical hallmark of apoptosis were performed on cultured and treated cells. ***Results:*** According to the findings the alcoholic extract of Dorema Glabrum seed can alter cells morphology and because of chromatin condensation and other changes they shrink and take a spherical shape, and lose their attachment too. So the plant extract inhibits cell growth albeit in a time and dose dependent manner and results in degradation of chromosomal DNA. ***Conclusion***: Our data well established the anti-proliferative effect of methanolic extract of Dorema Glabrum seed and clearly showed that the plant extract can induce apoptosis and not necrosis in vitro, but the mechanism of its activities remained unknown. These results demonstrated that Dorema Glabrum seed might be a novel and attractive therapeutic candidate for tumor treatment in clinical practices.

Introduction

Cancer with high death rate, second only to cardiac arrest comprises at least 100 different diseases. All cancer cells share one important characteristic; they are abnormal cells in which the processes regulating normal cell division are aberrant. Cell cycle and growth control are profoundly relevant to biological regulation of development and tissue renewal. Apoptosis (programmed cell death) was a term introduced in 1972 to distinguish a mode of cell death with characteristic morphology and apparently regulated, endogenously driven mechanism.[1,2] Defective apoptosis represents a major causative factor in the development and progression of cancer. Our understanding of the complexities of apoptosis and the mechanisms evolved by tumor cells to resist engagement of cell death have focused research efforts into the development of strategies designed to selectively induce apoptosis in cancer cells.[3-5]

There are considerable efforts to identify naturally occurring substances as new drugs in cancer therapy.[6-9] A number of chemotherapeutic agents, with properties including apoptosis induction and anti-angiogenesis, have been isolated from natural products and characterized to prevent the development of malignancies, such as curcumin from Curcuma longa, epicatechin gallate from tea, paclitaxel from Pacific yew[10] Emodin, a natural anthraquinone derivative from Rheum palmatum L[11] and Honokiol, a biphenyl extract from Magnolia obovata bark.[10] Understanding the modes of action of these compounds should provide useful information for their possible applications in cancer prevention and perhaps in cancer therapy.[12-13]

Approximately half of the drugs currently in clinical use are of natural origin.[7,14,15] Although herbal therapies are becoming increasingly popular worldwide, we know little about the molecular mechanisms and active ingredients in many of those therapeutic herbs.[7,16] Some of them tend to possess functional groups (providing hydrogen bond acceptor/donors, etc).[7]

Dorema glabrum is a species that grows in Transcaucasia (Nakhichevan and Armenia zone) and North West of Iran. The genus Dorema from Apiaceae family is represented by seven species in Iranian flora,

***Corresponding author:** Nadereh Rashtchizadeh and Behzad Baradaran, Tabriz University of Medical Sciences, Tabriz, Iran.
Emails: rashtchizadeh@yahoo.com, behzad_im@yahoo.com

among them Dorema glabrum Fisch. C.A. Mey, D. aucheri Boiss and D. ammonicum D. Don are endemic.[17] Dorema glabrum which grows in loamy or rocky slopes is a perennial herb. It is useful. as an herbal remedy or food additive in mentioned regions.[18] According to the common folk believes of Armenian and Azeri people, D glabrum can suppress different kinds of cancer. We aimed to study this matter by a scientific work; hence the effects of alcoholic extract of D. Glabrum seed on WEHI-164 cell line viability were investigated. Of course it should be mentioned in a preliminary work, antioxidant activity and anti-lipidemic effects were seen in the crude extract of the plant.[19]

In the present study cytotoxic effects of the extract of Dorema Glabrum seed on WEHI-164 cells were compared with its effects on L929 normal cells in contrast with the effects of Taxol as a positive control. Taxol which contains Paclitaxel as the main active compound is used in chemotherapy of cancer. Paclitaxel ($C_{47}H_{51}NO_{14}$, MW=853.9 Da) is yielded from Yew tree and its anticancer effects was known since 1971.[20,21]

Materials and Methods

Plant Material

Seeds of Dorema glabrum Fisch. C.A. Mey were collected during the fruiting stage from slopes of Aras River bank; Jolfa, Eastern Azerbaijan (38 30' 9.2", 45 27'36.2"; 1590 m, 15 km from Jolfa to St. Stephanus Church), Iran. Air dried and finely powdered seeds were subjected to extraction by refluxing Methanol in a soxhlet in order to obtain its ooze. Then the extract was dried using a Rotary Evaporator (Heidolph, Germany).

20 mg of dried extract were dissolved in 100 µl DMSO and diluted with 3.90 ml RPMI-1640 to give a concentration of 5000 µg/ml. The cells were treated with different concentrations (10, 30, 50, 100, 200, 300, and 400 µg/ml) of the extract.

Cell culture

WEHI-164 cells, mouse Fibrosarcoma cell line (NCBI Code: C200) and L929 cells, mouse normal adipose tissue cell line (NCBI Code: C161) were obtained from National Cell Bank of Iran (Pasteur Institute, Iran-Tehran). WEHI-164 cell line was originally established by M Rollinghoff and NL Warner from a fibrosarcoma induced by subcutaneous injections of 3-methylcholanthrene to Balb/c mice[22,23] and L929 cells, one of the first to be established in continuous culture, subclone of parental strain L, established by W R Earle in 1940. The L strain was derived from normal subcutaneous areolar and adipose tissue of a 100 day old male C3H/An mouse. These cells are $APRT^+$ (Adenine Phodphoribosyl Transferase) and $HPRT^+$ (Hypoxanthine-Guanine Phosphoribosyl Transferase).[24] The both cell lines were cultured in RPMI-1640 (Sigma, Germany, pH=7.2) containing 10% FCS (Fetal Calf Serum) and antibiotic (100 U/ml Penicillin, 100 µg/ml Streptomycine, Gibco), placed in 37 °C and 5% CO_2 in an incubator (Memert, Germany) overnight.

MTT Test

MTT assay is one of the most useful tests for investigating cells viability and cytotoxic effects of drugs, cosmetics and food additives. MTT (3-[4, 5-dimethyl-2-thiazolyl]-2, 5 diphenyl tetrazolium bromide) which is yellow and soluble in water, can be reduced by mitochondrial dehydrogenases of live cells to give a bluish purple and insoluble salt called Formosan that can easily and rapidly be quantitated by an ELISA plate reader at 570 nm.[25,26]

WEHI-164 and L929 cells were separately seeded, in a triplicate manner, in 96-well microplates (5000 cells/well) with RPMI-1640 containing 10% FCS (Fetal Calf Serum) and antibiotic (total volume of 200 µl), placed in 37 °C and 5% CO_2 in the incubator. After 6 hours both cells were treated with different concentrations (10, 30, 50 and 100, 200, 300, and 400 µg/ml) of alcoholic extract of Dorema glabrum seeds with different time periods (6, 24 and 36 hours). No plant extract was added to negative controls, but the same amount of DMSO was added to eliminate its intervening effects, if any. Positive control cells were treated with Taxol (Onco-time, Australia) as the same concentrations of plant extract in test cells. Of course prior to treatment the cells viability was determined by counting on a Neubauer slide (Hemocytometer) with the aid of Trypan blue. Trypan blue can penetrate into dead cells' membrane and colour them purple.

After desired time the supernatants of all wells were discarded and washed with PBS, then 100 µl of RPMI and 50 µl of MTT solution (2 mg/ml) were added to each well. Following incubation at 37 °C for 4 hours the liquid phase of wells were discarded again. After adding 200 µl DMSO and 25 µl Sorensen's glycine buffer (0.1 M glycine, 0.1 M NaCl, pH=10.5) the plates were incubated at 37 °C in the dark for another half an hour. At the end absorbencies of wells were determined at 570 nm wavelength using a microplate reader (Awareness technology, USA).

DNA fragmentation Assay

The biochemical hallmark of apoptosis is the fragmentation of the genomic DNA, an irreversible event that commits the cell to die and occurs before changes in plasma membrane permeability (prelytic DNA fragmentation). In many systems, this DNA fragmentation has been shown to result from activation of an endogenous Ca^{2+} and Mg^{2+} dependent nuclear endonuclease. This enzyme selectively cleaves DNA at sites located between nucleosomal units (linker DNA) generating mono and oligonucleosomal DNA fragments.[25] The DNA laddering technique is used to visualize the endonuclease cleavage products of apoptosis. This assay involves extraction of DNA from a lysed cell homogenate followed by agarose gel electrophoresis. This, results in a characteristic "DNA ladder" with each band in the ladder separated in size by approximately 180 base pairs. This methodology which is easy to perform, has a sensitivity of 1×10^6 cells (i.e., level of detection is as few as 1,000,000 cells), and is useful for tissues and cell cultures with high numbers of apoptotic cells per tissue mass or volume, respectively.[4]

DNA Extraction

Both cell lines, WEHI-164 and L929 were separately cultured in 6-well plates (1200000 cells/well) with RPMI-1640 supplemented by 10% FCS and antibiotic, placed in 37 °C and 5% CO_2 in the incubator. After 6 hours the cells were treated with different concentrations of plant extract (0, 30, 50 and 100 µg/ml) for different time periods (24 and 36 hours). Then the wells were washed with PBS buffer and cells were detached from the plates with the aid of Trypsin-EDTA (Gibco, Germany). The cells pellets were removed to falcon tube and 500 µl of lysis buffer were added. 10 µl of proteinase K (Fermentas, Life Sciences), 20 mg/ml were added, followed by incubation at 56 °C overnight. The next day 40 µl of saturated NaCl (5 M) were added and mixed completely and incubated at 4 °C for 10 minutes. After centrifugation in 12000 RPM for 20 minutes, their upper liquids were transferred to a fresh microtube and 1 ml of cold ethanol 100 % (stored in -20 °C) was added. The procedure was continued by incubation at -20 °C for 10 minutes, followed by centrifugation for 15 minutes in 12000 RPM. Then ethanol in upper phase was removed completely and 1 ml of ethanol 70 (kept in 4 °C) was added and mixed well by pipetting up and down. Next the samples were centrifuged again for 10 minutes in 12000 RPM, followed by removeing ethanol completely. After drying the samples in room temprature or 37 °C for 10-20 minutes, the pellets were dissolved in 100 µl distilled, deionised and sterile water or TE (Tris/EDTA). The samples concentrations were determined using a nanodrop UV spectrophotometer and equivalent amount of DNA samples diluted with the 6X DNA loading dye (supplied with the ladder) were subjected to 1.5 % agarose submarine electrophoresis in company with DNA ladder marker (Fermentas, Life Sciences, 1 kb DNA Ladder). Finally the fragmented DNAs bands were visualized by UV transilluminator (UVP, USA) following ethidium bromide staining.

Statistical analysis

All the data represented in this study are means±SEM of three identical experiments made in triplicate. Statistical significance was determined by independent T-test and p value ≤ 0.05 was considered significant. All analyses were conducted using the SPSS 20.

Results

Natural and live WEHI-164 cells are fusiform or spindle like (Figure 1A). But after treatment with Taxol or methanolic extract of Dorema glabrum seed they undergo morphological changes and because of chromatin condensation and other changes they shrinke and take a spherical shape (Figure 1B), characteristics of apoptotic cells.

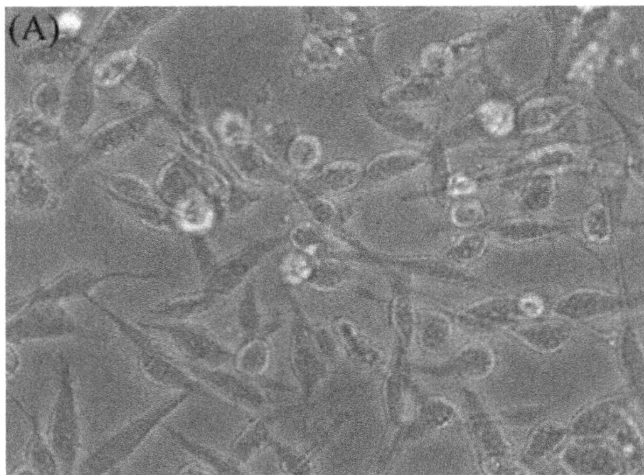

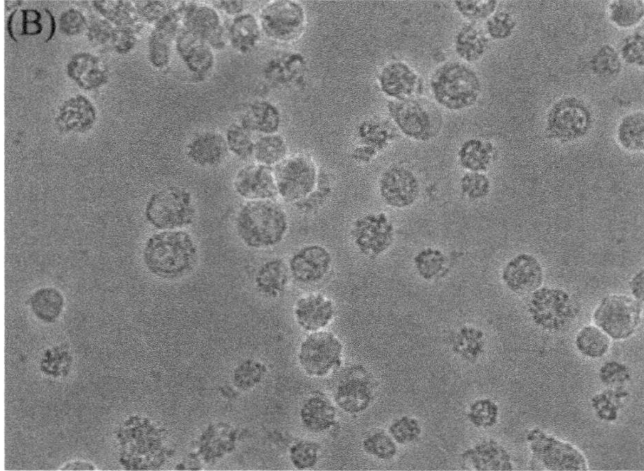

Figure 1. Panel A, Spindle like natural and live WEHI-164, 40X Panel B, Spherical apoptotic WEHI-164 cells, 40X.

Cells viability

Using Neubauer slide (Hemocytometer) and with the aid of Trypan blue the cells viability before treatment was determined >94%.

MTT Test

The antiproliferative effect of plant extract was determined by MTT method which showed a time and dose-dependent inhibition of the cell growth. Also effecivity of plant extract on both cell lines viabilities follows the same pattern as Taxol.

As the Figure 2 shows IC_{50} value, the concentration that causes 50% loss of cell viability, in WEHI-164 cell line is about 50 µg/ml in 36 hours for the plant extract. By contrast the plant extract had higher IC_{50} value (about 100 µg/ml in 36 hours) for normal L929 cells, meaning it is toxic to the normal cells in higher concentrations than WEHI-164 cells.

Statistical analysis using independent T-test was performed to show significant differences of cytotoxicity effects of 50 µg/ml plant extract in 36 hours to WEHI-164 and L929 cells. The test resulted in $P<0.0001$, meaning that 50 µg/ml plant extract affects cancerous cells viability more than normal cells.

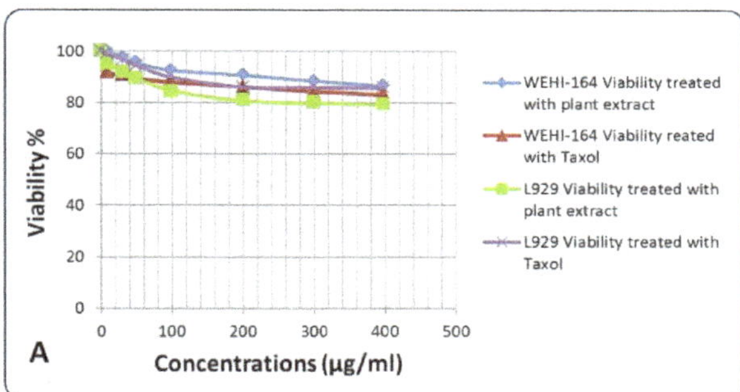

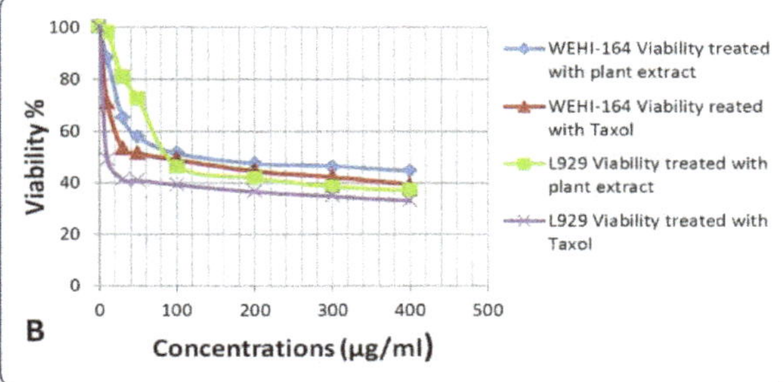

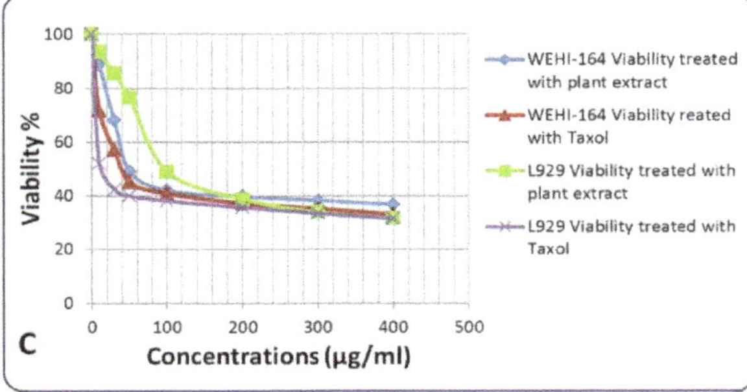

Figure 2. The viability of WEHI-164 and L929 cells treated with the different concentrations of plant extract in the different time periods in contrast with that of the cells treated with Taxol. A: Viability of cells after 6 hours, B: Viability of cells after 24 hours, C: Viability of cells after 36 hours

DNA fragmentation

DNA fragmentation can be analysed by the typical ''DNA ladder'' formation, for which DNA is extracted from the apoptotic cells and separated in an agarose gel. As shown in Figure 3 treatment with Dorema Glabrum seed extract resulted in degradation of chromosomal DNA into small internucleosomal fragments, a biochemical hallmark of cells undergoing apoptosis.

Discussion

Despite a period in which pharmaceutical companies cut back on their use of natural products in drug discovery, there are many promising drug candidates in the current development pipeline that are of herbal origin. After all, traditional cytotoxic chemotherapy although kills cancer cells by indirectly inducing apoptosis unfortunately, side effects are brutal, and most tumors become resistant.[27-29]

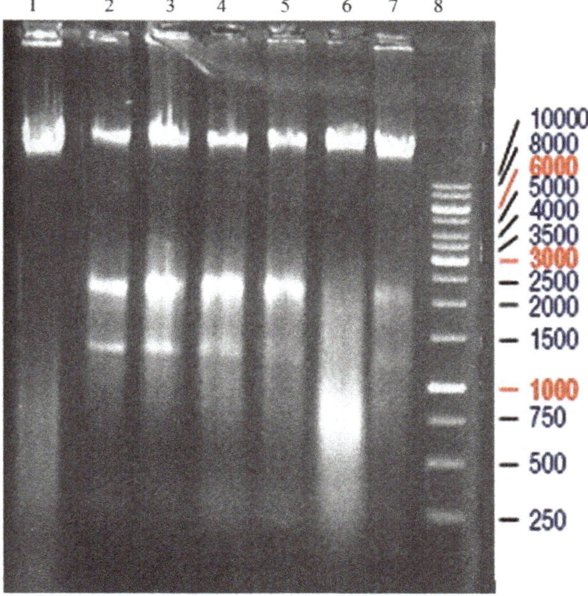

Figure 3. DNA ladder formation. From left Lane 1: negative control, Lane 2-4 treated cells with different concentrations (30, 50, 100 µg/ml) of plant extract in 24 hours, Lane 5-7 treated cells in 36 hours, and Lane 8 Ladder (1 kb).

To evaluate the effects of Dorema Glabrum seed extract on cell proliferation and identify its therapeutic potential we demonstrated, for the first time, the potent cytotoxic activity of different concentrations of methanolic extract of Dorema Glabrum seed against WEHI-164 Mouse Fibrosarcoma cell line and L929 normal cell line. A successful anticancer drug should kill or incapacitate cancer cells without causing excessive damages to normal cells, meaning minimum side effects. This ideal situation is reachable by inducing apoptosis in cancer cells. Cell cycle modulation by various natural and synthetic agents is gaining widespread attention in recent years.[13]

In the present study prior to treatment, first we determined cells viability by counting on a Neubauer slide (Hemocytometer) with the aid of Trypan blue. Trypan blue can penetrate into dead cells' membrane and colour them purple. The outcome was >94%. Then MTT assay was performed which showed that the methanolic extract of Dorema Glabrum seed causes growth inhibition in the WEHI-164 Mouse Fibrosarcoma cells in a dose and time dependent manner. But it appeared less toxic in low concentrations to normal or nonmalignant cells in vitro, because IC_{50} value of the plant extract for WEHI-164 cells is 50 µg/ml but for L929 cells is 100 µg/ml in 36 hours. So higher doses of plant extract were effective in L929 normal cells than in tumor cells. This claim was confirmed by statistical analysis using independent T-test that resulted in $P<0.0001$, meaning that the mean differences of cytotoxicity effects of 50 µg/ml plant extract in 36 hours to WEHI-164 and L929 cells are significant. 36 hours treatment was selected because in shorter times higher concentrations of plant extract were needed to cause 50% loss of cell viability. Since concentrations more than 50 µg/ml affect L929 cells viabilty too, it is preference to choose 36 hours treatment with 50 µg/ml plant extract in order to avoid massive damages to normal cells. Also we compared the effects of plant extract with the effects of Taxol, an anticancer and apoptosis inducer drug and it should be mentioned here that effects of plant extract on both cell lines followed the same pattern as Taxol effects on the cells (Figure 3).

Microscopic studies showed morphological changes of the cells too. Chromatin condensation, cell shrinkage and other alterations, characteristics of apoptotic cells, cause the morphology of treated cells with the plant extract, change from spindle like to spherical shape and also make them to lose their attachment (Figure 2). In conclusion the plant extract induced apoptosis and not necrosis in treated cells.

Also apoptosis induction was confirmed by DNA ladder technique. Treatment with the plant extract resulted in degradation of chromosomal DNA into smaller fragments (Figure 3), a biochemical hallmark of cells undergoing apoptosis.[4] Once more induction of apoptosis and not necrosis, by plant extract was confirmed, because electrophoresis of necrotic cells' DNA results in smear not ladder.

Conclussion

In conclusion our data, well established the anti-proliferative effects of methanolic extract of Dorema Glabrum seed and clearly showed that the plant extract can induce apoptosis and not necrosis in vitro, but its activities in vivo and mechanisms of its actions remained unknown. These results demonstrated that Dorema Glabrum seed with anti-proliferative properties, especially with IC_{50} value for cancerous cells lower than that of normal cells, might be a novel and attractive therapeutic candidate for tumor treatment in clinical practice.

Acknowledgements

Authors would like to thank Drug applied Research Center of Tabriz University of Medical sciences for its financial support.

Conflict of Interest

The authors report no conflicts of interest.

References

1. Wyllie AH. "where, O death, is thy sting?" a brief review of apoptosis biology. *Mol Neurobiol* 2010;42(1):4-9.
2. Igney FH, Krammer PH. Death and anti-death: tumour resistance to apoptosis. *Nat Rev Cancer* 2002;2(4):277-88.
3. Kasibhatla S, Tseng B. Why target apoptosis in cancer treatment? *Mol Cancer Ther* 2003;2(6):573-80.
4. Elmore S. Apoptosis: a review of programmed cell death. *Toxicol Pathol* 2007;35(4):495-516.
5. Cory S, Adams JM. The Bcl2 family: regulators of the cellular life-or-death switch. *Nat Rev Cancer* 2002;2(9):647-56.
6. Valiyari S, Baradaran B, Delazar A, Pasdaran A, Zare F. Dichloromethane and methanol extracts of scrophularia oxysepala induces apoptosis in MCF-7 human breast cancer cells. *Adv Pharm Bull* 2012;2(2):223-31.
7. Gao H, Lamusta J, Zhang WF, Salmonsen R, Liu Y, O'connell E, et al. Tumor Cell Selective Cytotoxicity and Apoptosis Induction by an Herbal Preparation from Brucea javanica. *N Am J Med Sci (Boston)* 2011;4(2):62-6.
8. Yamamoto M, Miura N, Ohtake N, Amagaya S, Ishige A, Sasaki H, et al. Genipin, a metabolite derived from the herbal medicine Inchin-ko-to, and suppression of Fas-induced lethal liver apoptosis in mice. *Gastroenterology* 2000;118(2):380-9.
9. Fau D, Lekehal M, Farrell G, Moreau A, Moulis C, Feldmann G, et al. Diterpenoids from germander, an herbal medicine, induce apoptosis in isolated rat hepatocytes. *Gastroenterology* 1997;113(4):1334-46.
10. Li Z, Liu Y, Zhao X, Pan X, Yin R, Huang C, et al. Honokiol, a natural therapeutic candidate, induces apoptosis and inhibits angiogenesis of ovarian tumor cells. *Eur J Obstet Gynecol Reprod Biol* 2008;140(1):95-102.
11. Su YT, Chang HL, Shyue SK, Hsu SL. Emodin induces apoptosis in human lung adenocarcinoma cells through a reactive oxygen species-dependent mitochondrial signaling pathway. *Biochem Pharmacol* 2005;70(2):229-41.
12. Yousefzadi M, Heidari M, Akbarpour M, Mirjalili MH, Zeinali A, Parsa M. In vitro cytotoxic activity of the essential oil of dorema ammoniacum D. Don. *Middle-East J Sci Res* 2011;7(4):511-4.
13. Abdolmohammadi MH, Fouladdel Sh, Shafiee A, Amin Gh, Ghaffari SM, Azizi E. Anticancer effects and cell cycle analysis on human breast cancer T47d cells treated with extracts of astrodaucus persicus (Boiss.) Drude in comparison to doxorubicin. *DARU* 2008;16(2):112-8.
14. Oubre AY, Carlson TJ, King SR, Reaven GM. From plant to patient: an ethnomedical approach to the identification of new drugs for the treatment of NIDDM. *Diabetologia* 1997;40(5):614-7.
15. Yano H, Mizoguchi A, Fukuda K, Haramaki M, Ogasawara S, Momosaki S, et al. The herbal medicine sho-saiko-to inhibits proliferation of cancer cell lines by inducing apoptosis and arrest at the G0/G1 phase. *Cancer Res* 1994;54(2):448-54.
16. Zahri S, Razavi SM, Niri FH, Mohammadi S. Induction of programmed cell death by Prangos

uloptera, a medicinal plant. *Biol Res* 2009;42(4):517-22.
17. Mozaffarian V. A Dictionary of iranian plant names. Tehran: Farhang Moaser; 1996.
18. Asnaashari S, Dadizadeh E, Talebpour AH, Eskandani M, Nazemiyeh H. Free radical scavenging potential and essential oil composition of the dorema glabrum fisch. C.A. mey roots from Iran. *BioImpacts* 2011;1(4):241-4.
19. Dehghan G, Fatholahi G, Sheikhzadeh N, Ahmadiasl N. Hypocholesteremic and antioxidant effects of Dorema glabrum extract in rats fed high cholesterol diet. 10th Iranian Congress of Biochemistry and the 3rd International Congress of Biochemistry and Molecular Biology; Tehran 2009.
20. Yuan H. Studies on the chemistry of paclitaxel [PhD Dissertation]. Virginia: Virginia Polytechnic Institute and State University; 1998.
21. Cavallaro G, Licciardi M, Caliceti P, Salmaso S, Giammona G. Synthesis, physico-chemical and biological characterization of a paclitaxel macromolecular prodrug. *Eur J Pharm Biopharm* 2004;58(1):151-9.
22. Cell lines service. 2013; Available from: http://www.cell-lines-service.de/content/e174/e157/e2006/e1712/index_eng.html.
23. Rollinghoff M, Warner NL. Specificity of in vivo tumor rejection assessed by mixing immune spleen cells with target and unrelated tumor cells. *Proc Soc Exp Biol Med* 1973;144(3):813-8.
24. Sigma-aldrich. 2013; Available from: http://www.sigmaaldrich.com/catalog/product/sigma/85011425?lang=en®ion=IR.
25. Wyllie AH. Apoptosis, cell death and cell proliferation. 3rd ed. Germany: Roche Applied Science; 2008.
26. Wan H, Williams R, Doherty P, Williams D. A study of the reproducibility of the MTT test. *J Mater Sci-Mater Med* 1994;5(3):154-9.
27. Jordan MA, Wilson L. Microtubules as a target for anticancer drugs. *Nat Rev Cancer* 2004;4(4):253-65.
28. Garber K. New apoptosis drugs face critical test. *Nat Biotechnol* 2005;23(4):409-11.
29. Kawabe T. G2 checkpoint abrogators as anticancer drugs. *Mol Cancer Ther* 2004;3(4):513-9.

Drug-Drug/Drug-Excipient Compatibility Studies on Curcumin using Non-Thermal Methods

Moorthi Chidambaram*, Kathiresan Krishnasamy

Department of Pharmacy, Annamalai University, Chidambaram, Tamil Nadu, India.

ARTICLEINFO

Keywords:
Compatibility Study
Curcumin
Piperine
Polymeric Nanoparticles
Quercetin
Silibinin

ABSTRACT

Purpose: Curcumin is a hydrophobic polyphenol isolated from dried rhizome of turmeric. Clinical usefulness of curcumin in the treatment of cancer is limited due to poor aqueous solubility, hydrolytic degradation, metabolism, and poor oral bioavailability. To overcome these limitations, we proposed to fabricate curcumin-piperine, curcumin-quercetin and curcumin-silibinin loaded polymeric nanoformulation. However, unfavourable combinations of drug-drug and drug-excipient may result in interaction and rises the safety concern. Hence, the present study was aimed to assess the interaction of curcumin with excipients used in nanoformulations.
Methods: Isothermal stress testing method was used to assess the compatibility of drug-drug/drug-excipient.
Results: The combination of curcumin-piperine, curcumin-quercetin, curcumin-silibinin and the combination of other excipients with curcumin, piperine, quercetin and silibinin have not shown any significant physical and chemical instability.
Conclusion: The study concludes that the curcumin, piperine, quercetin and silibinin is compatible with each other and with other excipients.

Introduction

Curcumin is a hydrophobic polyphenol isolated from dried rhizome of turmeric (*Curcuma Longa* Linn & zingiberaceae family), which is responsible for various pharmacological activities including anti-cancer, anti-oxidant, anti-bacterial, anti-fungal, anti-viral and anti-inflammatory and expected to have medicinal benefits in arthritis, psoriasis, diabetes, acquired immunodeficiency syndrome, cardiovascular diseases, multiple sclerosis, cancer and lung fibrosis.[1,2] However, clinical usefulness of curcumin in the treatment of cancer is limited due to poor aqueous solubility, hydrolytic degradation in alkaline pH, metabolism via glucuronidation and sulfation in the liver and in intestine, and poor oral bioavailability. These limitations results in decreased therapeutic efficacy or absence of therapeutic efficacy in *in-vivo* studies.[2] Though there are many novel approaches to overcome these limitations, nanotechnology (Particle size <1000 nm) is the most recent and offer significant improvement.[3,4] Hence, to overcome these limitations we proposed to fabricate curcumin-piperine, curcumin-quercetin and curcumin-silibinin loaded polymeric nanoformulation. However, unfavourable combinations of drug-drug and drug-excipient may result in interaction, which leads to physical instability or chemical instability. Physical instability refers to changes in the characteristics of a drug that do not involve chemical bond formation or breakage in the drug structure, which can be identified by changes in the organoleptic parameters such as appearance, form etc. Chemical instability refers to changes in the chemical structure of the drug molecule resulting in drug degradation, reduced drug content and formation of other molecule such as degradation products. Both physical and chemical instability may cause safety concerns. Hence, a thorough drug-drug/drug-excipient compatibility study is mandatory.[5] The present study was aimed to assess the physical and chemical instability of curcumin with various excipients to be used in the proposed nanoformulations.

Materials and Methods

Materials

Poly(butyl methacrylate-co-(2-dimethylaminoethyl) methacrylate-co-methyl methacrylate) polymer was obtained from Degussa, India. Curcumin, Piperine, Quercetin, Silibinin and Poloxamer 188 were obtained from Sigma-Aldrich, India. β-cyclodextrin was obtained from Himedia Laboratories, India.

Drug-drug/drug-excipient compatibility study

Isothermal stress testing method is used to assess the compatibility of drug-drug/drug-excipient.[6] Briefly, about 100 mg of pure drugs and excipients were

***Corresponding author:** Moorthi Chidambaram, Department of Pharmacy, Annamalai University, Chidambaram, Tamil Nadu, India.
Email: cmoorthitgodu@gmail.com

weighed separately and in combination as shown in Table 1. Individual drugs (Sample 1-4), individual excipients (Sample 5-7) and drug-drug/drug-excipient combinations (Sample 8-22) were transferred in to an appropriately labelled glass vial. Subsequently, 10 µL of ultra pure water (Milli-Q Academic, Milli-Pore) was added to each vial and mixed using a glass capillary, which was left inside the vial after mixing. Each vial was sealed properly and placed in hot air oven (T26/HAO-L, Technico) at 50°C for 4 weeks. To identify the physical instability, organoleptic parameters of samples (1-22) such as colour and texture were observed initially and at the end of 1st, 2nd, 3rd and 4th week. To identify the chemical instability, samples (1-22) were divided into two parts at the end of 4th week. First part of samples were used to record the Fourier-Transform Infrared (FT-IR) spectrum using FT-IR Spectrometer (Nicolet iS5, Thermo Scientific). Disappearance of absorption bands or reduction of the band intensity combined with the appearance of new bands give a clear evidence for interactions.[5,6] The second part of samples (sample 1-4 and 8-22) were separately mixed with 10 mL of methanol and sonicated (Ultrasonic cleaner, Lark) for 5 minutes followed by filtration through 0.22 µm membrane and analysed using the developed High Performance Liquid Chromatography (HPLC) methods in triplicate.[7-9]

Results and Discussion

The organoleptic parameters (colour and texture) of samples have not shown any significant visual changes throughout the storage period (Table 1). Hence, there were no physical instabilities in drug-drug/drug-excipient combinations.

Table 1. Summary of drug-drug/drug-excipient compatibility study

S.No.	Samples	Colour and Texture	Week 1 2 3 4	Assay (%)	% RSD
1	Curcumin*	Bright yellow-orange powder	NSVC	98.43	0.91
2	Piperine*	Faint yellow-off-white crystals	NSVC	98.98	1.23
3	Quercetin*	Yellow-green powder	NSVC	99.11	1.98
4	Silibinin*	White powder	NSVC	99.56	0.63
5	Polymer*	White powder	NSVC	-	-
6	Poloxamer 188*	White powder	NSVC	-	-
7	β-cyclodextrin*	White powder	NSVC	-	-
8	Curcumin + Piperine@	Bright yellow-orange powder	NSVC	97.91 & 98.17	1.39 & 0.86
9	Curcumin + Quercetin@	Yellowish green powder	NSVC	98.14 & 100.52	0.76 & 0.63
10	Curcumin + Silibinin@	Bright yellow powder	NSVC	99.02 & 98.71	0.49 & 1.59
11	Curcumin + Polymer@	Bright yellow powder	NSVC	100.17	1.79
12	Curcumin + Poloxamer@	Bright yellow powder	NSVC	99.49	0.61
13	Curcumin + β-cyclodextrin@	Bright yellow powder	NSVC	100.41	0.52
14	Piperine + Polymer@	White to off-white powder	NSVC	98.42	0.65
15	Piperine + Poloxamer@	White to off-white powder	NSVC	99.83	1.66
16	Piperine + β-cyclodextrin@	White to off-white powder	NSVC	100.10	0.73
17	Quercetin + Polymer@	Faint greenish powder	NSVC	98.29	1.19
18	Quercetin + Poloxamer 188@	Faint greenish powder	NSVC	97.84	1.21
19	Quercetin + β-cyclodextrin@	Faint greenish powder	NSVC	100.76	0.76
20	Silibinin + Polymer@	White powder	NSVC	99.56	0.63
21	Silibinin + Poloxamer 188@	White powder	NSVC	98.09	1.55
22	Silibinin + β-cyclodextrin@	White powder	NSVC	100.50	1.75

*Refers to 100 mg of samples; @Refers to 100 mg + 100 mg of samples in combination; NSVC: No significant visual changes; Polymer: Poly(butyl methacrylate-co-(2-dimethylaminoethyl) methacrylate-co-methyl methacrylate)

The FT-IR spectrum of samples (1-22) have shown characteristic absorption bands. Curcumin showed characteristic absorption bands at (a) 3726 and 3509 cm^{-1} (O-H stretch); (b) 2924 cm^{-1} (C-H stretch); (c) 1627 cm^{-1} (C=C stretch); (d) 1602 cm^{-1} (symmetric aromatic ring stretch); (e) 1509 cm^{-1} (C=O stretch); (f) 1429 cm^{-1} (C-H asymmetric stretch); (g) 1281, 1233, 1206, 1184 and 1153 cm^{-1} (C–O stretch); (h) 1026 cm^{-1} (C–O-C stretch); (i) 963 cm^{-1} (*trans*-CH vibration); and (j) 856 cm^{-1} (C-C skeleton vibration). Piperine showed characteristic absorption bands at (a) 3009 cm^{-1} (aromatic C-H stretch); (b) 2940 cm^{-1} (asymmetric & symmetric CH_2 stretch); (c) 2861 cm^{-1} (aliphatic C-H stretch); (d) 1633 cm^{-1} (-CO-N stretch); (e) 1611 cm^{-1} (symmetric & asymmetric C=C stretch); (f) 1584, 1510 and 1491 cm^{-1} (aromatic C=C stretch benzene ring); (g) 1448 cm^{-1} (CH_2 bend); (h) 1252 and 1194 cm^{-1} (asymmetrical =C-O-C stretch); (i) 1132 cm^{-1} (in-plane bend of phenyl C-H); (j) 1032 cm^{-1} (symmetrical =C-O-C stretch); (k) 930 cm^{-1} (C-O stretch); (l) 997 cm^{-1} (C-H bend of trans -CH=CH-); and (m) 847, 831 and 804 cm^{-1} (out-of-plane C-H bend). Quercetin showed characteristic absorption bands at (a) 3299 cm^{-1} (Phenolic OH stretch); (b) 1672 cm^{-1} (C=0 Aryl ketonic stretch); (c), 1615, 1550, 1512 and 1429 cm^{-1} (aromatic ring stretch); (d) 1360, 1316, 1244, 1212 cm^{-1} (-C-OH deformation vibration); and (e) 1165, 1141 and 1094 cm^{-1} (-C-OH stretch). Silibinin showed characteristic absorption bands at (a) 3606, 3455, 3137 and 2946 cm^{-1} (OH stretch); (b) 1873 and 1637 cm^{-1} (C=O stretch); (c) 1522, 1510, 1468 and 1435 cm^{-1} (skeleton vibration of aromatic C=C ring stretch); (d) 1366 cm^{-1} (OH in plane bend); (e) 1269, 1234, 1211 and 1189 cm^{-1} (C-O-C stretch); (f) 1166, 1143, 1128, 1082, 1041 and 1018 cm^{-1} (in plane = C-H bend); (g) 997, 956, 911 and 893 cm^{-1} (O-H out plane bend); and (h) 850, 834, 824, 812, 793, 774, 733, 703 and 668 cm^{-1} (in plane = C-H bend). Poly(butyl methacrylate-co-(2-dimethylaminoethyl) methacrylate-co-methyl methacrylate) showed characteristic absorption bands at (a) 2957 cm^{-1} (CH_X stretch); (b) 2822 and 2772 cm^{-1} (CH_3 stretch, dimethylamino groups); (c) 1731 cm^{-1} (C=O stretch); (d) 1457 and 1388 cm^{-1} (CH_X stretch); (e) 1272, 1241 and 1149 cm^{-1} (C=O stretch); (f) 1061 cm^{-1} (C-N stretch); and (g) 1017 and 966 cm^{-1} (CH_3 rocking). Poloaxmer 188 showed characteristic absorption bands at (a) 3445 cm^{-1} (O-H stretch); (b) 2874 cm^{-1} (C-H stretch); (c) 1467 cm^{-1} (C-H deformation); (d) 1348 cm^{-1} (in-plane OH bend); (e) 1282, 1250, 1108 and 951 cm^{-1} (C-O stretch); and (f) 842 cm^{-1} (C-C skeletal vibration. β-cyclodextrin showed characteristic absorption bands at (a) 3385 cm^{-1} (O-H stretch); (b) 2924 cm^{-1} (C-H stretch); (c) 1414 and 1368 cm^{-1} (C-H deformation vibration); (d) 1157, 1080 and 1028 cm^{-1} (C-O stretch); and (e) 947, 859, 755, 706 and 668 cm^{-1} (C-H deformation vibration). FT-IR spectrum of pure drug and excipients were displayed in Figure 1. Similarly, FT-IR spectrum of samples (8 to 22) showed characteristic absorption bands which were comparable with absorption bands of individual sample. Hence, there were no chemical instabilities in drug-drug/drug-excipient combinations.

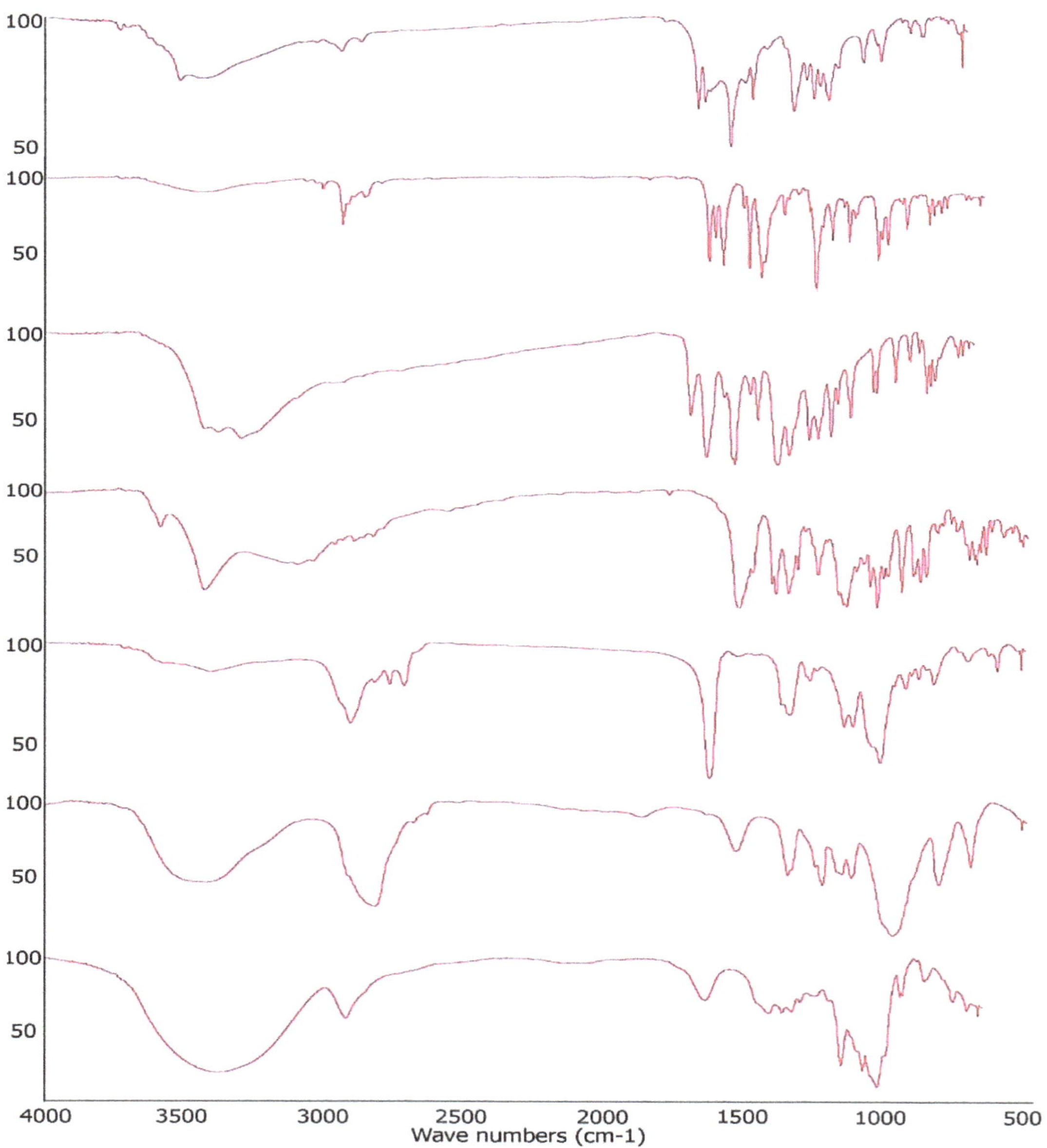

Figure 1. FT-IR spectrum of pure drugs and excipients

The assay of the samples (8-22) were well within ±2% of control samples (1-4) and the %RSD of assay was less than 2% (Table 1). Hence, there were no chemical instabilities in drug-drug/drug-excipient combinations.

Conclusion

The combination of curcumin-piperine, curcumin-quercetin, curcumin-silibinin and the combination of other excipients with curcumin, piperine, quercetin and silibinin have not shown any significant physical and chemical instability. Hence, the study concludes that the curcumin, piperine, quercetin and silibinin is compatible with each other and with other excipients.

Conflict of Interest

The authors report no conflicts of interest.

References

1. Moorthi C, Kiran K, Manavalan R, Kathiresan K. Preparation and characterization of curcumin-piperine dual drug loaded nanoparticles. *Asian Pac J Trop Biomed* 2012;2(11):841-8.
2. Moorthi C, Kathiresan K. Curcumin–Piperine/Curcumin–Quercetin/Curcumin–Silibinin dual drug-loaded nanoparticulate combination therapy: A novel approach to target and treat multidrug-resistant cancers. *J Med Hypotheses Ideas* 2013;7(1):15-20.
3. Moorthi C, Kathiresan K. Fabrication of dual drug loaded polymeric nanosuspension: Incorporating analytical hierarchy process and data envelopment analysis in the selection of a suitable method. *Int J Pharm Pharm Sci* 2013;5(2):499-504.
4. Moorthi C, Kathiresan K. A Step-by-step optimization process to fabricate narrow sized dual drug loaded polymeric nanoparticles using modified nanoprecipitation technique. *Nano Biomed Eng* 2013;5(3):107-15.
5. Narang AS, Desai D, Badawy S. Impact of excipient interactions on solid dosage form stability. *Pharm Res* 2012;29(10):2660-83.
6. Liltorp K, Larsen TG, Willumsen B, Holm R. Solid state compatibility studies with tablet excipients using non thermal methods. *J Pharm Biomed Anal* 2011;55(3):424-8.
7. Moorthi C, Senthil kumar C, Mohan S, Kiran K, Kathiresan K. Application of validated RP-HPLC-PDA method for the simultaneous estimation of curcumin and piperine in Eudragit E 100 nanoparticles. *J Pharm Res* 2013;7(3):224-9.
8. Moorthi C, Kathiresan K. Reversed phase high performance liquid chromatographic method for simultaneous estimation of curcumin and quercetin in pharmaceutical nanoformulation. *Int J Pharm Pharm Sci* 2013;5(3):622-5.
9. Moorthi C, Kathiresan K. Simultaneous estimation of curcumin and silibinin using validated RP-HPLC-PDA method and its application in pharmaceutical nanoformulation. *Int J Pharm Pharm Sci* 2013;5(3):475-8.

Analysis of Carotenoid Production by *Halorubrum* sp. TBZ126; an Extremely Halophilic Archeon from Urmia Lake

Davood Naziri[1,2], Masoud Hamidi[1,3], Salar Hassanzadeh[1], Vahideh Tarhriz[1], Bahram Maleki Zanjani[2], Hossein Nazemyieh[4], Mohammd Amin Hejazi[5]*, Mohammad Saeid Hejazi[1]*

[1] *Department of Pharmaceutical Biotechnology, Faculty of Pharmacy, Tabriz University of Medical Sciences, Tabriz, Iran.*

[2] *Department of Agricultural Biotechnology, Faculty of Agriculture, Zanjan University, Zanjan, Iran.*

[3] *Students' Research Committee, Tabriz University of Medical Sciences, Tabriz, Iran.*

[4] *Department of Pharmacognosy, Faculty of Pharmacy, Tabriz University of Medical Sciences, Tabriz, Iran.*

[5] *Branch for Northwest & West Region, Agricultural Biotechnology Research Institute of Iran (ABRII), Tabriz, Iran.*

ARTICLEINFO

Keywords:
Carotenoids
Halorubrum chaoviator
Bacterioruberin
Lycopene
ß-carotene

ABSTRACT

Purpose: Carotenoids are of great interest in many scientific disciplines because of their wide distribution, diverse functions and interesting properties. The present report describes a new natural source for carotenoid production.
Methods: *Halorubrum* sp., TBZ126, an extremely halophilic archaeon, was isolated from Urmia Lack following culture of water sample on marine agar medium and incubation at 30 °C. Then single colonies were cultivated in broth media. After that the cells were collected and carotenoids were extracted with acetone-methanol (7:3 v/v). The identification of carotenoids was performed by UV-VIS spectroscopy and confirmed by thin layer chromatography (TLC) in the presence of antimony pentachloride ($SbCl_5$). The production profile was analyzed using liquid-chromatography mass spectroscopy (LC-MS) techniques. Phenotypic characteristics of the isolate were carried out and the 16S rRNA gene was amplified using polymerase chain reaction (PCR).
Results: LC-MS analytical results revealed that produced carotenoids are bacterioruberin, lycopene and β-carotene. Bacterioruberin was found to be the predominant produced carotenoid. 16S rRNA analysis showed that TBZ126 has 100% similarity with *Halorubrum chaoviator* Halo-G[*T] (AM048786).
Conclusion: *Halorubrum* sp. TBZ126, isolated from Urmia Lake has high capacity in the production of carotenoids. This extremely halophilic archaeon could be considered as a prokaryotic candidate for carotenoid production source for future studies.

Introduction

Microorganisms are a great source of diverse natural products that are candidates for drug development, food and feed additives, and other industrial products.[1] Carotenoid pigments are one of these natural products responsible for the yellow, orange, red, and purple colors in a wide variety of plants, animals, and microorganisms.[2,3] These compounds are a group of more than 700 naturally occurring pigments. Animals are incapable of producing carotenoids and must obtain them from their diet. Lycopene, α-carotene, β-carotene, lutein, zeaxanthin, and β-cryptoxanthin are the most abundant in human plasma.[4]

Carotenoids have wide applications as colorants, feed additives, antioxidants, anti-tumor and heart disease prevention agents, precursors of vitamin A and enhancers of in vitro antibody production. Hence, they are widely applied in the food, medical, pharmaceutical, and cosmetic industries as dyes and functional ingredients.[2,3] *β*-carotene, astaxanthin, lutein, canthaxanthin, and lycopene are important examples.[5] Functions of the carotenoids are based on their molecular structures including molecular size, solubility, effective number of conjugated double bonds, and presence/absence of functional groups or cyclic ends.[6]

Chemical synthesis is one of the production methods for carotenoids. However, the consumer preference for natural products, as well as high costs, presence of by-products and damaging effects on the environment have together intensified efforts to identify alternative sources for chemical method. Accordingly different species of bacteria, molds, yeasts and algae have

***Corresponding authors:** Mohammad Saeid Hejazi, Faculty of Pharmacy, Tabriz University of Medical Sciences, Tabriz 51664, Iran.
Email: msaeidhejazi@yahoo.com; Mohamm Amin Hejazi, West & Northwest Agricultural Biotechnology Research Institute of Iran (ABRII), Tabriz, Iran. Email: aminhejazi@yahoo.com

attracted a great interest as alternative biosources.[7] The main reason for the interest in using microorganisms is the simplicity in increasing the production by environmental and genetic manipulation.[8] In addition, the production of natural colorants through fermentation has a number of advantages, such as cheaper production, higher yields, possibly easier extraction, less batch-to-batch variations and no seasonal variations. The production is flexible and can easily be controlled. Furthermore, the collection of microbial organisms is sustainable and has no negative impact on the environment.[9]

Halophilic archaea within the phylum Euryarchaeota are extreme halophiles and (mostly) aerobic, generally red-pigmented. The high-salt tolerance of haloarchaea enables their cultivation under non-sterile and thus cost-reducing conditions.[10,11] On the other hand, the process to obtain the carotenoids is simple because in lower NaCl concentrations cell lysis is induced[12] and consequently extraction could be conducted directly from the cells without any mechanical operation which is required in case of plants. Therefore, the study on production of carotenoids from halophilic haloarchaea could be considered as an alternative commercial source for carotenoids. Carotenoid pigments are particularly prominent in hypersaline ecosystems. Red and orangish color of hypersaline habitats is due to the presence of pigmented microorganisms, including *Dunaliella* , rich in β-carotene, Haloarchaea whose main production is bacterioruberin, and halophilic bacteria, such as *Salinibacter ruber* producing a carotenoid called salinixanthin.[12,13]

The most members of the family *Halobacteriaceae* including halophilic archaea have a high content of bacterioruberin, a 50-carbon open chain carotenoid. Other minor carotenoid compounds have been identified at low concentrations in halophilic archaea: lycopersene, cis- and trans-phytoene, cis- and transphytofluene, neo-β-carotene and neo-α-carotene. The low concentrations of these compounds suggest that they may be used as precursors for the synthesis of other carotenoids including lycopene, retinal and the members of the bacterioruberin group. Some species may also produce the ketocarotenoid canthaxanthin in addition to other carotenoids. Raman spectroscopy identified bacterioruberin as the major carotenoid in the halophilic archaea *Halobacterium salinarum* strains NRC-1 and R1, *Haloarcula sodomense*, and *Halorubrum vallismortis*.[13]

Following our previous report describing isolation and characterization of halophilic bacteria from Urmia Lake in northwest of Iran,[14] herein, we report isolation and characterization of a red haloarchaeon producing various carotenoids.

Materials and Methods

Isolation and growth conditions

Specimens were taken from water and soil of Urmia Lake, were delivered to the laboratory in sterilized containers and were cultured immediately on marine agar with various NaCl concentrations. Marine agar medium contained (per liter); $MgCl_2.7H_2O$, 8.8 g; Na_2SO_4, 3.24 g; $CaCl_2$, 1.8 g; KCl, 0.55 g; $NaHCO_3$, 0.16 g; KBr, 0.08 g; $SrCl_2$, 34.0 mg; H_3BO_3, 22.0 mg; Na_2O_3Si, 4.0 mg; NaF, 2.4 mg; $(NH_4)(NO_3)$,1.6 mg; Na_2HPO_4, 8.0 mg; peptone 5 g; yeast extract, 1 g; agar, 15.0 g and various NaCl concentrations (0-25% w/v). The pH of medium was adjusted at 7.5 before autoclaving. For this purpose, 400 μl of water samples were inoculated on the medium and incubated at 30 °C. Colony growth was first observed after about 7 days. To obtain pure cultures, single red colonies were picked from the plates and were used for Gram-staining and stock preparation, by growing in marine broth in an orbital shaker (Shaking Incubator VS-8480, Korea). Marine broth contained (per liter); $MgCl_2.7H_2O$ 5.9 g; $MgSO_4$, 3.24 g; $CaCl_2$, 1.8 g; KCl, 0.55 g; $NaHCO_3$, 0.16 g; KBr, 0.08 g; $SrCl_2$, 34.0 mg; H_3BO_3, 22.0 mg; Na_2O_3Si, 4.0 mg; NaF, 2.4 mg; $(NH_4)(NO_3)$, 1.6 mg; Na_2HPO_4, 8.0 mg; peptone 5 g and yeast extract 1 g and various NaCl concentrations (0-25% w/v). The pH of culture medium was adjusted at 7.5 before autoclaving. Axenic cultures were stored at −70°C in marine broth supplemented with 30% glycerol.

Extraction of genomic DNA and sequencing of 16S rRNA

DNA was extracted using Corbin "Genomic DNA isolation" protocol with some modification.[15] Briefly, cells were lysed by freeze-thaw cycles in liquid nitrogen and then suspended in solution I [Tris 10 mM (pH 7.4), EDTA 1 mM, sodium dodecyl sulphate (SDS) 0.5%, proteinase K 0.1 mg/ml] and lysed by incubation at 37 °C for 1 h. Then, the solution II [0.8 M NaCl and 1% CTAB] was added to the lysates and incubated at 65°C for 20 min and finally genomic DNA was extracted with equal volume of chloroform-isoamylalcohol (24:1 v/v). Nucleic acids were precipitated from the aqueous phase with 0.6 volume of isopropanol. The 16S rRNA gene was amplified using polymerase chain reaction (PCR) using 20F (5′-TCCGGTTGATCCTGCCG-3′)[16] and 1530R (5′-AGGAGGTGATCCAACCGCA-3′)[17] primers. PCR was performed using a thermal cycler (eppendorf) with a 50-μl reaction containing 1.5 μl $MgCl_2$, 1 μl of each dNTP, 0.5 μl of each primer, 5 μl PCR buffer, 36.5 μl H_2O and 1 U of Taq DNA polymerase (Cinnagen, Iran). Initial denaturation was carried out for 3 min at 95 °C. It was followed by 35 cycles of denaturation at 94 °C for 30 sec, annealing at 45 °C for 40 sec and extension at 72 °C for 1.5 min with a further 10 min extension at 72 °C. The amplified DNA fragment was separated using 1% agarose gel electrophoresis, then the DNA fragment was extracted from gel and sequenced by Faza Biotechnology Co. The sequence was compared with reference 16S rRNA gene sequences available in NCBI GenBank database BLAST using blastn and megablast softwares and EzTaxon-e server (http://eztaxon-e.ezbiocloud.net).[18]

Physiological characterization of the isolate

Gram-staining was performed as described by Gerhardt et al.[19] and confirmed according to Dussault.[20] To investigate basic physiological characteristics of the isolate, Mac Faddin[21] and Barrow et al.[22] methods were used for the following tests: oxidase and catalase reactions, phenylalanine deaminase, nitrate reduction, hydrolysis of urea, gelatin, starch, Tween 80 and tyrsosin, H_2S and indol production from L-cysteine and tryptophan, respectively. To examine nitrate reduction, 0.2% (w/v) KNO_3 was added to the liquid media. Gelatin and starch hydrolysis were tested by flooding cultures on solid media containing 1% (w/v) gelatin and starch, respectively. Hydrolysis of Tween 80 was tested on solid media supplemented with 1% (w/v) Tween 80. Tyrosine hydrolysis was evaluated by appearance of a clear zone on marine agar medium culture containing 5 g/l tyrosine. H_2S production was tested in liquid media supplemented with 0.01% (w/v) of L-cysteine. The indicator used in this experiment was a band of paper impregnated with lead-acetate placed in the neck of the tube.

Pigments extraction and analysis

To extract carotenoids, 100 ml of marine broth cultures were centrifuged at 8,000 rpm for 10 min at 4 °C. The supernatant was separated and a mixture of acetone-methanol (7:3 v/v)[23] containing butylhydroxytoluene (BHT) (0.1%; as antioxidant) was added to the pellet. The pelleted cells were then frozen and thawed using liquid nitrogen to facilitate extraction and followed by centrifugation at 10,000 × *g* for 10 min at 4 °C. Successive extractions carried out until both solvent and cells were colorless. The solvent was evaporated under a stream of nitrogen and the pigments were dissolved in 10 ml of acetone (containing 0.1% BHT). Samples were wrapped with aluminum foil to protect them from light. The extracts were stored under nitrogen at -70 °C. Extraction procedures and analysis tests were conducted in dark conditions.

UV-Visible Spectroscopy

Extraction solution UV spectra were recorded at 200-700 nm using a spectrophotometer (Shimadzu UV-1800 Series, Kyoto, Japan). The approximate content of total carotenoids was determined by measuring the optical density of the sample in 495 (λ_{max} of our extraction solution). The total amount of carotenoids was calculated according to Davies.[23]

Thin-Layer Chromatography

In order to confirm carotenoid pigments contained in the extract, thin-layer chromatography (TLC) was used. For this analysis, the acetone extract was placed on a TLC silica gel GF254 plate (Merck, Darmstadt, Germany) and developed in hexane:acetone (7:3). After development, the individual spots were identified by visibility and spraying with a saturated solution of antimony pentachloride ($SbCl_5$) in chloroform (1:10 v/v).

Liquid chromatography–mass spectrometry (LC-MS)

The extraction solution was centrifuged, and the supernatant was filtered through cellulose acetate filters (25 mm, 0.45 mm; VWR International). Samples were handled on ice and wrapped with aluminum foil to reduce isomerisation and oxidation of carotenoids by light irradiation. Chromatographic separation was performed on an Agilent 1200 series HPLC system including a quaternary pump and a degasser equipped with a G1315B Diode Array Detector. The accompanying Agilent LC Chemstation was employed for instrument control, data acquisition and processing. HPLC analysis was performed using Eurosphere RP-column (100-5 C18 column, 300×4.6 mm Knauer, Germany) by isocratic elution with a flow rate of 0.8 ml/min. The mobile phase was acetonitrile-dichloromethane-methanol (70:20:10 v/v/v), 20 mM ammonium acetate and 0.1% triethylamine. The temperature was maintained at 20 °C and UV detection was performed at 450 nm. Both the extracts and standards were injected (injection volume: 20 μL) into the reverse phase column and identifications of all trans-isomers were carried out using comparison of retention times and UV spectra of the extracts with standard mixture. The experiment was conducted in triplicate. The mass spectra were recorded in the positive ion mode in the mass range from 300 to 2000 m/z. The mass spectrometer parameters were set as follows: Nebulizer pressure was 40 psi, drying gas flow was 20 liter/min and gas temperature was 250 °C. The capillary voltage was 5000 V. Ions were monitored in the scan mode. The identification of carotenoids were performed by comparing retention time, UV spectra and characteristics of the mass spectra (protonated molecule ($[M+H]^+$) and its MS/MS fragments. All of the carotenoids were monitored at 450 nm with a UV-visible detector.

Results

Morphologic and genotypic characteristics

Cells were Gram-negative and rod-shaped. Strain TBZ126 formed circular and red colonies on marine agar. Strain TBZ126 didn't grow in the presence of NaCl and could tolerate NaCl up to 30% at 30 °C. It did not grow in acidic medium but tolerated alkaline medium (pH=10). 16S rRNA gene sequence analysis revealed that strain TBZ126 belongs to *Halorubrum* genus and has 100% similarity with *Halorubrum chaoviator* Halo-G^T.[24]

Physiological and biochemical characterization

Catalase and oxidase tests were positive and negative, respectively. Nitrate was not reduced to nitrite and indole was produced. Hydrolysis of gelatin and starch were found to be positive whereas Tween 80 was not hydrolysed. Urease activity was found to be positive. Phenylalanine deaminase was negative. H_2S formation was positive. Results of physiological and biochemical characteristics of *Halorubrum* sp. TBZ126 are summarized in Table 1.

Table 1. Physiological and biochemical characteristics of *Halorubrum* sp. TBZ126. +: positive reaction; -: negative reaction.

Characteristic	TBZ126
Gram-staining	-
Cell shape	Rod
Colony	Circle- red
Growth in the absence of NaCl	-
Catalase	+
Oxidase	-
Tyrosin Hydrolysis	-
Nitrate reduction	-
Gelatin Hydrolysis	+
Tween 80 Hydrolysis	-
Starch Hydrolysis	+
Urease	+
Indol	+
H_2S	+
Phenylalanine deaminase	-

UV-VIS spectrum of carotenoids and total carotenoid content

Pigments solution in acetone mixture showed characteristic absorptions of carotenoids (Figure 1).[25,26] Britton described that bacterioruberin and its derivatives exhibited the characteristic spectral peaks of red carotenoids at nearly identical absorption maxima at 467, 493, and 527 nm for three fingered peaks and at 370 and 385 nm for two cis peaks.[27] As seen in Figure 1, the pigments in the extract solution showed absorption peaks at 469 nm, 494 nm and 526 nm, indicating bacterioruberin is the main component in the extracted sample. The total carotenoid content of *Halorubrum* sp. TBZ126 was found to be 11280 µg/l.

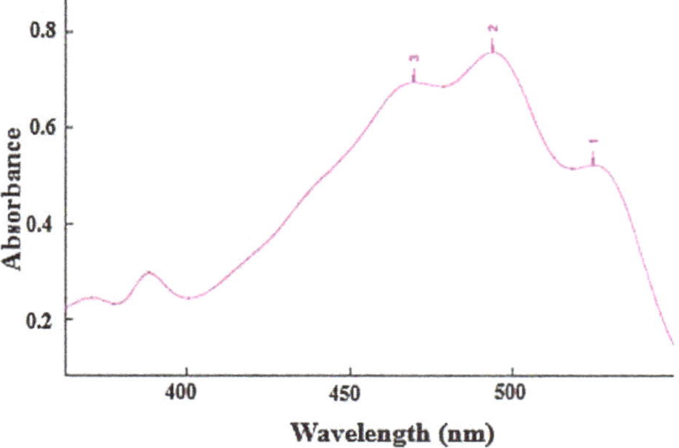

Figure 1. UV-VIS spectrum of acetone extract from *Halorubrum* sp. TBZ126. The extract corresponds to 100 ml of culture in marine broth medium and 1 ml of the extract was diluted to 10 ml with acetone to give a reading in the spectrophotometer between 0.5 and 0.8 at the wavelength of the middle main absorption maximum of the extract (495 nm). The pigments in the extract solution showed absorption peaks at 469 nm, 494 nm and 526 nm.

Thin-Layer Chromatography

After development of TLC test, four spots were visible. Staining the plate with antimony pentachloride ($SbCl_5$) in chloroform showed only one blue spot[23] confirming the presence of carotenoids in the extraction solution.

Liquid chromatography–mass spectrometry (LC-MS)

HPLC analysis of TBZ126 carotenoids revealed 5 distinctive peaks (Figure 2). Carotenoid production is composed of bacterioruberin (peak 1), all-trans-lycopene (peak 2), 13-cis-lycopene (peak 3), all-trans-β-carotenes (peak 4), and all-cis-β-carotene (peak 5).

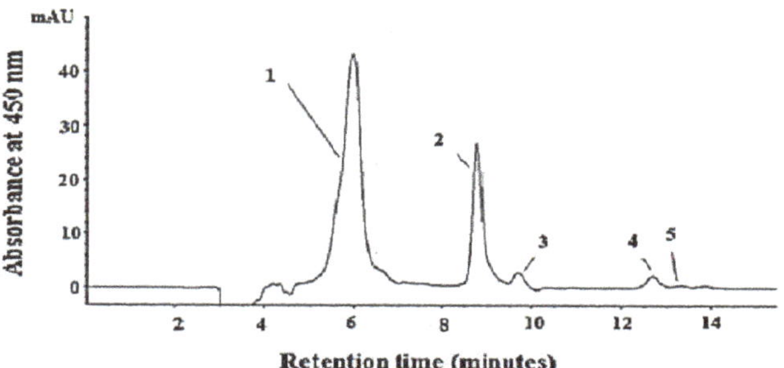

Figure 2. Reverse-phase liquid chromatography of the major carotenoids of *Halorubrum* sp. TBZ126. Column: 100-5 C18 column (300 by 4.6 mm, Knauer, Germany). Eluent: acetonitrile-dichloromethane-methanol (70:20:10, vol/vol/vol). Flow rate: 0.8 ml/min. Detection: 450 nm. Peak identities: peak 1, bacterioruberin; peak 2, all-trans lycopenes; peaks 3, 13-cis-lycopene; peak 4, all-trans- β-carotenes; peak 5, all-cis- β-carotenes.

The peaks of all trans-isomers of lycopene and β-carotene were identified by comparing the retention times of authentic standards and the UV spectra. Since most of the major cis-isomers of the carotenoids are not available in the market, they were identified by their UV absorption characteristics and also by comparing the obtained chromatograms with the fully investigated isomers of lycopene and β-carotene reported by Müller et al.[28] Bacterioruberin was identified by comparing the UV and mass spectra with those reported in literature.[29,30] The maximum absorption wavelengths for the carotenoids of interest, detected by diode array detector are 466 nm, 495 nm and 528 nm for bacterioruberin, 448 nm, 474 nm and 505 nm for Lycopene and 425 nm, 455 nm and 482 nm for β-carotene. The UV-VIS spectrum of this main carotenoids present in TBZ126 extract detected by diode array detector are presented in Figure 3. Because the ionization mode was positive, most of the m/z data were $[M+H]^+$ and the mass data of compounds identified are given in Table 2. Derived from the mass fragmentation interpretation, bacterioruberin, lycopene and β-carotene were identified in TBZ126 extract.

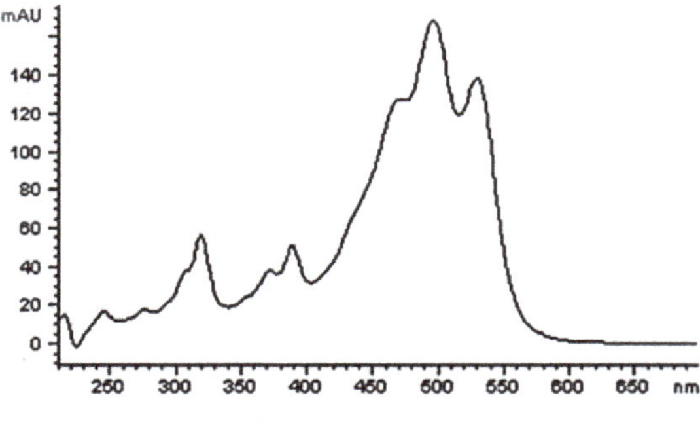

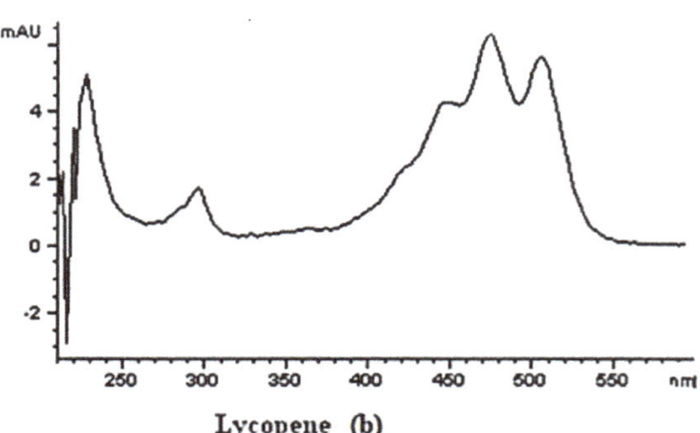

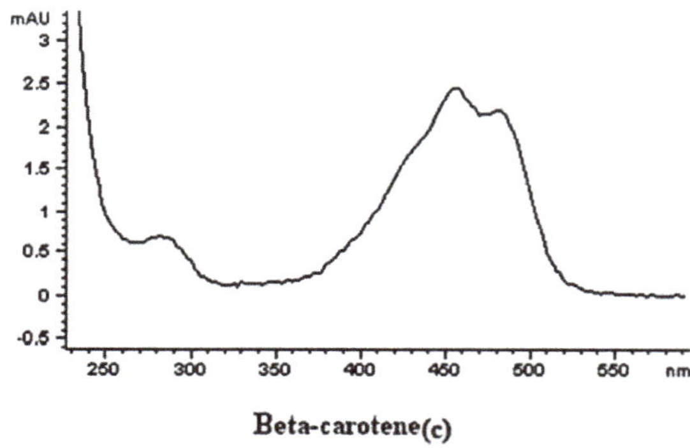

Figure 3. UV–visible absorption spectra of the carotenoids extracted from *Halorubrum* sp. TBZ126. bacterioruberin (a), lycopene (b) and β-carotene (c) detected by G1315B Diode Array Detector. The maximum absorption wavelengths for the carotenoids of interest are 466 nm, 495 nm and 528 nm for bacterioruberin, 448 nm, 474 nm and 505 nm for Lycopene and 425 nm, 455 nm and 482 nm for β-carotene.

Discussion

The carotenoid pigments are favorable ingredients owing to high biological activities and potential health benefits with many functions in nutraceuticals, cosmetics and feed industries.[31] The use of microorganisms in biotechnology to produce carotenoids is approving by consumer and can help meet the growing demand for these bioactive compounds in the food, feed, and pharmaceutical industries. The major advantages of the biological production of carotenoids are the wide range of their biosynthetic capability and ability to produce only the naturally occurring stereoisomers.[32] The marine environment is estimated to be home to more than 80 % of life and yet it remains largely unexplored. Marine microorganisms are an intact source for pigments that can have wide range of applications. In a general evaluation of several thousand colonies isolated from marine sources it was found that 31.3 % were yellow, 15.2 % orange, 9.9 % brown and 5.4 % red or pink.[33] However, there are not many reports available on investigation on marine microorganisms as source of natural pigments mainly carotenoids and there is little information in the literature about the carotenoid profile of extremophile microorganisms. In the present study we reported for the first time a new extremely halophilic archaeon isolated from Urmia Lack called *Halorubrum* sp. TBZ126 capable to produce carotenoid pigments.

Carotenoid-producing microorganisms have been isolated from various extreme environments, such as very low temperatures, high salinity, strong light, acidic and alkaline, and thermophilic conditions. One may hypothesize, based on these evidences, that the oxidative stresses in extreme environments are selective factors associated with pigmented microorganisms, which are able to synthesize antioxidants (i.e., carotenoids) to protect their vital molecules (e.g., proteins and nucleic acids). Carotenoids give the microbial colonies their distinctive color.[32]

Table 2. Identification of carotenoids from *Halorubrum* sp. TBZ126 extract elucidated by ESI ion mode showing their molecular mass and molecular formula.

Identification of carotenoids	Molecular formula	Approximate molecular mass (Dalton)	Fragmentation mass (m/z)	MS/MS fragment ion (m/z)
Bacterioruberin	$C_{50}H_{76}O_4$	740	741	723 $[M+H-18]^+$ 705 $[M+H-18-18]^+$ 683 $[M+H-58]^+$
Lycopene	$C_{40}H_{56}$	536	537	444 $[M+H-92]^+$
β-carotene	$C_{40}H_{56}$	536	537	444 $[M+H-92]^+$

Although there are several reports about carotenoid profile of eubacteria, fewer papers describe carotenoid production from archaea.[34] Marshall et al. mentioned that bacterioruberin is a ubiquitous and abundant pinkish-red pigment in moderately to extremely halophilic archaea.[35] Jehlicka et al. identified bacterioruberin by Resonance Raman spectroscopy as the major carotenoid in the halophilic archaea *Halobacterium salinarum* strains NRC-1 and R1, *Haloarcula sodomense*, and *Halorubrum vallismortis*. Kelly et al. showed that bacterioruberin was the main carotenoid (85 % of total) of *Halobacterium salinarium* (an extremely halophilic marine archaeon).[29] Ronnekleiv and colleagues reported that *Heloferax vokanii* contained the (2S,2′S)-bacterioruberin (82% of total carotenoid), monoanydrobacterioruberin (7%), (2S,2′S)-bisanhydrobacterioruberin (3%), 3,4-dihydromonoanhydrobacterioruberin (2%) and two undecaene $C_{50}H_{74}O_4$ carotenoids (each 2%), the C_{45}-carotenoid (2S)-2-isopentenyl-3,4-dehydrorhodopin (1%) and lycopene (0.3%).[30] Mandelli et al. studied carotenoid production by the extremophile microorganisms *Halococcus morrhuae*, *Halobacterium salinarium* and *Thermus filiformis*. The major carotenoid was all-trans-bacterioruberin, accounting for 69% of the carotenoids in *Halococcus morrhuae* and 68% in *Halobacterium salinarium.*[36]

Halorubrum sp. TBZ126, a Gram-negative, aerobic, rod-shaped and extremely halophilic archaeon was isolated from Urmia Lake in Azerbaijan region of Iran. 16S rRNA gene sequence showed that TBZ126 is a new extremely halophilic archaeon related to *Halorubrum chaoviator* Halo-G^{*T} (AM048786). To choose the appropriate solvent for carotenoid extraction, acetone, methanol, hexane and acetone/methanol (7:3 v/v) were examined, individually with the best recoveries for acetone/methanol (7:3 v/v). The simplicity of carotenoid extraction with acetone/methanol (7:3 v/v) at room temperature gives the strain an advantage over for instance yeast cells which need either be disrupted by mechanical means or treated with DMSO before carotenoid extraction is possible and might prove useful in a future production process. Today the most widely used method for the analysis of carotenoids is reversed phased HPLC equipped with diode array detection (DAD) and MS detection (LC-DAD-MS).[37]

As shown in Figure 2, the present reverse phase isocratic HPLC method was separated three main carotenoids with good resolution and in a short time (14min). The retention times of Lycopene and β-carotene in the sample were in a good agreement with authentic standards. The UV–Vis spectra of the carotenoids also serve as a helpful source for their identification and the DAD allows the UV–Vis spectrum of each component to be determined on line. Both the wavelengths of maximum absorption (λmax) and the shape of the spectra are feature of each carotenoid.

From the results, it can be concluded that the produced carotenoids of *Halorubrum* sp. TBZ126 isolated from Urmia Lake, the largest saline lake in the Middle East and the second largest salt water lake on the Earth, were bacterioruberin, lycopene and β-carotene.

Conclusion

As a consequence, this study introduced and opens the way for employment of a novel prokaryotic source of carotenoid production for future use in the pharmaceutical and food industries. Further reports on enhanced carotenoid production in the optimized condition are in program.

Conflict of Interest

The authors report no conflicts of interest.

References

1. Stafsnes MH, Dybwad M, Brunsvik A, Bruheim P. Large scale MALDI-TOF MS based taxa identification to identify novel pigment producers in a marine bacterial culture collection. *Antonie Van Leeuwenhoek* 2013;103(3):603-15.
2. Li Z, Sun M, Li Q, Li A, Zhang C. Profiling of carotenoids in six microalgae (Eustigmatophyceae) and assessment of their beta-carotene productions in bubble column photobioreactor. *Biotechnol Lett* 2012;34(11):2049-53.
3. Cabral MMS, Cence K, Zeni J, Tsai SM, Durrer A, Foltran LL, et al. Carotenoids production from a newly isolated Sporidiobolus pararoseus strain by submerged fermentation. *Eur Food Res Technol* 2011;233(1):159-66.
4. Peng J, Yuan JP, Wu CF, Wang JH. Fucoxanthin, a marine carotenoid present in brown seaweeds and diatoms: metabolism and bioactivities relevant to human health. *Mar Drugs* 2011;9(10):1806-28.
5. Mantzouridou F, Tsimidou MZ, Roukas T. Performance of crude olive pomace oil and soybean oil during carotenoid production by Blakeslea trispora in submerged fermentation *J Agric Food Chem* 2006;54(7):2575-81.
6. Furubayashi M, Umeno D. Directed Evolution of Carotenoid Synthases for the Production of Unnatural Carotenoids. In: Barredo J, editor. Microbial Carotenoids from Bacteria and Microalgae : Methods and Protocols. USA: Springer; 2012. P. 245-53.
7. Perez-Fons L, Steiger S, Khaneja R, Bramley PM, Cutting SM, Sandmann G, et al. Identification and the developmental formation of carotenoid pigments in the yellow/orange Bacillus spore-formers. *Biochim Biophys Acta* 2011;1811(3):177-85.
8. Zeni J, Colet R, Cence K, Tiggemann L, Toniazzo G, Cansian R, et al. Screening of microorganisms for production of carotenoids Selección de microorganismos para la producción de carotenoides. *CyTA -J Food* 2011;9(2):160-6.
9. Wang B, Lin L, Lu L, Chen W. Optimization of β-carotene production by a newly isolated Serratia marcescens strain. *Electron J Biotechn* 2012;15(6):1-3.
10. Manikandan M, Pasic L, Kannan V. Optimization of growth media for obtaining high-cell density cultures of halophilic archaea (family Halobacteriaceae) by response surface methodology. *Bioresour Technol* 2009;100(12):3107-12.

11. Andrei AS, Banciu HL, Oren A. Living with salt: metabolic and phylogenetic diversity of archaea inhabiting saline ecosystems. *FEMS Microbiol Lett* 2012;330(1):1-9.
12. El-Banna AaE-R, El-Razek AMA, El-Mahdy AR. Isolation, identification and screening of carotenoid-producing strains of Rhodotorula glutinis. *Food Nutr (Roma)* 2012;3(5):627-33.
13. Jehlicka J, Edwards HG, Oren A. Bacterioruberin and salinixanthin carotenoids of extremely halophilic Archaea and Bacteria: a Raman spectroscopic study. *Spectrochim Acta A Mol Biomol Spectrosc* 2013;106:99-103.
14. Vahed SZ, Forouhandeh H, Hassanzadeh S, Klenk HP, Hejazi MA, Hejazi MS. Isolation and characterization of halophilic bacteria from Urmia Lake in Iran. *Mikrobiologiia* 2011;80(6):826-33.
15. Corbin DR, Greenplate JT, Wong EY, Purcell JP. Cloning of an insecticidal cholesterol oxidase gene and its expression in bacteria and in plant protoplasts. *Appl Environ Microbiol* 1994;60(12):4239-44.
16. Enache M, Itoh T, Kamekura M, Teodosiu G, Dumitru L. Haloferax prahovense sp. nov., an extremely halophilic archaeon isolated from a Romanian salt lake. *Int J Syst Evol Microbiol* 2007;57(Pt 2):393-7.
17. Spangler R, Goddard NL, Thaler DS. Optimizing Taq polymerase concentration for improved signal-to-noise in the broad range detection of low abundance bacteria. *PLoS One* 2009;4(9):e7010.
18. Kim OS, Cho YJ, Lee K, Yoon SH, Kim M, Na H, et al. Introducing EzTaxon-e: a prokaryotic 16S rRNA gene sequence database with phylotypes that represent uncultured species. *Int J Syst Evol Microbiol* 2012;62(Pt 3):716-21.
19. Gerhardt P, Murray RGE, Wood WA, Krieg NR. Methods for General and Molecular Bacteriology. Washington, DC: American Society for Microbiology; 1994.
20. Dussault HP. An improved technique for staining red halophilic bacteria. *J Bacteriol* 1955;70(4):484-5.
21. Mac Faddin JF. Biochemical tests for identification of medical bacteria. Philadelphia: Lippincott Williams & Wilkins; 1976.
22. Barrow G, Feltham RKA. Cowan and Steel's manual for the identification of medical bacteria. Cambridge: Cambridge university press; 2004.
23. Davies BH. Chemistry and biochemistry of plant pigments. London: Academic Press; 1976.
24. Mancinelli RL, Landheim R, Sanchez-Porro C, Dornmayr-Pfaffenhuemer M, Gruber C, Legat A, et al. Halorubrum chaoviator sp. nov., a haloarchaeon isolated from sea salt in Baja California, Mexico, Western Australia and Naxos, Greece. *Int J Syst Evol Microbiol* 2009;59(Pt 8):1908-13.
25. Wang Y, Wang J, Liu Z, Zhao J, Zhou S, editors. Identification of a Gordonia sp. strain producing carotenoids. 2011 International Symposium on IT in Medicine and Education (ITME 2011); 2011; China.
26. De La Vega M, Diaz E, Vila M, Leon R. Isolation of a new strain of Picochlorum sp and characterization of its potential biotechnological applications. *Biotechnol Prog* 2011;27(6):1535-43.
27. Britton G, Liaaen-Jensen S, Pfander H. Carotenoids. Volume 1B: Spectroscopy. Basel: Birkhäuser Verlag AG; 1995.
28. Miller A, Pietsch B, Faccin N, Schierle J, Waysek EH. Method for the determination of lycopene in supplements and raw material by reversed-phase liquid chromatography: single-laboratory validation. *J AOAC Int* 2008;91(6):1284-97.
29. Kelly M, Norgard S, Liaaen-Jensen S. Bacterial carotenoids. 31. C50-carotenoids 5. Carotenoids of Halobacterium salinarium, especially bacterioruberin. *Acta Chem Scand* 1970;24(6):2169-82.
30. Ronnekleiv M, Liaaen-Jensen S. Bacterial carotenoids 53, C50-carotenoids 23; carotenoids of Haloferax volcanii versus other halophilic bacteria. *Biochem Syst Ecol* 1995;23(6):627-34.
31. Gharibzahedi SMT, Razavi SH, Mousavi SM, Moayedi V. High efficiency canthaxanthin production by a novel mutant isolated from Dietzia natronolimnaea HS-1 using central composite design analysis. *Ind Crop Prod* 2012;40:345-54.
32. Asker D, Awad TS, Beppu T, Ueda K. Isolation, characterization, and diversity of novel radiotolerant carotenoid-producing bacteria. *Methods Mol Biol* 2012;892:21-60.
33. Zobell CE, Feltham CB. Preliminary studies on the distribution and characteristics of marine bacteria. Berkeley: University of California Press; 1934.
34. Takano H, Asker D, Beppu T, Ueda K. Genetic control for light-induced carotenoid production in non-phototrophic bacteria. *J Ind Microbiol Biotechnol* 2006;33(2):88-
35. Marshall CP, Leuko S, Coyle CM, Walter MR, Burns BP, Neilan BA. Carotenoid analysis of halophilic archaea by resonance Raman spectroscopy. *Astrobiology* 2007;7(4):631-43.
36. Mandelli F, Miranda VS, Rodrigues E, Mercadante AZ. Identification of carotenoids with high antioxidant capacity produced by extremophile microorganisms. *World J Microbiol Biotechnol* 2012;28(4):1781-90.
37. Breeman RBV. Peer Reviewed: Innovations in Carotenoid Analysis Using LC/MS. *Anal Chem* 1996;68(9):299A-304A.

Characterization of Non-Terpenoids in *Marrubium crassidens* Boiss. Essential Oil

Sanaz Hamedeyazdan[1], Solmaz Asnaashari[2], Fatemeh Fathiazad[3]*

[1] *Student's Research Committee, Faculty of Pharmacy, Tabriz University of Medical Sciences, Tabriz, Iran.*

[2] *Drug Applied Research Center, Tabriz University of Medical Sciences, Tabriz, Iran.*

[3] *Department of Pharmacognosy, Faculty of Pharmacy, Tabriz University of Medical Sciences, Tabriz, Iran.*

ARTICLEINFO

Keywords:
Marrubium crassidens
Lamiaceae
Oil-poor species
GC-MS
Acetophenone
Tolualdehyde

ABSTRACT

Purpose: *Marrubium crassidens,* a plant belonging to the family Lamiaceae, was studied for its volatile components present in the aerial parts of the plant during the flowering stage. ***Methods:*** The essential oil of the plant obtained through hydrodistillation of the dried plant material was assessed for its chemical composition by GC/MS and GC-FID analyses. ***Results:*** Twenty-five compounds were identified, which constituted 94.3% of the total oil composition. The major components were identified as, m-tolualdehyde (23.3%), acetophenone (15.8%), nonacosane (13.1%), docosane (7.2%), o-tolualdehyde (4.1%), β-caryophyllene (3.8%) and caryophyllene oxide (3.4%). Non-terpenoids with 75.7% were the most abundant components of the essential oil. ***Conclusion:*** Overall, *M. crassidens* essential oil revealed to include rather higher proportions of non-terpenoid compounds compared with other species of genus *Marrubium*.

Introduction

The family Lamiaceae with about 220 genera and almost 4000 species worldwide has always been the leader sources for culinary, vegetable and medicinal plants.[1,2] In this regard, *Marrubium* a genus of about 40 species of flowering plants in this family has been holding a place of value in different cultures and herbal medicine with some known healing attributes.[3,4] Cytotoxicity, immunomodulating, vasorelaxant, antispasmodic, hypolipidemic, hypoglycemic, and analgesic activities are some of the famous properties for species of genus *Marrubium* that have been reported by several studies.[5-14] Although *Marrubium* species are mainly recognized for their non-volatile compounds, like diterpenes, polyphenols, steroids, phenylpropanoid glycosides and flavonoids, they happen to produce small amounts of essential oil and thus they are called as oil-poor species.[15-17] Generally, essential oils from *Marrubium sp.* consist mostly of sesquiterpenes and studies concerning their antimicrobial and antioxidant activities are sparse.[18-24] Nevertheless in our previous study on *M. persicum*, it was described substantially as a species distinct in chemical composition of the essential oil rich in non-terpenoid compounds from other species of *Marrubium*. According to the chemical diversity of essential oils within a genus indicating both quantitative and qualitative diversity in the composition of the essential oils, searching for the variety of naturally occurring volatile constituents in the essential oil of a plant appears to be of value. So as, based on flora Iranica, *M. crassidens,* endemic to the countries; Armenia, Azerbaijan, Turkey and Iran[25] was selected to be further analyzed for its volatile constituents from the aerial parts of the plant that is grown in Azarbaijan province in Iran.

Materials and Methods

Plant material

Aerial parts of *Marrubium crassidens* were collected during the flowering stage from Chichaklou in East Azarbaijan province, in June 2011. A voucher specimen of the plant (Tbz-Fph-719) representing this collection has been deposited at the Herbarium of the Faculty of Pharmacy, Tabriz University of Medical science, Iran.

Essential oil extraction

Air-dried plant material of the aerial parts of *M. crassidens* was subjected to hydrodistillation using a Clevenger-type apparatus (Clevenger, 1928). Since

***Corresponding author:** Fatemeh Fathiazad, Department of Pharmacognosy, Faculty of Pharmacy, Tabriz University of Medical Sciences, Tabriz, Iran. Email: fathiazad@tbzmed.ac.ir

the oil content was low in quantity, the distillation time was prolonged (3h) and xylene was used as an absorbing medium. The obtained essential oil was stored in sealed glass vial at 4-5 °C prior to analysis.

Gas Chromatography-Mass Spectrometry (GC-MS)

The essential oil was analyzed by GC-MS using a Shimadzu GC-MS-QP 5050A gas chromatograph fitted with a DB1 (methyl phenyl sylonane, 60 m x 0.25 mm i.d., 0.25 μm film thickness) capillary column. The GC was set at the following conditions with helium as the carrier gas; flow rate of 1.3 mL/min; linear velocity: 29.6 cm/s; Split ratio, 1:29; column temperature, 2 min in 60 °C, 50-260 °C at 3 °C/min; injector temperature, 240 °C, and 1 μL of volume injection of the essential oil. The MS operating parameters were as follows: ionization potential, 70 eV; ion source temperature; 270 °C; quadrupole 100 °C, Solvent delay 2 min, scan speed 2000 amu/s and scan range 30-600 amu, EV voltage 3000 volts.

Identification of the compounds

The identification of compounds was based on direct comparison of the retention indices and mass spectral data with those for the standards and by computer matching with the Wiley 229, Nist 107, Nist 21 Library, as well as by comparing the fragmentation patterns of the mass spectra with those reported in the literature.[26] For quantification purpose, relative area percentages were obtained by FID without the use of correction factors, where the FID detector condition was set on a duplicate of the same column applying the same operational conditions.

Results and Discussions

The GC–MS analysis of the small amount of essential oil obtained through hydrodistillation led to the identification of 25 different components, representing 94.3% of the total oil constituents. All the identified compounds were arranged in order of their elution from the DB1-MS column and the retention indices whereas their percentage compositions were summarized in Table 1.

Table 1. Chemical constituent of the essential oil from aerial parts of *M. crassidens*.

No.	RI[a]	Compounds	Area (%)
1	906	n-Nonane	2.1
2	933	Benzaldehyde	0.5
3	936	α-Pinene	1.8
4	966	1-Octen-3-ol	2.8
5	1004	Decane	0.3
6	1025	Limonene	0.6
7	1037	Acetophenone	15.8
8	1041	m-Tolualdehyde	23.3
9	1053	o-Tolualdehyde	4.1
10	1381	α-Cubebene	0.7
11	1424	β-Caryophyllene	3.8
12	1450	β-Farnesene	1.5
13	1457	α-Humulene	0.4
14	1482	Germacrene D	2.6
15	1488	β-Selinene	0.6
16	1497	Bicyclogermacrene	1.9
17	1520	δ-Cadinene	0.4
18	1571	Spathulenol	0.9
19	1578	Caryophyllene oxide	3.4
20	1834	Hexahydrofarnesyl acetone	1.9
21	1945	Eicosanoic acid	0.7
22	1989	Docosane	7.2
23	2592	Hexacosane [b]	2.0
24	2793	Octacosane [b]	1.9
25	2892	Nonacosane [b]	13.1
Total			**94.3**
Non-terpenoids			**75.7**
Monoterpene hydrocarbons			**2.4**
Sesquiterpene hydrocarbones			**11.9**
Oxygenated sesquiterpenes			**4.3**

[a] RI is the Retention Index relative to C8–C24 n-alkanes on the DB-1 column.
[b] This compound was compared with an authentic sample.

It was established that the essential oil of *M. crassidens* was a complex mixture of mostly non-terpenoids (75.7%), sesquiterpene hydrocarbons (11.9%), oxygenated sesquiterpenes (4.3%) and monoterpene hydrocarbons (2.4%). In spite of the absence of oxygenated monoterpenes, something to be expected in study of *Marrubium* species essential oil, our sample was characterized by the presence of alkanes, alkanoic acid derivatives and ketones in great amounts. As regards, m-tolualdehyde with 23.3%, and acetophenone with 15.8% were the two basic constituents present among the non-isoprenoid compounds of the essential oil. Moreover, β-caryophyllene (3.8%), germacrene D (2.6%), and bicyclogermacrene (1.9%) were the leader sesquiterpene hydrocarbons that were present in the *M. crassidens* essential oil. The only identified two monoterpenes in the essential oil were α-pinene, and limonene with the relative percentages of 1.8 and 0.6%, respectively. Besides, caryophyllene oxide with 3.4% and spathulenol with 0.9% were the only components of the oxygenated sesquiterpen compound grouping.

Having reviewed previously reports of the essential oils from genus *Marrubium*, it was established that *Marrubium* species possess rather low amounts of aliphatic and non-terpenoid fractions in essential oils, in contrary to our findings.[22-24,27] Owing to the fact that the production of terpenoid and non-isoprenoid compounds diverges early in the pathway of anabolic plant secondary compound synthesis,[28,29] necessitates fundamental studies in advance especially in practical applications of the essential oils in fragrance and flavor industries, as well as in the pharmaceutical and chemical industries. In order to distinguish between the differences observed in the essential oil constituents of *M. crassidens* with other species of genus *Marrubium* additional studies could be of advantageous in determining the intrinsic (genetic, growth stage, etc.) and extrinsic (climatic, seasonal, environmental distillation processes, etc.) conditions affecting the relative biosynthesis pathways of the essential oils.

Conclusion

On the whole, *M. crassidens* in agreement with previous reports for other *Marrubium* species seems to be poor in essential oil content while it shares some similarities and also differences in constituents of the essential oil. Meanwhile, presence of relatively higher amounts of non-terpenoids; acetophenone with different isomers of tolualdehyde in the *M. crassidens* essential oil has been reported for the first time in this study for this plant.

Acknowledgments

The authors would like to thank Drug Applied Research Center of Tabriz University of Medical Sciences for recording the mass spectra. Financial support of this work by the Research Vice-Chancellor of Tabriz University of Medical Sciences is faithfully acknowledged. This article was written based on a data set of PhD. thesis, registered in Tabriz University of Medical Sciences (5/4/6651- NO. 71).

Conflict of Interest

The authors report no conflict of interest in this study.

References

1. Hadley SK, Petry JJ. Medicinal herbs: a primer for primary care. *Hosp Pract (1995)* 1999;34(6):105-6, 109-12, 115-6 passim.
2. Naghibi F, Mosaddegh M, Mohammadi Motamed S, Ghorbani A. Labiatae Family in folk Medicine in Iran: from Ethnobotany to Pharmacology. *Iran J Pharm Res* 2005;2:63-79.
3. Paula De Oliveira A, Santin JR, Lemos M, Klein Junior LC, Couto AG, Meyre Da Silva Bittencourt C, et al. Gastroprotective activity of methanol extract and marrubiin obtained from leaves of Marrubium vulgare L. (Lamiaceae). *J Pharm Pharmacol* 2011;63(9):1230-7.
4. Meyre-Silva C, Cechinel-Filho V. A review of the chemical and pharmacological aspects of the genus marrubium. *Curr Pharm Des* 2010;16(31):3503-18.
5. Boudjelal A, Henchiri C, Siracusa L, Sari M, Ruberto G. Compositional analysis and in vivo anti-diabetic activity of wild Algerian Marrubium vulgare L. infusion. *Fitoterapia* 2012;83(2):286-92.
6. Hamedeyazdan S, Fathiazad F, Sharifi S, Nazemiyeh H. Antiproliferative activity of Marrubium persicum extract in the MCF-7 human breast cancer cell line. *Asian Pac J Cancer Prev* 2012;13(11):5843-8.
7. Zaabat N, Hay AE, Michalet S, Darbour N, Bayet C, Skandrani I, et al. Antioxidant and antigenotoxic properties of compounds isolated from Marrubium deserti de Noe. *Food Chem Toxicol* 2011;49(12):3328-35.
8. Meyre-Silva C, Yunes RA, Schlemper V, Campos-Buzzi F, Cechinel-Filho V. Analgesic potential of marrubiin derivatives, a bioactive diterpene present in Marrubium vulgare (Lamiaceae). *Farmaco* 2005;60(4):321-6.
9. Rigano D, Aviello G, Bruno M, Formisano C, Rosselli S, Capasso R, et al. Antispasmodic effects and structure-activity relationships of labdane diterpenoids from Marrubium globosum ssp. libanoticum. *J Nat Prod* 2009;72(8):1477-81.
10. El Bardai S, Lyoussi B, Wibo M, Morel N. Pharmacological evidence of hypotensive activity of Marrubium vulgare and Foeniculum vulgare in spontaneously hypertensive rat. *Clin Exp Hypertens* 2001;23(4):329-43.
11. Karioti A, Skopeliti M, Tsitsilonis O, Heilmann J, Skaltsa H. Cytotoxicity and immunomodulating characteristics of labdane diterpenes from Marrubium cylleneum and Marrubium velutinum. *Phytochemistry* 2007;68(11):1587-94.
12. Berrougui H, Isabelle M, Cherki M, Khalil A. *Marrubium vulgare* extract inhibits human-LDL oxidation and enhances HDL-mediated cholesterol efflux in THP-1 macrophage. *Life Sci* 2006;80(2):105-12.

13. Boudjelal A, Henchiri C, Siracusa L, Sari M, Ruberto G. Compositional analysis and in vivo anti-diabetic activity of wild Algerian Marrubium vulgare L. infusion. *Fitoterapia* 2012;83(2):286-92.
14. Argyropoulou A, Samara P, Tsitsilonis O, Skaltsa H. Polar constituents of Marrubium thessalum Boiss. & Heldr. (Lamiaceae) and their cytotoxic/cytostatic activity. *Phytother Res* 2012;26(12):1800-6.
15. Calis I, Hosny M, Khalifa T, Ruedi P. Phenylpropanoid glycosides from Marrubium alysson. *Phytochemistry* 1992;31(10):3624-6.
16. Karioti A, Skaltsa H, Heilmann J, Sticher O. Acylated flavonoid and phenylethanoid glycosides from Marrubium velutinum. *Phytochemistry* 2003;64(2):655-60.
17. Argyropoulou C, Skaltsa H. Identification of essential oil components of Marrubium thessalum Boiss. & Heldr., growing wild in Greece. *Nat Prod Res* 2012;26(7):593-9.
18. Semnani KM, Saeedi M, Babanezhad E. The essential oil composition of *Marrubium vulgare* L. from Iran. *J Essent Oil Res* 2008;20(6):488-90.
19. Tajbakhsh M, Khalilzadeh A, Rineh A, Balou J. Essential oils of *Marrubium anisodon* C. Koch and *Marrubium propinquum* Fisch. et C.A. Mey., growing wild in Iran. *J Essent Oil Res* 2008:161-2.
20. Petrovic S, Pavlovic M, Maksimovic Z, Milenkovic M, Couladis M, Tzakouc O, et al. Composition and antimicrobial activity of Marrubium incanum Desr. (Lamiaceae) essential oil. *Nat Prod Commun* 2009;4(3):431-4.
21. Laouer H, Yabrir B, Djeridane A, Yousfi M, Beldovini N, Lamamra M. Composition, antioxidant and antimicrobial activities of the essential oil of Marrubium deserti. *Nat Prod Commun* 2009;4(8):1133-8.
22. Nagy M, Svajdlenka E. Comparison of essential oils from *Marrubium vulgare* L. and *M. peregrinum* L. *J Essent Oil Res* 1998;10:585-7.
23. Demirci B, Baser KGC, Kirimer N. Composition of the essential oil of *Marrubium bourgaei* ssp. caricum P.H. Davis. *J Essent Oil Res* 2004;16:133-4.
24. Javidnia K, Miri R, Soltani M, Khosravi AR. Constituents of the Essential Oil of *Marrubium astracanicum* Jacq. from Iran. *J Essent Oil Res* 2007;19:559-61.
25. Mozaffarian V. A Dictionary of Iranian Plant Names. Tehran, Iran: Farhang Moaser Publication; 2004.
26. Adams RP. Identification of Essential oil Components by Gas Chromatography/ Quadrupole Mass Spectroscopy. Carol Stream, IL: Allured Publ Corp; 2004.
27. Zarai Z, Kadri A, Ben Chobba I, Ben Mansour R, Bekir A, Mejdoub H, et al. The in-vitro evaluation of antibacterial, antifungal and cytotoxic properties of Marrubium vulgare L. essential oil grown in Tunisia. *Lipids Health Dis* 2011;10:161.
28. Ganjewala D, Luthra R. Essential oil biosynthesis and regulation in the genus Cymbopogon. *Nat Prod Commun* 2010;5(1):163-72.
29. Lawrence BM. Essential oils. Carol Strem, IL: Allured Publishing Corp; 1992.

31

Formulation, Evaluation and Optimization of Pectin- Bora Rice Beads for Colon Targeted Drug Delivery System

Kuldeep Hemraj Ramteke[1]*, Lilakant Nath[2]

[1] *Modern College of Pharmacy (for Ladies), Moshi, Pune, Maharashtra.*

[2] *Department of Pharmaceutical Sciences, Dibrugarh University, Dibrugagh, Assam.*

ARTICLEINFO

Keywords:
Bora Rice
Glipizide
Pectin
Factorial design
In Vivo study

ABSTRACT

Purpose: The purpose of this research was to established new polysaccharide for the colon targeted drug delivery system, its formulation and *in vitro* and *in vivo* evaluation.
Methods: Microspheres containing pectin and bora rice were prepared by ionotropic gelation technique using zinc acetate as cross linking agent and model drug used was glipizide. A 3^2 full factorial design was employed to study the effect of independent variables, polymer to drug ratio (A), and concentration of cross linking agent (B) on dependent variables, particle size, swelling index, drug entrapment efficiency and percentage drug release.
Results: Results of trial batches indicated that polymer to drug ratio and concentration of cross linking agent affects characteristics of beads. Beads were discrete, spherical and free flowing. Beads exhibited small particle size and showed higher percentage of drug entrapment efficiency. The optimized batch P2 exhibited satisfactory drug entrapment efficiency 68% and drug release was also controlled for more than 24 hours. The polymer to drug ratio had a more significant effect on the dependent variables. *In vivo* gamma scintigraphy study of optimized pectin-bora rice beads demonstrated degradation of beads whenever they reached to the colon.
Conclusion: Bora rice is potential polysaccharide for colon targeted drug delivery system.

Introduction

Colonic drug delivery is intended for the local treatment of ulcerative colitis, irritable bowel syndrome and can potentially be used for colon cancer or the administration of drugs that are adversely affected by the upper gastro-intestinal (GI) tract.[1] The colon is an ideal site for protein and peptide absorption.[2] Acidic and enzymatic degradation are major obstacles in the oral administration of peptide drugs, but by targeting to the colon the proteolysis can be minimized. There has been considerable research in the design of colonic delivery systems and targeting has been achieved by several ways.[3] The primary approaches to the colonic delivery of the drugs included prodrugs, coating with pH-sensitive and time-dependent polymers. Nevertheless, these parameters i.e. pH and time can vary from one individual to the next and also according to the pathological and dietary conditions. So these systems can lead to premature and non-specific drug delivery in the colon and they have limited success. Precise colonic drug delivery requires that the triggering mechanism in the delivery system only response to the physiological conditions particular to the colon. Polysaccharides are widely used in oral dtug delivery systems because of the simplicity to obtained the desired drug delivery system and drug release profile, by the control of cross-linking, insolubility of crosslinked beads in gastric environment and and broad regulatory acceptance. The includes sodium alginate, pectin, chitosan, xantan gum, guar gum, starch, dextran and gellan.[4]

Pectin is a predominately linear polymer of mainly α-(1-4)- linked to D-galacturonic acid residues interrupted by 1, 2-linked L-rhamnase residues. Pectin is a polysaccharide found in the cell walls of plants.[5] The rationale for the development of a polysaccharide based delivery system for colon is the ability of the colonic microflora to degrade various types of polysaccharides that escape small bowel digestion. Pectins are polysaccharides and consist of linear polymers of d-galacturonic acid residues with varying degrees of methyl ester substituents. The degree of esterification (DE) and degree of amidation (DA), which are both expressed as a percentage of carboxyl groups (esterified or amidated), are important means to classify pectin. It is totally degraded by colonic bacteria but is not digested in the upper GI tract.[6] One

***Corresponding author:** Kuldeep Hemraj Ramteke, Department of Pharmaceutics, Modern College of Pharmacy (for ladies), Moshi, Dist-Pune, Maharashtra, India. Email: dr.kuldeepramteke@gmail.com

interesting approach is to use calcium salts of pectin because calcium binding reduces the solubility and induces non-covalent associations of carbohydrate chains through "egg – box" complex.[7,8] Bora rice is a natural polysaccharide having higher concentration of amylopectin (>98%) than that of the starch due to which it is more resistant to the gastric fluid of the upper GIT and at the same time it is degraded in the colon. Though bora rice can be used as a very good substitute for other starch in the development of colon targeted drug delivery system, it becomes important to establish the bora rice polysaccharide as controlled release polymer. Glipizide is a second-generation sulfonylurea that can acutely lower the blood glucose level in humans by stimulating the release of insulin from the pancreas and is typically prescribed to treat type II diabetes (non-insulin dependent diabetes mellitus). Its short biological half-life (2-4 hr) necessitates it to be administered 2.5 to 10 mg per day in 2 to 3 doses.[9] It shows pH dependent solubility thus, the development of controlled release dosage form would be much more advantageous than the conventional tablets.[10,11]

Materials and Methods

Materials

Glipizide was obtained as a gift sample from Standmed Pharmaceuticals, Kolkata, Amidated low methoxy pectin (PT) (DE≈25% and DA≈21%) was purchased from Loba chem., Mumbai, Bora rice (BR) was purchased from the local market of Dibrugarh, Calcium chloride dehydrated ($CaCl_2$), Barium chloride ($BaCl_2$) and Zinc acetate {$Zn(CH_3COO)_2$} was purchased from SD fine chemicals, Mumbai. All other chemicals and reagents used were of analytical grade.

Methods

Formulation of trial batches of Pectin-Bora Rice (PT-BR) hydrogel beads of glipizide

The standard ionotropic gelation technique[12,13] was used for the preparation of the hydrogel beads with slight modification as described below:

Aqueous dispersion of Pectin-Bora Rice (1:2) was prepared and kept overnight. Appropriate amount of the model drug glipizide (2:1 polymer:drug) was dispersed in the PT-BR dispersion until an uniform dispersion was obtained. The bubble free dispersion was added drop wise, through a disposable syringe (nozzle of 1.0 mm inner diameter) to a 200 ml of a gently agitated solution of the crosslinking agents i.e. [$CaCl_2$, $BaCl_2$ and Zn $(CH_3COO)_2$] at room temperature separately as shown in Table 1. The distance of falling of the drops was 5 cm. The gelled particles thus formed were allowed to remain in the crosslinking solution up to different duration of time period. The particles were subsequently washed with purified water, in order to remove Cl^- and excess of Ca^{2+}, Ba^{2+} and Zn^{2+} ions and separated by filtration. The particles were air dried for 24 hr and stored in a desiccator at room temperature.

Similarly pectin beads (PB) were also prepared by using pectin alone without bora rice by the above gelation technique.

Table 1. Formulation of trial batches of drug loaded PT-BR beads.

Batch Code	PT-BR ratio (%w/w)	Polymer:Drug ratio(%w/w)	Cross linking agent	Conc. of cross-linking agent (%w/v)	Curing time (hr)
T1	1:2	2:1	$CaCl_2$	2	2
T2	1:2	2:1	$CaCl_2$	4	4
T3	1:2	2:1	$CaCl_2$	6	6
T4	1:2	2:1	$BaCl_2$	2	2
T5	1:2	2:1	$BaCl_2$	4	4
T6	1:2	2:1	$BaCl_2$	6	6
T7	1:2	2:1	Zn $(CH_3COO)_2$	2	2
T8	1:2	2:1	Zn $(CH_3COO)_2$	4	4
T9	1:2	2:1	Zn $(CH_3COO)_2$	6	6
PB	3:0	2:1	Zn $(CH_3COO)_2$	6	6

Formulation of factorial design batches of PT-BR hydrogel beads of glipizide

The response surface approach involving 3^2 randomized full factorial design was adopted for optimization purpose. In this design, two factors each was evaluated at three levels and experimental trial were performed at all nine possible combinations, as presented in Table 2. Polymer:Drug ratio (A) and % of zinc acetate (B) were selected as independent variables. The percentage of drug release, entrapment efficiency, particle size and swelling index were selected as four dependent variables.

Evaluation of trial and factorial design batches of PT-BR beads

Entrapment efficiency (EE):[14] Hydrogel beads equivalent to 5 mg of glipizide were crushed in a glass mortar-pestle and the powdered beads were suspended in 50 ml phosphate buffer (pH 7.4). After 24 hr the solution was sonicate for 1 hr, filtered and the filtrate was analyzed by a UV spectrophotometer (Shimadzu UV-1601 UV/VIS double beam spectrophotometer) method at the wavelength of 276 nm for the drug content. The drug entrapment efficiency was calculated as per the following formula:

% EE = (Estimated drug content/Theoretical drug content) × 100

The drug entrapment efficiency of the beads of T7 to T9 of trial batches and formulations P1 to P9 of factorial batches have been determined.

Table 2. Formulation of 3^2 full factorial design batches of PT-BR beads of glipizide.

Batch code	Variable level (A)	Variable level (B)	Polymer to Drug ratio (% w/w)	Conc. of cross-linking agent (% w/v)
P1	-1	-1	1:1	2
P2	-1	0	1:1	4
P3	-1	1	1:1	6
P4	0	-1	2:1	2
P5	0	0	2:1	4
P6	0	1	2:1	6
P7	1	-1	3:1	2
P8	1	0	3:1	4
P9	1	1	3:1	6

Micromeritic properties of drug loaded PT-BR beads:[15]
Bulk density: Apparent bulk density (D_b) was determined by pouring the beads into a graduated cylinder. The bulk volume (V_b) and weight of the beads (M) was determined. The bulk density was calculated using the formula

$$D_b = V_b/M$$

Tapped density: The measuring cylinder containing a known mass of beads was tapped for 100 times. The minimum volume (V_t) occupied in the cylinder and weight (M) of the beads was measured. The tapped density (D_t) was calculated by following formula

$$D_t = V_t/M$$

Angle of repose: Angle of repose was determined using funnel method. The beads were poured through a funnel that was raised vertically on the plane surface until a maximum cone hight (h) was obtained. Radius of the heap (r) was measured and the angle of repose (θ) was calculated using following formula

$$\theta = \tan^{-1}(h/r)$$

Swelling Index:[16] A known weight (100 mg) of various glipizide loaded PT-BR beads were placed in phosphate buffer, pH 7.4 and allowed to swell at 37 °C ± 0.5 °C in the USP type II dissolution rate test apparatus (Electrolab TDT-06T, India). The beads were periodically removed and blotted with filter paper; then gain in weight (after correcting for drug loss) of the beads were measured until attainment of constant weight. The swelling index (SI) was calculated using the following formula:

$$\mathbf{SI = (w_g - w_0)/w_0}$$

SI= Swelling index

w_g = Final weight of beads

w_0 = Initial weight of beads

Particle size analysis*:* Particle size of beads was determined by optical microscopy method. Approximately 100 particles were counted by using calibrated occular micrometer in an optical microscope (Nikon, DR-06M, Japan).

Kinetics of drug release: Different mathematical models i.e. zero order, first order and Higuchi equations were applied for describing the kinetics of the drug release process from controlled released colon targeted glipizide beads, the most suited being the one which fitted best the experimental results. The data obtained from *in-vitro* drug release studies were used to calculate the correlation coefficient (R) value between 'cumulative amount of drug released and time' for zero order, 'log cumulative percentage of drug remaining and time' for first order and 'cumulative percentage of drug released and square root of time' for Higuchi's model. The best fit model was considered to that one which had maximum 'R' value (~ 1).

In vitro dissolution rate study of trial and factorial design batches beads:
Preparation of 4.0% w/v rat cecal material:[17] Male albino rats were taken weighing 200 - 250 g and maintained at normal diet and administered orally 1 ml of 2.0% w/v aqueous dispersion of PT:BR (1:1) daily for 7 days for induction of reductive and hydrolytic enzymes like β-glucoronidase, β-xylosidase, β-galactosidase, α-arabinosidase, nitroreductase, azoreductase, deaminase and urea hydrosylase in the colonic bacteria of the animals. The experiment was conducted in the laboratory of Jay Research Foundation (JRF), Vapi, Gujrat on the permission of the IAEC of JRF with their CPCSEA registration number 35/1999 CPCSEA. Six rats were asphyxiated using carbon dioxide. Their abdomens were opened, the cecal were traced, legated at both ends, dissected, and immediately transferred into previously weighed beaker containing 100 ml of phosphate buffer PBS, pH 7.4 previously bubbled with CO_2. The cecal content in the beaker, was weighed and required volume of PBS, pH 7.4 was added to provide desired concentration (4.0% w/v) of the rat cecal material in the buffer. Then the suspension was filtered through cotton wool and was used as simulated colonic fluid. Because the cecum is naturally anaerobic, all of these operations were carried out under anaerobic condition i.e. in presence of CO_2.

In vitro drug release (DR) study of beads of trial and factorial design batches in 4.0 % w/v rat cecal medium: The *in vitro* drug release study was carried out using USP XXIV paddle type apparatus (Electrolab, TDT-06T, India) at 37 ± 0.5 °C and at 75 rpm using 500 ml of phosphate buffer (pH 7.4) containing 4.0 %w/v rat cecal material as a dissolution medium. Hydrogel beads equivalent to 5 mg of glipizide were used for the test. Samples (5ml) were withdrawn at predetermined time intervals replacing equal volume of fresh dissolution medium. The samples were transferred into a series of 10 ml volumetric flask, diluted suitably with PBS, pH 7.4 and centrifuged. The supernatant was filtered through 0.45 μm membrane filter and the filtrate was analyzed in a UV spectrophotometer at 276 nm wavelength using a blank prepared exactly the same way without the drug.

Solid state characterization of factorial design batches: *FTIR study*: Mixed glipizide, BR, PT-BR beads powder and drug loaded PT-BR beads powder with KBr individually. KBr pallets were prepared by using KBr press. FTIR spectra of Glipizide, PT-BR beads and drug loaded PT-BR beads were obtained in KBr pellets using a JASCO model 5300, Italy FTIR spectrophotometer in the range of 4000 to 400 cm^{-1}.

XRD study: X-ray powder diffractograms of glipizide, bora rice, pectin-bora rice placebo beads and drug loaded PT-BR beads were recorded on powder X-ray diffractometer (Bruker AXS D8 Advance, Germany). The samples were irradiated with monochromatized Cu Kα radiation (1.54060 °A) and analyzed between 10 and 40, 2θ (Degree). The voltage and current used were 30 kV and 30 mA, respectively. The range and chart speed were 2 X 10^3 cps and 10mm/2θ, respectively.

Thermal Studies: Thermograms of samples were obtained by a Prkin-Elmer Differential Scanning Colorimeter. Samples of 10mg were accurately weighed into aluminum pans and then hermetically sealed with aluminum lids. The thermograms of samples were obtained at a scanning rate of 10 °C/ min over a temperature range of 50 to 250 °C under the flow of nitrogen gas at a rate of 20 ml/min.

Shape and Surface morphology: Surface and shape morphology of PT-BR beads were evaluated by means of Tabletop microscopy (TM) (HITACHI TM1000). The samples of TM were prepared by lightly sprinkling the beads on a double adhesive tape, which struck to an aluminum stub.

In vivo Gamma Scintigraphy study of the optimized factorial design batch formulation of glipizide: Three Wistar rats, weighing 200 – 250 g were taken for the study. The animals were fasted for 12 hr prior to commencement of the experiment. Radiolabled (>90%) beads (50 mg) of formulation P9 was administered orally to the animals with the help of feeding tube, followed by sufficient volume of drinking water. All four legs of rat were tied over a piece of plywood and the location of the formulation in GI tract was monitored keeping the subject in front of gamma camera. The total radiation dosimetry for each rat was 0.1 mSv.

Scintigraphy image was captured using a Siemens E-Cam gamma camera fitted with a LEHR collimator. The image schedule was as follows: 1 minute, 15 minutes and 450 minutes after dosing. During the gamma scintigraphy scanning, the animals were freed and allowed to move and carry out normal activity. The experiment was conducted in the laboratory of Bombay Veterinary College (BVC), Mumbai, (Maharashtra) permitted by the IAEC of BVC with the CPCSEA registration number BVC/IAEC/23/2010.

Stability study of the optimized factorial design batch formulation of glipizide: Accelerated stability study was conducted on the optimized formulation P9. The samples were stored at 40 °C ± 2 °C and 75% ± 5% RH for 3 months period. The sample was withdrawn periodically and subjected to dissolution rate determination.

For the comparison of release profiles of the samples of stability studies, "difference factor", f_1 and "similarity factor", f_2 were calculated.[18] The difference factor (f_1) measures the percent error between the two curves over all time points and was calculated using following equation.

$$f1 = \frac{\sum_{j=1}^{n} |R_j - T_j|}{\sum_{j=1}^{n} R_j}$$

Where, 'n' is the number of sampling points, R_j and T_j are the percent dissolved of the reference and test samples at each time point j respectively. The two release profiles are considered to be similar, if f_1 value is lower than 15 (between 0 and 15).

The similarity factor (f_2) is a logarithmic transformation of the sum of squared error of differences between the test T_j and the reference sample R_j over all time points. It was calculated as follows.

$$f_2 = 50 \log \{ [1 + (1/n) \sum_{j=1}^{n} W_j |Rj - T_j|]^2 \times 100 \}$$

Where, w_j is an optional weight factor and other terms are as defined earlier.

Statistical analysis and modeling: Analysis of variance (ANOVA) was used for the analysis of regression coefficient, predicted equations and case statistics. The experimental results of response surface methodology (RSM) were fitted via the response surface regression procedure, using the following second order polynomial equation:

$$Y = \beta_0 + \sum \beta_i X_i + \sum \beta_{ii} X_i^2 + \sum \beta_{ij} X_i X_j$$

Where Y is the predicted response, X_i and X_j are independent variables, β_0 is the intercept term, β_i is the linear coefficient, β_{ii} is the quadratic coefficient and β_{ij} is the interaction coefficient.

However, in this study, the independent variables are coded as A and B. Thus the second order polynomial equation is represented as follows

$$Y = \beta_0 + \beta_1 A + \beta_2 B + \beta_{12} AB + \beta_{11} A^2 + \beta_{22} B^2$$

The main effects (A and B) represent the average result of changing one factor at a time from its low to high value. The interaction terms A and B show how the response changes when 2 factors were simultaneously changed. The polynomial terms (β_{12} and β_{22}) are included to investigate non-linearity.

Model graphs were obtained by using the Design Expert software (Design Expert 8.0) to analyze the effect of variables individually and its interaction to determine their optimum level. The point prediction method was used for optimization of the levels of each variable for maximum response.

Results and Discussion

Formulation of PT-BR hydrogel beads of glipizide

The formulae of the trial batches and the factorial design batches of drug loaded PT-BR hydrogel beads have been shown in Table 1 and 2 respectively. Calcium chloride, barium chloride and zinc acetate were selected as cross-linking agent for PT-BR beads for trial batches formulation. Cross-linking time selected was 4 hr. The curing time was selected as more the time showed better cross linking and hence the release was retarded. The cross-linking agent calcium chloride did not give proper strength to the beads which might be due to the addition of bora rice. In case of barium chloride, PT-BR cross-linked with Ba^{++} ions where pallets were formed instead of beads. This effect might be due the presence of bora rice in pectin gel suspension, pectin loses its cross-linking property to some extend as calcium and barium ions forms the weak linkage with carboxyl groups in the pectin chain during "egg-box" formation.[19] Zinc cations produced an extensive cross-linking and less permeable pectinate matrix than calcium and barium cations. Thus, it can be concluded that zinc forms stronger network due to its interaction with pectin with a higher binding affinity and selectivity than calcium and barium. Therefore zinc cross-linked PT-BR beads are more suitable than calcium and barium cross-linked beads for the use as a colonic delivery carrier. Also, zinc formed spherical beads with PT-BR. Hence for factorial design batches zinc acetate was selected as cross-linking agent.

Evaluation of trial batch PT-BR hydrogel beads of glipizide

Evaluation parameters of the trial batch PT-BR beads have been produced in the Table 3 and Figure 1. Formulation T7 showed 100 % drug release within 20 hr. T7 showed larger particle size, and lesser entrapment efficiency as compared to formulation T8 and T9. The complete release of the drug within 20 hr from the formulation T7 might be due to less concentration of cross-linking agent (2.0 %w/v) and lesser exposure time (2 hr) to the cross-linking solution. On other hand as cross-linking concentration and exposure time was increased in the formulation T8 to 4.0 %w/v and 4 hr respectively 100% drug released was recorded within 24 hr and drug entrapment efficiency was found to be 52.65% which is an acceptable value. In case of formulation T9 where the concentration of cross-linking agent was 6.0 %w/v with the exposure time of 6 hr the drug release has been recorded as 100% within 24 hr similar to the formulation T8. Therefore, as the same results have been obtained out of the formulation T8 and T9 we have selected the formulation T8 for the factorial design batches with a lesser concentration of cross-linking agent (4.0 %w/v) and exposure time 4 hr than that of the formulation T9 which contained more amount of cross-linking agent.

Table 3. Evaluation parameters of trial batch PT-BR beads.

Batch code	% Drug Release (24 hr) (± SD)	Particle size (mm) (± SD)	Drug Entrapment Efficiency (%) (± SD)	Swelling index (± SD)
T7	100.23 ± 1.25 **(20 hr)**	1.289 ± 0.23	41.46 ± 0.25	0.743 ± 0.074
T8	100.65 ± 1.57 **(24 hr)**	1.135 ± 0.12	52.65 ± 0.16	1.068 ± 0.018
T9	100.42 ± 1.43 **(24 hr)**	1.132 ± 0.11	51.21± 0.20	1.077 ± 0.012
PB	100.16 ± 1.16 **(12 hr)**	0.864 ± 0.43	51.67 ± 0.83	0.732 ± 0.047

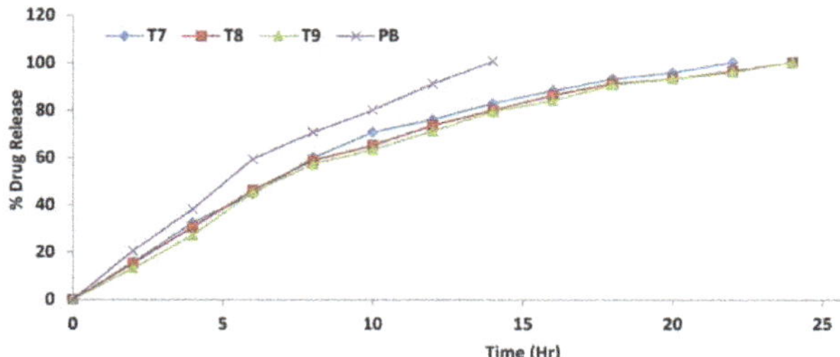

Figure 1. In vitro dissolution study of trial batches PT-BR beads (T7, T8, T9 and PB Beads)

The beads prepared from only the pectin gel, formulation PB, showed 100% drug release within 12 hr even at higher concentration of cross-linking agent (6.0 %w/v) with the larger exposure time (6 hr) when compared to the beads containing bora rice and pectin i.e. T7, T8 and T9.

Evaluation of factorial design batches of PT-BR beads of glipizide

On the basis of the preliminary trials a 3^2 full factorial design was adopted to study the effect of independent variables (i.e polymer to drug ratio [A] and cross-linking concentration [B] on dependent variables, percent drug release, entrapment efficiency, particle size and swelling index. The result is presented in Table 4 and Figure 2. From the result it is clear that the release profile of factorial design batch beads were in the order of P1>P2>P3>P4>P5>P6>P7>P8>P9. The concentration of cross-linking agent and polymer influence the control of drug release for 24 hr. The concentration of cross-linking agent is inversely proportional to drug release, particle size and swelling index but it is directly proportional to the drug entrapment efficiency which might be due the formation of more dense network with pectin and bora rice. On the other hand the effect of polymer concentration is also inversely proportional to the drug release and directly proportional to the particle size, drug entrapment efficiency and swelling index which might be due to the presence of the bora rice in the formulation.

Formulation P9 showed 91.06% of drug release within 24 hr and highest drug entrapment efficiency i.e. 68.21% among all other formulations (P1 to P9), hence formulation P9 was selected for the further studies.

Table 4. Evaluation parameters of factorial design batch PT–BR beads of glipizide.

Batch code	% Drug Release (± SD) (12 hr)	% Drug release (± SD) (24hr)	Particle size (mm) (± SD)	Entrapment Efficiency (%) (± SD)	Swelling index (± SD)
P1	76.01 ± 1.25	100.89 ± 1.48 **(20 hr)**	1.117 ± 0.21	43.23 ± 0.18	0.843 ± 0.034
P2	71.67 ± 1.32	99.40± 1.34 **(22 hr)**	1.113 ± 0.14	44.15 ± 0.13	0.723 ± 0.026
P3	69.03 ± 1.56	99.60 ± 1.22 **(22 hr)**	1.107 ± 0.12	45.22 ± 0.15	0.657 ± 0.031
P4	66.4 ± 1.12	100.85 ± 1.63	1.142 ± 0.17	50.07 ± 0.26	1.172 ± 0.017
P5	64.17 ± 1.57	100.65 ± 1.14	1.135 ± 0.13	52.65 ± 0.16	1.068 ± 0.018
P6	60.85 ± 1.32	100.10 ± 1.58	1.128 ± 0.22	54.23 ± 0.12	0.947 ± 0.014
P7	63.22 ± 1.61	96.26 ± 1.26	1.182 ± 0.14	65.04 ± 0.15	1.456 ± 0.02
P8	62.37 ± 1.32	94.38 ± 1.32	1.163 ± 0.21	66.14 ± 0.2	1.343 ± 0.018
P9	59.11 ± 1.16	91.06 ± 1.40	1.156 ± 0.13	68.21 ± 0.14	1.278 ± 0.022

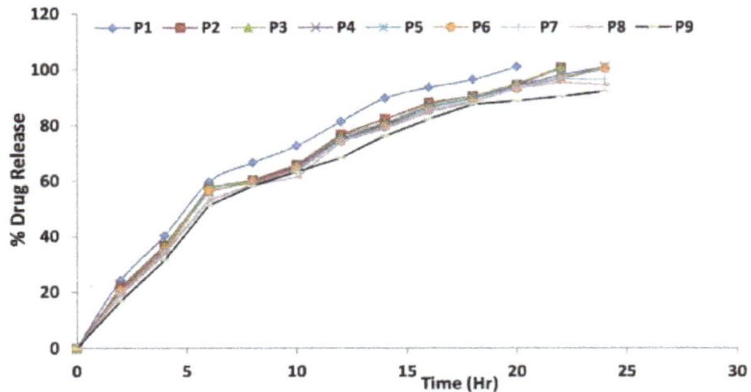

Figure 2. In Vitro dissolution study of factorial design batches PT-BR beads (P1 to P9)

Micromeretic properties of PT–BR beads

The values of bulk density, tapped density and angle of repose have been depicted in Table 5 for trial and factorial design batches of PT–BR beads. The flow properties of material considered as excellent, good, poor, very poor if the angle of repose (θ) value is <20°, 25° to 30°, 30° to 40° and >40° respectively. The angle of repose, 31.37° to 36.54° of trial and factorial design batch beads indicated that the beads possess poor flow property which might be due to less spherical structure of the PT–BR beads.

Table 5. Micromeretic properties of trial and factorial design batch PT–BR beads.

Batch Code	Bulk Density (g/cc) (± SD)	Tapped Density (g/cc) (± SD)	Angle of Repose (θ^0) (± SD)
T7	0.986 ± 0.072	1.05 ± 0.068	36.54 ± 2.56
T8	0.854 ± 0.034	1.10 ± 0.076	32.34 ± 1.95
T9	0.861 ± 0.044	1.19 ± 0.061	33.24 ± 1.78
P1	0.842 ± 0.065	1.45 ± 0.12	33.54 ± 2.47
P2	0.835 ± 0.09	1.36 ± 0.086	32.55 ± 2.13
P3	0.865 ± 0.057	1.49 ± 0.083	33.74 ± 1.95
P4	0.851 ± 0.078	1.47 ± 0.08	32.62 ± 2.12
P5	0.854 ± 0.034	1.10 ± 0.076	32.34 ± 1.95
P6	0.852 ± 0.019	1.124 ± 0.036	31.56 ± 1.87
P7	0.859 ± 0.045	1.120 ± 0.033	31.42 ± 2.06
P8	0.856 ± 0.025	1.123 ± 0.023	32.12 ± 1.76
P9	0.843 ± 0.015	1.118 ± 0.034	31.37 ± 2.09

Kinetics of drug release

The release rate constant was calculated from the slope of appropriate equations and the correlation coefficient (R) was determined for all the formulations (Table 6). The release profile and the entrapment efficiency of formulation P9 was found to be satisfactory in comparison to other formulation, the discussion on the kinetics of other formulations was not considered further.

In vitro drug release of P9 was best explained by k-peppas equation with highest linearity (R_p=0.9985), followed by Higuchi's equation, (R_h=0.9836) and First order (R_1=0.981). This indicates that the drug was diffused from polymeric matrix. The drug release was found to be very closed to Higuchi kinetics which indicates that the drug diffuses at a comparatively slower rate as the distance of diffusion increases.

Table 6. Analysis of *in vitro* dissolution data of factorial design batches of PT-BR beads.

Batch Code		P1	P2	P3	P4	P5	P6	P7	P8	P9
Zero order	R_0	0.906	0.8868	0.9106	0.937	0.9464	0.9501	0.9517	0.9659	0.9611
	K_0	6.1021	5.239	5.0995	4.7935	4.7642	4.6717	4.4993	4.3133	4.2492
1st order	R_1	0.9506	0.8746	0.8256	0.8367	0.8476	0.8734	0.9474	0.9541	0.981
	K_1	-0.1423	-0.1476	-0.1439	-0.1458	-0.1421	-0.1432	-0.1034	-0.0915	-0.0853
Higuchi	R_h	0.9933	0.9925	0.9955	0.9914	0.9893	0.9871	0.9862	0.9806	0.9836
	K_h	22.07	20.885	20.261	19.760	19.604	19.204	18.489	17.661	17.424
k-peppas	R_p	0.9961	0.9963	0.9925	0.9961	0.9974	0.9963	0.997	0.9983	0.9985
	K_p	18.28	17.679	16.011	15.185	13.809	13.376	11.986	10.084	10.071
	n_p	0.5787	0.5652	0.5908	0.5954	0.628	0.6317	0.6586	0.7047	0.701

Mechanism of drug release

The K_p value of P1 to P9 decreases and n_p value increases (Table 6) as the concentration of PT-BR polymer and cross-linking agent increases which reveled that the rate of drug release decreases as the concentration of PT-BR polymer and cross-linking agent increase in the formulation (Table 4).

The n_p value indicated the mechanism of drug release from beads of P1 to P9. All the formulation showed n_p value >0.5 and <1 during the entire period of drug release (24 hr) as shown in Table 6. This indicated that the drug release from the beads followed non-fickian diffusion. Anomalous diffusion of drug release mechanism signifies a coupling of the diffusion and erosion mechanism i.e. the drug release is controlled by more than one process. Hence the drug release from formulation P9 (n_p = 0.701) is controlled by both diffusion and erosion process in 24 hr study.

Solid state characterization of factorial design batches of PT–BR beads

FTIR study

FTIR spectra of glipizide, bora rice, PT-BR beads and drug loaded PT-BR beads are shown in Figure 3.

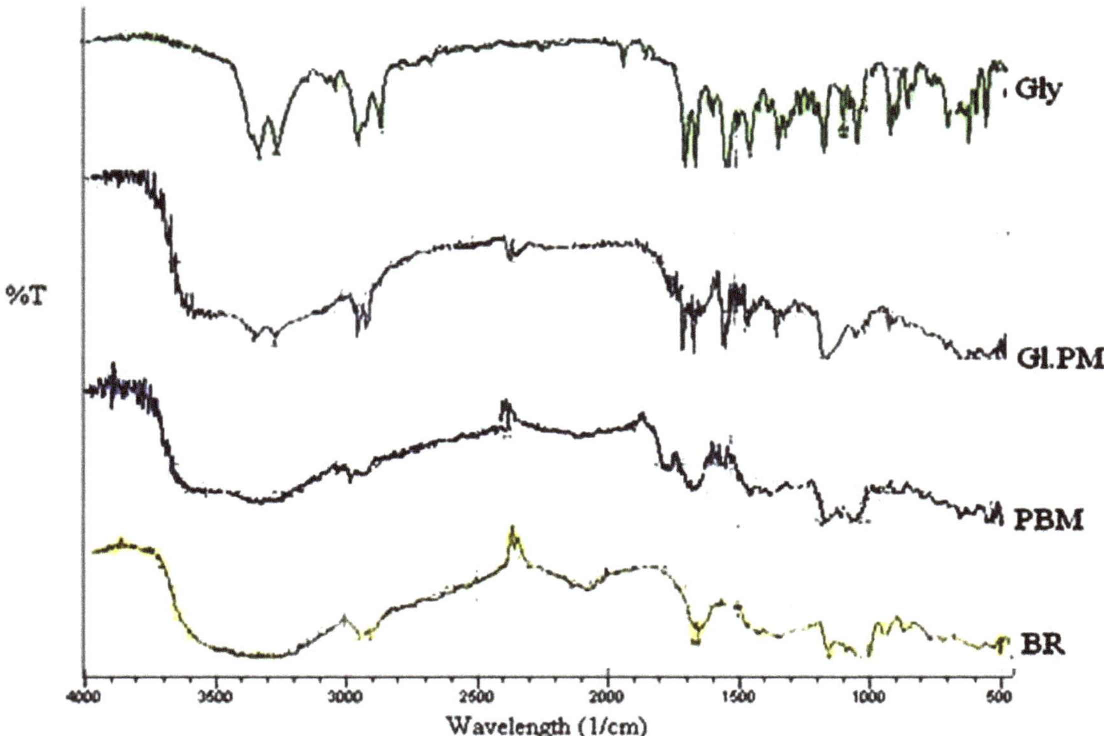

Figure 3. FTIR spectra of Glipizide (Gly), Glipizide loaded PT-BR beads (Gl.PM), PT-BR beads without drug (PBM), Bora Rice (BR)

Glipizide showed prominent peaks at 1651, 3480, 3030, 1690, and 2943 due to the presence of C=N aliphatic groups, N-H stretching, aromatic –CH stretching, C=O stretching and C-H_2 aliphatic respectively. The same peaks were also observed in the formulation of drug loaded PT-BR beads indicating the stable nature of the drug during encapsulation.

XRD study

X-ray diffraction analysis of the PT-BR placebo beads and drug loaded PT-BR beads were performed to charaterize the physical state of the loaded drug in the polymeric matrix.[20] The characteristics X-ray diffraction spectra of pure drug (glipizide), bora rice, placebo PT-BR beads and drug loaded PT-BR beads are presented in the Figure 4. Characteristic crystalline peaks of glipizide were observed at 2θ of 14.5, 16.8, 19.5, 23.3, 26.7 and 29.5, indicating the presence of crystalline glipizide. XRD spectra of Bora rice and placebo PT–BR beads did not show any peaks which indicates its amorphous nature. Glipizide loaded PT-BR beads shows some peaks but not as the intensity of glipizide. Hence it revealed that the glipizide was present in the drug loaded pectin-bora rice beads in dispersed form.

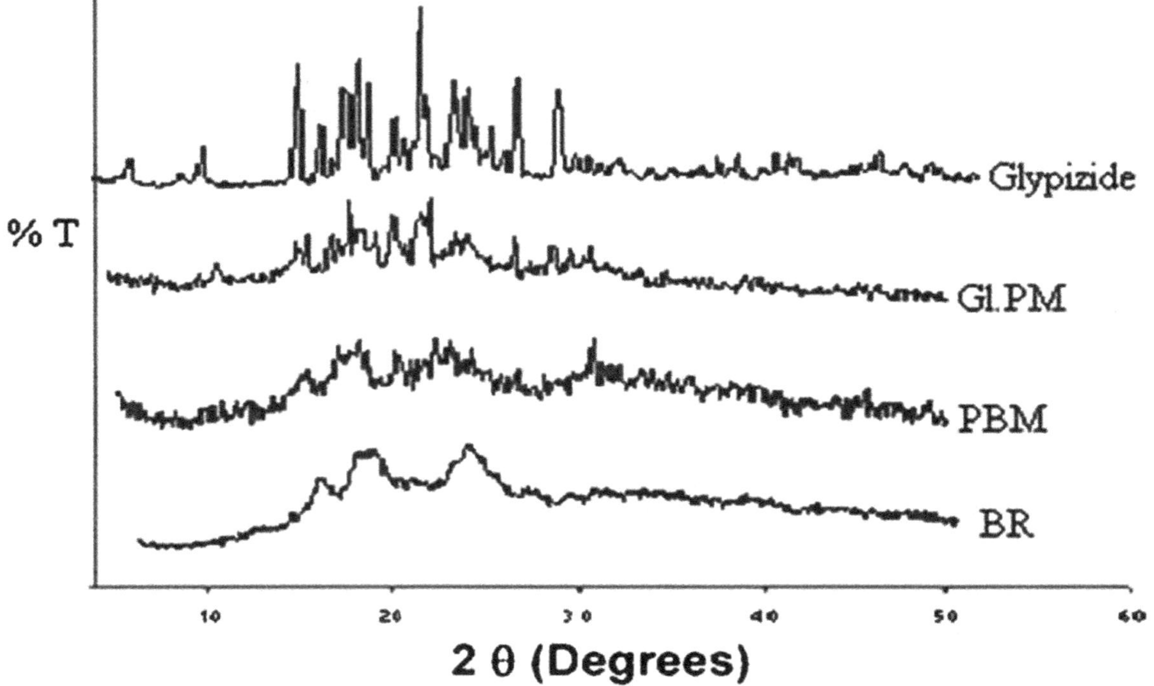

Figure 4. XRD spectra of Glipizide, Glipizide loaded PT-BR beads (Gl.PM), PT-BR beads without drug (PBM), Bora Rice (BR)

DSC study

DSC study was performed to check the possible interaction of glipizide with other excipients the PT–BR beads. The comparision of DSC thermograpm of placebo PT–BR beads and drug loaded PT–BR beads along with glipizide and pectin are presented in Figure 5. Glipizide gave a sharp endothermic peak at 212.90 °C and the drug loaded PT–BR beads (Gl.PM) shows a peak at 209.65 °C which indicated that there were no any interaction between the glipizide and PT-BR polymer.

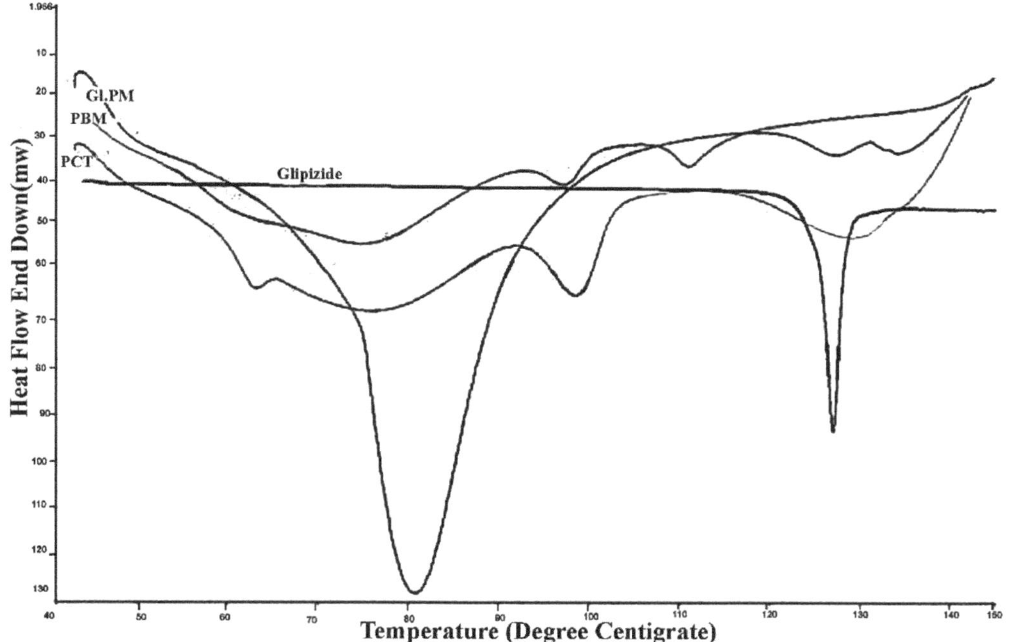

Figure 5. DSC thermogram of Glipizide, Glipizide loaded PT-BR beads (Gl.PM), PT-BR beads without drug (PBM), Pectin (PCT)

The broad hemp of Gl.PM, PBM and PCT in the range of 100 to 120 °C indicated the presence of moisture in the formulation. PBM showed two peaks at 147.63 °C and 162.38 °C, and PCT showed one peak at 146.43 °C which may be due to presence of impurity in the pectin.

Shape and Surface Morphology

As shown in the Figure 6 Tabletop microscopy revealed that PT-BR beads were discrete and spherical in shape with rough and porous outer surface at higher magnification because of adherence of drug crystals on the surface of beads.

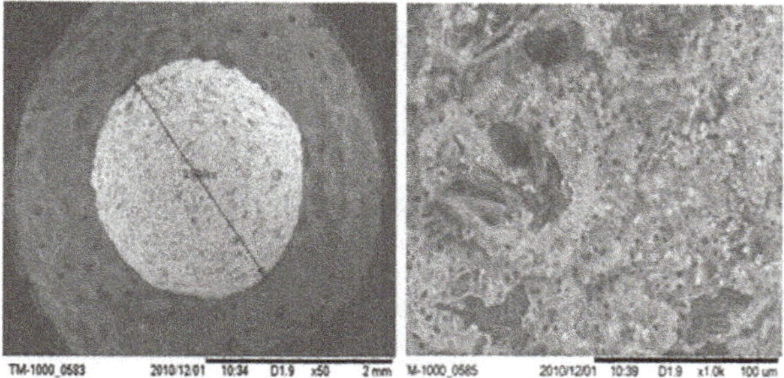

Figure 6. TM Photograph of glipizide loaded PT-BR beads

In vivo gamma scintigraphy study of the optimized factorial design batch formulation of glipizide

As shown in Figure 7 gamma scintigraphy study in rat showed that the beads were intact in the hostile environment of the stomach but whenever they reached to the colonic region they start degradation due to presence of anaerobic bacteria present in the colon.

Stability study of the optimized factorial design batch formulation of glipizide

The optimized formulation (P9) was evaluated for difference factor (f_1) and similarity factor (f_2) of dissolution rate study after 3 months of storage at accelerated condition (40 °C ± 2 °C and 75% ± 5% RH), the results of which are shown in Table 7 and Figure 8. The dissolution profile of the formulation at initial stage was considered as reference for calculation of dissimilarity factor (f_1) and similarity factor (f_2). When the value of f_2 lies between 50 to 100 and f_1 is less than 15, the two dissolution profiles (test and reference) are considered to be similar. The results obtained (Table 7) revealed that the dissolution profile of formulations after 3 months of storage at accelerated condition was similar with the initial dissolution profile of formulation. Based on the results it was considered that the formulation is stable after 3 months of storage at accelerated stability conditions.

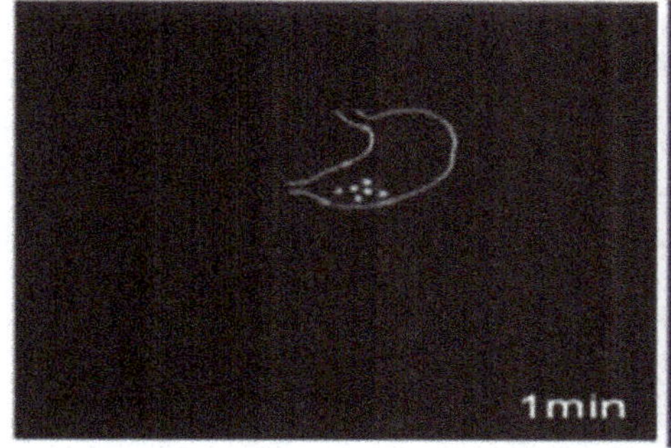

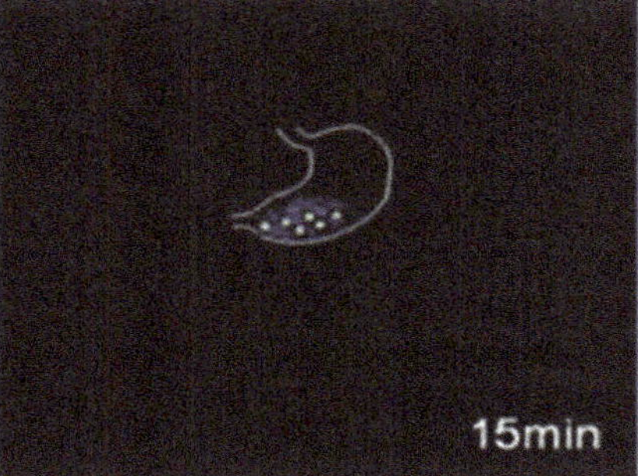

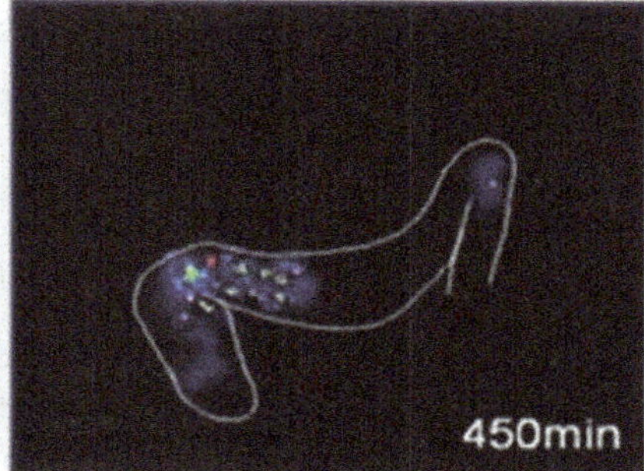

Figure 7. Gamma scintigraphy showed p9 instead of P9

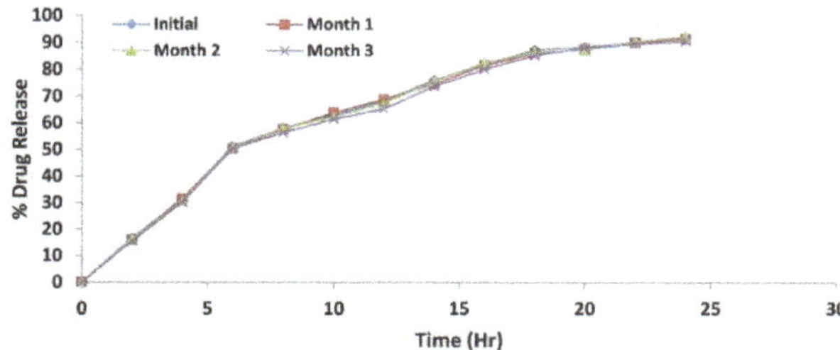

Figure 8. In vitro dissolution profile of the optimized formulation (P9) after subjected to stability study (Initial, Month 1, Month 2 and Month 3)

Table 7. Evaluation of PT-BR beads (P9) after 3 months of storage at 40 °C ± 2 °C and 75% RH ± 5 % RH.

Parameter	Initial	One month	Two months	Three months
f_1 value*	---	2.43	3.21	4.65
f_2 value*	---	85.32	78.56	73.48

*Initial sample (0 month) was taken as reference to calculate f_1 and f_2 values

Statistical Analysis and Modeling

The application of response surface methodology (RSM) offers an empirical relationship between the response variable DR_{12hr}, Entrapment Efficiency (EE), Particle Size, Swelling Index and the test variables under conditions. Quadratic model (partial sum squares type-III) was selected for all the RSM studies. By applying multiple regression analysis on the experimental data, the response variable DR_{12hrs} and the test variables A (Polymer to Drug ratio) and B (% of Zinc acetate) were related by second order polynomial equation.

Final equation in terms of coded factors:

$$\text{Drug Release (12 hr)} = 63.81 - 5.34A - 2.77B + 3.09A^2$$

Final equation in terms of actual factors:

$$\text{Drug Release (12 hr)} = +92.38034 - 17.69509(\text{PT-BR}) - 1.38462(\text{CLA}) + 3.08898(\text{PT-}\text{BR}^2)$$

It is observed from the coefficient estimation table and above equations that coefficient of 'A' and 'B' bears a negative sign. It signifies that on increasing the concentration of PT-BR and $Zn(CH_3COO)_2$ the DR_{12hrs} was decreased.

By applying multiple regression analysis on the experimental data, the response variable EE and the test variables A (Polymer to Drug ratio) and B (% of Zinc acetate) were related by second order polynomial equation.

Final equation in terms of coded factors:

$$\text{Entrapment Efficiency (\%)} = +52.00+11.17A+1.50B+0.25AB+3.17A^2$$

Final Equation in Terms of Actual Factors:

$$\text{Entrapment Efficiency (\%)} = +40.33333 +2.0000 (\text{PT-BR}) +0.50000 (\text{CLA})+0.1250 (\text{PT-BR} \times \text{CLA})+3.16667 (\text{PT-BR}^2)$$

It is observed from the coefficient estimation table and above equations that coefficient of 'A' and 'B' bears a positive sign. It signifies that on increasing the concentration of PT-BR and $Zn(CH_3COO)_2$ the EE was increased.

By applying multiple regression analysis on the experimental data, the response variable Particle Size and the test variables A (Polymer to Drug ratio) and B (% of Zinc acetate) were related by second order polynomial equation.

Final equation in terms of coded factors:

$$\text{Partical size (mm)} = +1.13+0.027A - 8.333E - 003B - 4.000E - 003AB+4.667E - 003A^2$$

Final Equation in Terms of Actual Factors:

$$\text{Partical size (mm)} = +1.09967 +0.016667(\text{PT-BR})-1.66667E-004(\text{CLA})-2.00000E-003(\text{PT-BR} \times \text{CLA})+4.66667E-003(\text{PT-BR}^2)$$

It is observed from the coefficient estimation table and above equations that coefficient of 'A' bears a positive sign indicating that when the PT-BR polymer concentration increased, particle size was also increased. Coefficient of 'B' bears negative sign indicated that concentration of $Zn(CH_3COO)_2$ is inversely proportional to particle size. It signifies that on increasing the concentration of PT-BR the particle size was increased and on increasing the concentration of $Zn(CH_3COO)_2$ the particle size was decreased.

By applying multiple regression analysis on the experimental data, the response variable Swelling Index and the test variables A (Polymer to Drug ratio) and B (% of Zinc acetate) were related by second order polynomial equation.

Final equation in terms of coded factors:

$$\text{Swelling Index} = +1.06 +0.31A -0.098 B +2.000E-003 AB -0.012A^2$$

Final Equation in Terms of Actual Factors:

$$\text{Swelling Index} = +0.59933 +0.35433(\text{PT-BR})-0.051083(\text{CLA})+1.00000E-003(\text{PT-BR} \times \text{CLA})-0.012333(\text{PT-BR})$$

It is observed from the coefficient estimation table and above equations that coefficient of 'A' bears a positive sign indicating that when the PT-BR polymer concentration increased, swelling index also increased. Coefficient of 'B' bears negative sign indicated that concentration of $Zn(CH_3COO)_2$ is inversely proportional to swelling index. It signifies that on increasing the concentration of PT-BR the swelling index was increased and on increasing the concentration of $Zn(CH_3COO)_2$ the swelling index was decreased.

Conclusion

The results of study clearly indicate that there is a great potential in delivery of glipizide to the colonic region. Study showed that the manipulation of polymer concentration and cross linking agent influence particle size of beads, sphericity and flow property of beads. From the above study it concluded that high concentration of Bora Rice will retard the drug release, may be due to high content of amylopectin present in the bora rice. Formulation P9 is the best formulation for controlling the drug release to the colon. Hence from the above study it concluded that high amylopectin containing bora rice, natural polysaccharide showed potential for controlled release colon targeting drug delivery.

Conflict of Interest

The authors declare that they have no conflict of interest.

References

1. Yang L, Chu JS, Fix JA. Colon-specific drug delivery: new approaches and in vitro/in vivo evaluation. *Int J Pharm* 2002;235(1-2):1-15.
2. Swarbrick J, Boylan JC. Encyclopedia of Pharmaceutical Technology. 2nd ed. New York: Marcel Dekker; 2002.
3. Vandamme F, Lenourry A, Charrueau C, Chaumeil JC. The use of polysaccharides to target drugs to the colon. *Carbohyd Polym* 2002;48(3):219-31.
4. Pawar AP, Gadhe AR, Venkatachalam P, Sher P, Mahadik KR. Effect of core and surface cross-linking on the entrapment of metronidazole in pectin beads. *Acta Pharm* 2008;58(1):78-85.
5. Sinha VR, Kumria R. Polysaccharides in colon-specific drug delivery. *Int J Pharm* 2001;224(1-2):19-38.
6. Liu L, Fishman ML, Kost J, Hicks KB. Pectin-based systems for colon-specific drug delivery via oral route. *Biomaterials* 2003;24(19):3333-43.
7. Sriamornsak P. Investigation of pectin as a carrier for oral delivery of proteins using calcium pectinate gel beads. *Int J Pharm* 1998;169(2):213-20.
8. Sriamornsak P, Nunthanid J. Calcium pectinage gel beads for controlled release drug delivery: I. Preparation and in vitro release studies. *Int J Pharm* 1998;160(2):207-12.
9. Foster RH, Plosker GL. Glipizide. A review of the pharmacoeconomic implications of the extended-release formulation in type 2 diabetes mellitus. *Pharmacoeconomics* 2000;18(3):289-306.
10. Thombre AG, Denoto AR, Gibbes DC. Delivery of glipizide from asymmetric membrane capsules using encapsulated excipients. *J Control Release* 1999;60(2-3):333-41.

11. Chowdary KP, Balatripura G. Design and evaluation of mucoadhesive controlled release oral tablets of glipizide. *Indian J Pharm Sci* 2003;65(6):591-4.
12. Aydin Z, Akburga J. Preparation and evaluation of pectin beads. *Int J Pharm* 1996;137(1):133-6.
13. Bourgeois S, Gernet M, Andremont A, Fattal E. Design and characterization of pectin beads for the colon delivery. Paper presented at: Fourth Word Meeting ADRITELF/PGI/APV 2002 Sept; Florence.
14. Bigucci F, Luppi B, Monaco L, Cerchiara T, Zecchi V. Pectin-based microspheres for colon-specific delivery of vancomycin. *J Pharm Pharmacol* 2009;61(1):41-6.
15. United States Pharmacopeia XXVII/National Formulary 22. Rockville, MD, USA: United States Pharmacopeial Convention; 2004.
16. El-Gibaly I. Oral delayed-release system based on Zn-pectinate gel (ZPG) microparticles as an alternative carrier to calcium pectinate beads for colonic drug delivery. *Int J Pharm* 2002;232(1-2):199-211.
17. Paharia A, Yadav AK, Rai G, Jain SK, Pancholi SS, Agrawal GP. Eudragit-coated pectin microspheres of 5-fluorouracil for colon targeting. *AAPS Pharm Sci Tech* 2007;8(1):12.
18. Moore J, Flanner H. Mathematical comparison of dissolution profiles. *Pharma Tech* 1996;20:64-74.
19. Dupuis G, Chambin O, Genelot C, Champion D, Pourcelot Y. Colonic drug delivery: influence of cross-linking agent on pectin beads properties and role of the shell capsule type. *Drug Dev Ind Pharm* 2006;32(7):847-55.
20. Desai KG. Preparation and characteristics of high-amylose corn starch/pectin blend microparticles: a technical note. *AAPS Pharm Sci Tech* 2005;6(2):E202-8.

Validated Spectrophotometric Quantification of Aripiprazole in Pharmaceutical Formulations by using Multivariate Technique

Kandikonda Sandeep[1]*, Madhusudhanareddy Induri[2], Muvvala Sudhakar[3]

[1] *Department of Pharmaceutical Analysis, Malla Reddy College of Pharmacy, Maisammaguda, Dhulapally, Secunderabad, Andhra Pradesh, India-500014.*

[2] *Department of Pharmaceutical Chemistry, Malla Reddy College of Pharmacy, Maisammaguda, Dhulapally, Secunderabad, Andhra Pradesh, India-500014.*

[3] *Department of Pharmaceutics, Malla Reddy College of Pharmacy, Maisammaguda, Dhulapally, Secunderabad, Andhra Pradesh, India-500014.*

ARTICLEINFO

Keywords:
Aripiprazole
Tablets
UV-Spectrophotometry
Multivariate Technique

ABSTRACT

Purpose: An accurate and precise UV spectrophotometric method with multivariate calibration technique for the determination of aripiprazole in pharmaceutical formulations has been described. ***Methods:*** This technique is based on the use of the linear regression equations by using the relationship between concentration and absorbance at five different wavelengths. The aripiprazole shows absorption maxima at 255 nm and obeyed Beer's law in the range of 5-30 µg/mL. ***Results:*** The results were treated statistically and were found highly accurate, precise and reproducible. This statistical approach gives optimum results for the eliminating fluctuations coming from instrumental or experimental conditions. ***Conclusion:*** It was concluded that the proposed method is simple, easy to apply, economical and could be used as an alternative to the existing spectrophotometric and non-spectrophotometric methods for the routine analysis of aripiprazole in pharmaceutical formulations.

Introduction

Aripiprazole is a sixth and a recent second generation anti-psychotic drug with chemical formula 7-[4-[4-(2, 3-dichlorophenyl) -1-piprazinyl] butoxy] -3,4-dihydro-(1H) -quinolinone belonging to the class of benzisoxazole. It is used in the treatment of Schizophrenia and bipolar disorder associated episodes as like acute, manic and mixed.[1,2] It has the partial agonist effect towards 5-HT1A-receptor, dopamine D_2 receptor and antagonistic effect on 5-HT2- receptor.[3]

A survey of pertinent literature revealed that few analytical methods reported for determination of aripiprazole in pharmaceutical dosage forms and biological samples include HPLC[4-11] and spectrophotometric[12,13] methods. Till date no multivariate spectrophotometric method for the estimation of aripiprazole is reported. Multivariate calibration refers to the process of constructing a mathematical model that relates a property such as content or identity to the absorbance of a set of known reference samples at more than one wavelength.[14] If the absorbance of an analyte (Z) is measured at five wavelengths set, straight line equation can be written as; $A_\lambda = aX(Cz+k)$ where A_λ represent the absorbance of the analyte, A is the slope and k is the intercept of the linear regression function of the analyte. C_Z represents the concentration of analyte. At five selected wavelengths, the equation system can also be summed as; $A_T = aX (C_Z + b) X (C_Z +c) X (C_Z + d) X (C_Z +e) X (C_Z +K_T)$, which can be simplified to $A_T = C_Z (a+b+c+d+e) +K_T$ where a, b, c, d, e are the slopes, A_T and K_T represents the sum of absorbance obtained and sum of intercepts of regression equations at five-wavelength set respectively. The concentration of the Z analyte in a mixture can be calculated by using the Eqn. $C_Z = A_T - K_T /(a+b+c+d+e)$.[15,16] This paper describes the application of UV spectral multivariate calibration technique having simple mathematical content for the quantitative determination of aripiprazole in pharmaceutical formulation.

Materials and Methods

Chemicals

The aripiprazole (Figure 1) reference standard (assigned purity 99.59%) was kindly supplied by Hetero Drugs Limited (Hyderabad). The commercial pharmaceutical formulations were obtained from local Pharmacies.

***Corresponding author:** Kandikonda Sandeep, Department of Pharmaceutical Analysis, Malla Reddy College of Pharmacy, Maisammaguda, Dhulapally, Secunderabad, Andhra Pradesh, India-500014. Email: sandeep.kandikonda5@gmail.com

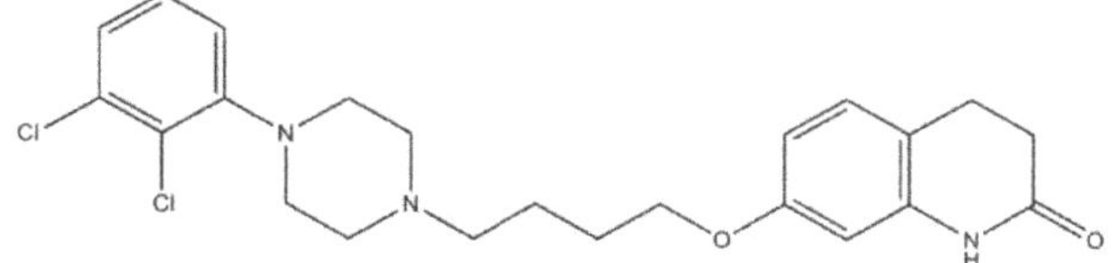

Figure 1. Structure of aripiprazole

Instrumentation

The multivariate technique was performed in 1.0cm quartz cells using T60U UV-Visible spectrophotometer (PG Instruments Ltd., England) with a fixed 2nm spectral bandwidth and UV-Win5 software v5.1.1 was used for all absorbance measurements.

Preparation of Standard Solutions

The standard solution (1000 µg/mL) was prepared by accurately weighed 100 mg of aripiprazole in 100 mL volumetric flask containing 50 mL of ethanol and sonicated for about 5 min, and then the volume was made up to the mark with ethanol. From this 10 mL was pipette out into a 100 mL volumetric flask and volume was made up to the mark with ethanol to get final concentration of 100 µg/mL.

Preparation of sample solution

For analysis of marketing formulations, twenty tablets were weighed accurately and powdered. The powder equivalent to 100mg of the drug weighed accurately and transferred to 100mL volumetric flask containing 50mL of ethanol. The mixture was sonicated to dissolve, make up the volume with ethanol. The above solutions were filtered through Whatmann filter paper and the solution was transferred into volumetric flask, and was made up to the mark with ethanol to obtain a final concentration of 20 µg/mL. All determinations were conducted with six replicates.

Method Validation

The method was validated according to International Conference on Harmonization (ICH) Q2B guidelines[17] for validation of analytical procedure to determine the linearity, limit of detection, limit of quantitation, accuracy and precisions.

Results and Discussion

Aripiprazole was estimated by proposed multivariate UV spectrophotometric method in tablets. It was completely soluble in ethanol and hence ethanol was selected as the solvent for aripiprazole to obtain UV spectrum in the range of 220-400 nm. After the evaluation of the spectrum, aripiprazole presented maximum absorbance at 255 nm (Figure 2).

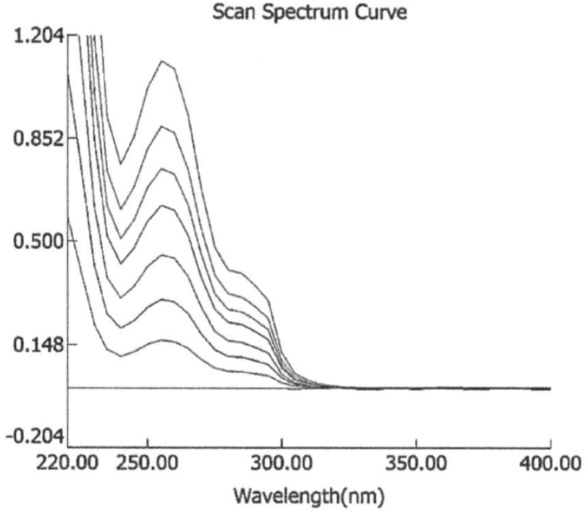

Figure 2. Absorbance spectrum of aripiprazole

A validation sets consisting of six solutions in working range of 5-30 µg/mL were freshly prepared and scanned in the UV region. The absorbance was recorded and plotted calibration curve against concentration, which followed the Beer's law and gave a straight line (Table 1). In order to improve this correlation and minimize instrumental fluctuations, absorbances of these solutions were measured over a range surrounding 255 nm i.e., 251, 253, 257,259 nm. The calibration curves of aripiprazole at different wavelengths is shown in Figure 3.

Table 1. Calibration data of the proposed method

Parameters		Results				
		At 251nm	At 253nm	At 255nm	At 257nm	At 259nm
Beer's law range (µg/mL)		5-30	5-30	5-30	5-30	5-30
Molar extinction coefficient (1/mol/cm)		0.0313	0.0304	0.0299	0.0297	0.0289
Sandell's sensitivity (µg/cm^2)		0.032	0.0329	0.0334	0.0337	0.0347
Limit of detection (µg/mL)		0.29	0.22	0.3	0.23	0.2
Limit of quantitation (µg/mL)		0.87	0.68	0.91	0.69	0.61
Regression equation	Intercept (a)	0.0059	0.0067	0.0071	0.0072	0.0047
	Slope (b)	0.0305	0.0296	0.0292	0.0288	0.0283
	Correlation coefficient (r^2)	0.9993	0.9994	0.9992	0.9996	0.9992

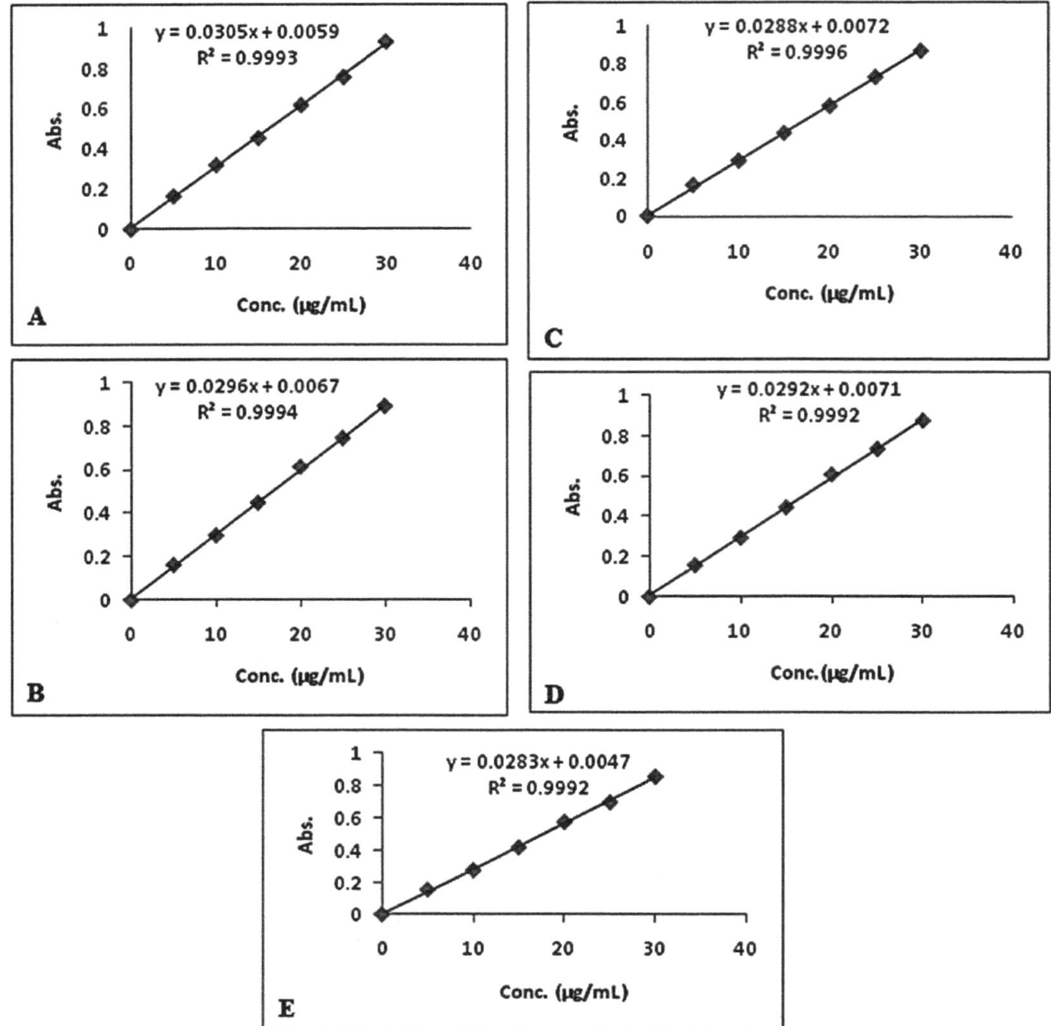

Figure 3. Calibration curve of aripiprazole A) at 255 nm, B) at 257 nm, C) at 259 nm, D) at 251 nm and E) at 253 nm

The accuracy of the method was evaluated through the recovery studies. Recovery studies were carried out by addition of a known quantity of pure drug solution to pre analyzed sample solution at three different concentration levels (50, 100 and 150%). The percentage recovery values were found to be 98.27-102.01 with %RSD of <2% (Table 2), which indicates that the proposed method was accurate.

Table 2. Accuracy of the proposed method (standard addition technique)

Amount (%) of drug added to analyte	Theoretical content (µg/mL)	Conc. found (Mean± SD)*	%RSD	% Recovery range
50	5	5.02±0.8	0.8	99.6-101.2
100	10	10.19±0.2082	0.2	101.7-102.01
150	15	14.76±0.13	0.14	98.27-98.53

Precision was determined as intra-assay and inter-assay, in accordance with ICH guidelines. The intra-day and inter-day precision were determined by analyzing the samples of aripiprazole at a concentration of 10, 20 and 30µg/mL. The results of intra-day and inter-day precision studies were shown in Table 3. The low %RSD values obtained from the analysis of tablets indicated that the method was highly precise.

Table 3. Precision data of proposed method

Analyte Conc. (µg/mL)	Intra-assay precision		Inter-assay precision	
	*Mean ±SD	%RSD	*Mean ±SD	%RSD
10	100.26±0.5565	0.56	99.21±0.6906	0.7
20	99.94±0.1704	0.17	99.41±0.1852	0.19
30	100.32±0.83	0.83	100.43±1.3009	1.3

*Triplicate results

The developed methods were applied to the quantification of aripiprazole in tablet dosage forms available in the local market. The results were tabulated in Table 4. It can be seen that, the results obtained by proposed method was very much similar to that of established methods.

Table 4. Assay results of aripiprazole in tablet dosage forms

Brand Name	Label Claim (mg)	Assay	SD	%RSD
ARIP MT	10	99.75	0.2833	0.28
APICORD	10	99.44	1.0192	1.02
ARIA	10	99.36	0.6526	0.66
ARIPAT	10	100.01	0.3562	0.36

* Average of six determinations

Conclusion

The proposed method is rapid, accurate, precise and sensitive for the quantification of aripiprazole from its pharmaceutical dosage forms by the multivariate spectrophotometric method. The method relies on the use of simple working procedure comparable to that achieved by sophisticated and expensive technique like HPLC, and hence this method can be routinely employed in quality control for analysis of aripiprazole in tablets.

Conflict of Interest

The authors report no conflicts of interest.

References

1. Merck. The Merck Index, 12th ed. USA: Merck and Co; 1996.
2. Deleon A, Patel NC, Crismon ML. Aripiprazole: a comprehensive review of its pharmacology, clinical efficacy, and tolerability. *Clin Ther* 2004;26(5):649-66.
3. Michel B. Aripiprazole: a new treatment for schizophrenia. *Future Neurol* 2006;1(4):373-88.
4. Rao DV, Shetty S, Satheesh K, Radhakrishnanand P, Himabindu V. A stability indicating RPLC method for aripiprazole. *Indian J Anal Chem* 2008;7:444-53.
5. Shimokawa Y, Akiyama H, Kashiyama E, Koga T, Miyamoto G. High performance liquid chromatographic methods for the determination of aripiprazole with ultraviolet detection in rat plasma and brain: application to the pharmacokinetic study. *J Chromatogr B Analyt Technol Biomed Life Sci* 2005;821(1):8-14.
6. Vijaya kumar M, Muley PR. Determination of aripiprazole in bulk drug and solid dosage forms by RP-HPLC method. *Indian Pharm* 2005;4:71-5.
7. Koduri SV, Buchireddy SR, Madhusudhan G, Mukkanti K, Srinivasulu P. Stress degradation Studies on aripiprazole and development of a validated stability indicating LC method. *Chromatographia* 2008;68:635-40.
8. Lancelin F, Djebrani K, Tabaouti K, Kraoul L, Brovedani S, Paubel P, et al. Development and validation of a high-performance liquid chromatography method using diode array detection for the simultaneous quantification of aripiprazole and dehydro-aripiprazole in human plasma. *J Chromatogr B Analyt Technol Biomed Life Sci* 2008;867(1):15-9.
9. Akamine Y, Yasui-Furukori N, Kojima M, Inoue Y, Uno T. A sensitive column-switching HPLC method for aripiprazole and dehydroaripiprazole and its application to human pharmacokinetic studies. *J Sep Sci* 2010;33(21):3292-8.
10. Babu GR, Rao JS, Kumar KS, Reddy PJ. Stability indicating liquid chromatographic method for aripiprazole. *Asian J Pharm Anal* 2011;1(1):3-7.
11. Bhanotu B, Srinath P, Kedarnath J. Development, Estimation and Validation of Aripiprazole in Bulk and Its Pharmaceutical Formulation by HPLC Method. *Int J Chem Tech Res* 2012;4(1):124-8.
12. Kalaichelvi R, Thangabalan B, Srinivasarao D, Jayachandran E. UV Spectrophotometric Determination of Aripiprazole in Bulk and Pharmaceutical Formulation. *E-J Chem* 2009;6(S1):S87-S90.
13. Jain R, Kashaw SK, Jain R, Mishra P, Kohli DV. Visible spectrophotometric method for the determination of aripiprazole in tablets. *Indian J Pharm Sci* 2011;73(1):74-6.
14. Sena MM, Poppi RJ. N-way PLS applied to simultaneous spectrophotometric determination of acetylsalicylic acid, paracetamol and caffeine. *J Pharm Biomed Anal* 2004;34(1):27-34.
15. Arayne MS, Sultana N, Bahadur SS. Multivariate calibrations in UV spectrophotometric analysis. *Pak J Pharm Sci* 2007;20(2):163-74.
16. Arayne MS, Sultana N, Siddiqui FA. Optimization of levofloxacin analysis by RP-HPLC using multivariate calibration technique. *Pak J Pharm Sci* 2007;20(2):100-6.
17. International Conference on Harmonization (ICH) of Technical Requirements for Registration of Pharmaceuticals for Human Use Guideline on Validation of Analytical Procedure-Methodology ICH. Geneva, Switzerland 1996.

Permissions

All chapters in this book were first published in APB, by Tabriz University of Medical Sciences; hereby published with permission under the Creative Commons Attribution License or equivalent. Every chapter published in this book has been scrutinized by our experts. Their significance has been extensively debated. The topics covered herein carry significant findings which will fuel the growth of the discipline. They may even be implemented as practical applications or may be referred to as a beginning point for another development.

The contributors of this book come from diverse backgrounds, making this book a truly international effort. This book will bring forth new frontiers with its revolutionizing research information and detailed analysis of the nascent developments around the world.

We would like to thank all the contributing authors for lending their expertise to make the book truly unique. They have played a crucial role in the development of this book. Without their invaluable contributions this book wouldn't have been possible. They have made vital efforts to compile up to date information on the varied aspects of this subject to make this book a valuable addition to the collection of many professionals and students.

This book was conceptualized with the vision of imparting up-to-date information and advanced data in this field. To ensure the same, a matchless editorial board was set up. Every individual on the board went through rigorous rounds of assessment to prove their worth. After which they invested a large part of their time researching and compiling the most relevant data for our readers.

The editorial board has been involved in producing this book since its inception. They have spent rigorous hours researching and exploring the diverse topics which have resulted in the successful publishing of this book. They have passed on their knowledge of decades through this book. To expedite this challenging task, the publisher supported the team at every step. A small team of assistant editors was also appointed to further simplify the editing procedure and attain best results for the readers.

Apart from the editorial board, the designing team has also invested a significant amount of their time in understanding the subject and creating the most relevant covers. They scrutinized every image to scout for the most suitable representation of the subject and create an appropriate cover for the book.

The publishing team has been an ardent support to the editorial, designing and production team. Their endless efforts to recruit the best for this project, has resulted in the accomplishment of this book. They are a veteran in the field of academics and their pool of knowledge is as vast as their experience in printing. Their expertise and guidance has proved useful at every step. Their uncompromising quality standards have made this book an exceptional effort. Their encouragement from time to time has been an inspiration for everyone.

The publisher and the editorial board hope that this book will prove to be a valuable piece of knowledge for researchers, students, practitioners and scholars across the globe.

List of Contributors

Ahad Bavili Tabrizi
Department of Medicinal Chemistry, Faculty of Pharmacy & Biotechnology Research Center, Tabriz University of Medical Sciences, Tabriz, Iran

Nakisa Seyyedeh Tutunchi
Students' Research Committee, Tabriz University of Medical Sciences, Tabriz, Iran

Adeleh Divsalar
Department of Biological Sciences, Kharazmi University, Tehran, Iran

Soheila Bolandnazar
Department of Biological Sciences, Kharazmi University, Tehran, Iran
Biotechnology Research Center, Tabriz University of Medical Sciences, Tabriz, Iran

Hadi Valizadeh
Research Center for Pharmaceutical Nanotechnology and Faculty of Pharmacy, Tabriz University of Medical Sciences, Tabriz, Iran

Arash Khodaei
Department of biological sciences, Institute for Advanced Studies in Basic Sciences, Zanjan, Iran

Parvin Zakeri-Milani
Drug Applied Research Center and Faculty of Pharmacy, Tabriz University of Medical Sciences, Tabriz, Iran

Xican Li and Yanping Huang
School of Chinese Herbal Medicine, Guangzhou University of Chinese Medicine, Waihuang East Road No.232, Guangzhou Higher Education Mega Center, 510006, Guangzhou, China

Dongfeng Chen
School of Basic Medical Science, Guangzhou University of Chinese Medicine, Guangzhou, 510006, China

Veni Bharti and Neeru Vasudeva
Department of Pharmaceutical Sciences, Guru Jambheshwer University of Science and Technology, Hisar, Haryana, India

Joginder Singh Dhuhan
Department of Biotechnology, Chaudhary Devilal University, Sirsa, Haryana, India

Sepide Mahluji, Vahide Ebrahimzade Attari and Laleh Payahoo
Student Research Committee, Tabriz University of Medical Science, Tabriz, Iran

Alireza Ostadrahimi
Nutrition Research Center, Tabriz University of Medical Sciences, Tabriz, Iran

Majid Mobasser
Endocrinology and Metabolism Section, Department of Medicine, Imam Reza Hospital, Tabriz, Iran

Hossain Hemayet and Ismet Ara Jahan
BCSIR Laboratories, Dhaka, Bangladesh Council of Scientific and Industrial Research, Dhaka-1205, Bangladesh

Howlader Sariful Islam
Department of Pharmacy, World University of Bangladesh, Dhaka-1205, Bangladesh

Dey Shubhra Kanti, Hira Arpona and Ahmed Arif
Pharmacy Discipline, Life Science School, Khulna University, Khulna-9208, Bangladesh

Ama Udu Ibiam
Department of Biochemistry, Faculty of Biological Sciences, Ebonyi State University, PMB 053, Abakaliki, Nigeria

Emmanuel Ike Ugwuja
Department of Chemical Pathology, Faculty of Clinical Medicine, Ebonyi State University, PMB 053 Abakaliki, Nigeria

Christ Ejeogo
Department of Biochemistry, Institute of Management and Technology (IMT), Enugu, Nigeria

Okechukwu Ugwu
Department of Biotechnology, Faculty of Biological Sciences, Ebonyi State University, PMB 053, Abakaliki, Nigeria

Mina Ghahramanian Golzar, Zohre Ataie, Hadi Ebrahimi and Fariba Mirzaie
Neuroscience Research Centre (NSRC), Tabriz University of Medical Sciences, Tabriz, Iran

Shirin Babri
Neuroscience Research Centre (NSRC), Tabriz University of Medical Sciences, Tabriz, Iran
Neuroscience Research Centre (NSRC), Tabriz University of Medical Sciences, Tabriz, Iran

Gisou Mohaddes
Neuroscience Research Centre (NSRC), Tabriz University of Medical Sciences, Tabriz, Iran
Neuroscience Research Centre, Shahid Beheshti Universiy of Medical Sciences, Tehran, Iran

Manoj Kumar
Department of Pharmaceutical Sciences, Guru Jambheshwar University of Science and Technology, Hisar-125001, India

Sunil Sharma
Pharmacology Divisions, Department of Pharmaceutical Sciences,Guru Jambheshwar University of Science and Technology, Hisar-125001, India

Neeru Vasudeva
harmacognosy Divisions, Department of Pharmaceutical Sciences,Guru Jambheshwar University of Science and Technology, Hisar-125001, India

Fatemeh Fathiazad
Department of Pharmacognosy, Faculty of Pharmacy, Tabriz University of Medical Sciences, Iran

Sanaz Hamedeyazdan
Student's Research Committee, Faculty of pharmacy, Tabriz University of Medical Sciences, Iran

Mohamad Karim Khosropanah
Department of Biology, Faculty of Science, Islamic Azad University of Sanandaj, Sanandaj, Iran

Arash Khaki
Department of Veterinary Pathology, Tabriz Branch, Islamic Azad University, Tabriz, Iran

Abbas Akhgari, Zohreh Heshmati and Behzad Sharif Makhmalzadeh
Nanotechnology Research Center and School of Pharmacy, Ahvaz Jundishapur University of Medical Sciences, Ahvaz, Iran

Deepak Ganjewala and Ashish Kumar Gupta
Amity Institute of Biotechnology, Amity University Uttar Pradesh, Sector-125, Noida-201303 (UP), India

Abolfazl Aslani and Fatemeh Fattahi
Department of Pharmaceutics, School of Pharmacy and Novel Drug Delivery Systems Research Center, Isfahan University of Medical Sciences, Isfahan, Iran

Raju Asirvatham
Department of Pharmacology, Shri Rawatpura Sarkar Institute of Pharmacy, Datia, Mathya Pradesh, India

Arockiasamy Josphin Maria Christina
Department of Pharmacology, AIMST University, Malaysia

Anita Murali
MS Ramaiah College of Pharmacy, Banglore, India

Veni Bharti and Neeru Vasudeva
Department of Pharmaceutical Sciences, Guru Jambheshwer University of Science and Technology, Hisar, Haryana, India

Xican Li and Weikang Chen
School of Chinese Herbal Medicine, Guangzhou University of Chinese Medicine, Guangzhou, China

Dongfeng Chen
School of Basic Medical Science, Guangzhou University of Chinese Medicine, Guangzhou, China

Abbas Delazar, Sanaz Hamedeyazdan, Hossein Babaei, Yousef Javadzadeh, Solmaz Asnaashari, Sadeighe Bamdad Moghadam and Shahriar Barzegar Jalali
Drug Applied Research Centre and School of Pharmacy, Tabriz University of Medical Sciences, Tabriz 51664, Iran

Satyajit D. Sarker
Department of Pharmacy, School of Applied Sciences, University of Wolverhampton, MM Building, Molineux Street, Wolverhampton WV1 SB, UK

Lutfun Nahar
Drug Discovery and Design Research Division, Department of Pharmacy, School of Applied Sciences, University of Wolverhampton, City Campus, MA Building, Wulfruna Street, Wolverhampton WV1 1LY, UK

Masoud Modaresi
School of Pharmacy, Kermanshah University of Medical Sciences, Kermanshah, Kermanshah 67346, Iran

Jannatun Tazri, Md. Mizanur Rahman Moghal, Syed Masudur Rahman Dewan and Wahiduzzaman Noor
Department of Pharmacy, Noakhali Science and Technology University, Sonapur, Noakhali-3814, Bangladesh

Nor Mohammad
Department of Chemistry, University of Chittagong, Chittagong-4331, Bangladesh

Jamal Mohammadian
Department of Clinical Biochemistry, Division of Medical Biotechnology, Faculty of Medicine, Tabriz University of Medical Sciences, Tabriz, Iran

Sima Mansoori-Derakhshan and Mahmoud Shekari-Khaniani
Department of Medical Genetics, Faculty of Medicine, Tabriz University of Medical Sciences, Tabriz, Iran

Masood Mohammadian
East Azerbaijan Agriculture and Jahad Organization, Tabriz, Iran

Khaled Nabih Rashed
Pharmacognosy Department, National Research Centre, Dokki, Giza, Egypt

Monica Butnariu
Chemistry and Vegetal Biochemistry, Banat's University of Agricultural Sciences and Veterinary Medicine from Timisoara, Calea Aradului, Timisoara 300645, Romania

Jing Lin, Yaoxiang Gao, Haiming Li, Lulu Zhang and Xican Li
School of Chinese Herbal Medicine, Guangzhou University of Chinese Medicine, Guangzhou, 510006, China

Mohammadali Torbati
Students' Research Committee, Faculty of Pharmacy, Tabriz University of Medical Sciences, Iran

Hossein Nazemiyeh and Fatemeh Fathiazad
Department of Pharmacognosy, Faculty of Pharmacy, Tabriz University of Medical Sciences, Iran

Farzaneh Lotfipour and Mahboob Nemati
Pharmaceutical and Food Control, Faculty of Pharmacy, Tabriz University of Medical Sciences, Iran

Solmaz Asnaashari
Drug Applied Research Centre, Tabriz University of Medical Sciences, Iran

Riaz Uddin, Moni Rani Saha and Raushanara Akter
Department of Pharmacy, Stamford University Bangladesh, Dhaka-1217, Bangladesh

Nusrat Subhan
School of Biomedical Sciences, Charles Sturt University, Wagga Wagga (NSW), Australia

Hemayet Hossain and Ismet Ara Jahan
BCSIR Laboratories, Bangladesh Council of Scientific and Industrial Research (BCSIR), Dhaka-1205, Bangladesh

Ashraful Alam
Department of Pharmacy, North-South University, Dhaka-1229, Bangladesh

Mohammadreza Abbaspour, Negar Jalayer and Behzad Sharif Makhmalzadeh
Nanotechnology Research Center and school of Pharmacy, Ahvaz Jundishapur University of Medical Sciences, Ahvaz, Iran

Mitra Jelvehgari
Drug Applied Research Center and Faculty of Pharmacy, Tabriz University of Medical Sciences, Tabriz, Iran

Hadi Valizadeh
Biotechnology Research Center and Faculty of Pharmacy, Tabriz University of Medical Sciences, Tabriz, Iran

Ramin Jalali Motlagh
Student Research Committee, Tabriz University of Medical Sciences, Tabriz, Iran

Hassan Montazam
Islamic Azad University of Bonab Unit, Bonab, Iran

Mahnaz Kesmati, Maysam Mard-Soltani and Lotfolah Khajehpour
Department of Biology, Faculty of Science, Shahid Chamran University, Ahvaz, Iran

Nadereh Rashtchizadeh and Jalal Abdolalizadeh
Drug Applied Research Center, Tabriz University of Medical Sciences, Tabriz, Iran

Maryam Bannazadeh Amirkhiz
Drug Applied Research Center, Tabriz University of Medical Sciences, Tabriz, Iran
student of Tabriz International University of Medical Sciences (Aras), Tabriz University of Medical Sciences, Tabriz, Iran

Hosein Nazemieh
Research Center for Pharmaceutical Nanotechnology, Tabriz University of Medical Sciences, Tabriz, Iran

Leila Mohammadnejad and Behzad Baradaran
Immonuology Research Center, Tabriz University of Medical Sciences, Tabriz, Iran

Moorthi Chidambaram and Kathiresan Krishnasamy
Department of Pharmacy, Annamalai University, Chidambaram, Tamil Nadu, India

Salar Hassanzadeh, Vahideh Tarhriz and Mohammad Saeid Hejazi
Department of Pharmaceutical Biotechnology, Faculty of Pharmacy, Tabriz University of Medical Sciences, Tabriz, Iran

Davood Naziri
Department of Pharmaceutical Biotechnology, Faculty of Pharmacy, Tabriz University of Medical Sciences, Tabriz, Iran
Department of Agricultural Biotechnology, Faculty of Agriculture, Zanjan University, Zanjan, Iran

Masoud Hamidi
Department of Pharmaceutical Biotechnology, Faculty of Pharmacy, Tabriz University of Medical Sciences, Tabriz, Iran
Students' Research Committee, Tabriz University of Medical Sciences, Tabriz, Iran

Bahram Maleki Zanjani
Department of Agricultural Biotechnology, Faculty of Agriculture, Zanjan University, Zanjan, Iran

Hossein Nazemyieh
Department of Pharmacognosy, Faculty of Pharmacy, Tabriz University of Medical Sciences, Tabriz, Iran

Mohammd Amin Hejazi
Branch for Northwest & West Region, Agricultural Biotechnology Research Institute of Iran (ABRII), Tabriz, Iran

Sanaz Hamedeyazdan
Student's Research Committee, Faculty of Pharmacy, Tabriz University of Medical Sciences, Tabriz, Iran

Solmaz Asnaashari
Drug Applied Research Center, Tabriz University of Medical Sciences, Tabriz, Iran

Fatemeh Fathiazad
Department of Pharmacognosy, Faculty of Pharmacy, Tabriz University of Medical Sciences, Tabriz, Iran

Kuldeep Hemraj Ramteke
Modern College of Pharmacy (for Ladies), Moshi, Pune, Maharashtra

Lilakant Nath
Department of Pharmaceutical Sciences, Dibrugarh University, Dibrugagh, Assam

Kandikonda Sandeep
Department of Pharmaceutical Analysis, Malla Reddy College of Pharmacy, Maisammaguda, Dhulapally, Secunderabad, Andhra Pradesh, India-500014

Madhusudhanareddy Induri
Department of Pharmaceutical Chemistry, Malla Reddy College of Pharmacy, Maisammaguda, Dhulapally, Secunderabad, Andhra Pradesh, India-500014

Muvvala Sudhakar
Department of Pharmaceutics, Malla Reddy College of Pharmacy, Maisammaguda, Dhulapally, Secunderabad, Andhra Pradesh, India-500014

Index

www.ingramcontent.com/pod-product-compliance
Lightning Source LLC
Chambersburg PA
CBHW080644200326
41458CB00013B/4725
9781639275458